Integrative Systemic Therapy

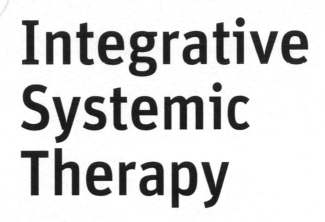

Integrative Systemic Therapy

**Metaframeworks
for Problem Solving
With Individuals,
Couples, and Families**

William M. Pinsof, Douglas C. Breunlin,

William P. Russell, Jay L. Lebow,

Cheryl Rampage, and Anthony L. Chambers

AMERICAN PSYCHOLOGICAL ASSOCIATION
Washington, DC

Published by
American Psychological Association
750 First Street, NE
Washington, DC 20002
www.apa.org

APA Order Department
P.O. Box 92984
Washington, DC 20090-2984
Tel: (800) 374-2721; Direct: (202) 336-5510
Fax: (202) 336-5502; TDD/TTY: (202) 336-6123
Online: www.apa.org/pubs/books
E-mail: order@apa.org

In the U.K., Europe, Africa, and the Middle East, copies may be ordered from
Eurospan Group
c/o Pegasus Drive
Stratton Business Park
Biggleswade Bedfordshire
SG18 8TQ United Kingdom
Phone: +44 (0) 1767 604972
Fax: +44 (0) 1767 601640
Online: https://www.eurospanbookstore.com/apa
E-mail: eurospan@turpin-distribution.com

Typeset in Goudy by Circle Graphics, Inc., Columbia, MD

Printer: Gasch Printing, Odenton, MD
Cover Designer: Beth Schlenoff Design, Bethesda, MD; Mercury Publishing Services, Inc., Rockville, MD

Library of Congress Cataloging-in-Publication Data
Names: Pinsof, William M., author. | Breunlin, Douglas C., author. | Russell, William P., author. | Lebow, Jay, author. | Rampage, Cheryl, author. | Chambers, Anthony L., author.
Title: Integrative systemic therapy : metaframeworks for problem solving with individuals, couples, and families / William M. Pinsof, Douglas C. Breunlin, William P. Russell, Jay L. Lebow, Cheryl Rampage, and Anthony L. Chambers.
Description: First edition. | Washington, DC : American Psychological Association, [2018] | Includes bibliographical references and index.
Identifiers: LCCN 2017013558 | ISBN 9781433828126 | ISBN 143382812X
Subjects: LCSH: Systemic therapy (Family therapy)
Classification: LCC RC488.5 .P57 2018 | DDC 616.89/156—dc23 LC record available at https://lccn.loc.gov/2017013558

British Library Cataloguing-in-Publication Data
A CIP record is available from the British Library.

Printed in the United States of America
First Edition

http://dx.doi.org/10.1037/0000055-000

To the thousands of students who have trained at The Family Institute
since 1967, whose questions and curiosity fueled the development
of our ideas about systems and therapy; to our colleagues who have
supported and challenged us to make integrative systemic therapy
better, more comprehensive, and more comprehensible;
and last, to the thousands of clients with whom we have worked
over more than 40 years, who have entrusted us with their
hearts and souls and in the process made us
smarter, wiser, and better.

CONTENTS

PREFACE

There are two ideas, or more accurately, two passionate beliefs, at the core of this book. The first is that the field of psychotherapy has to move beyond specific models (empirically supported or not) to a comprehensive and integrative framework that simultaneously incorporates and transcends those models. This belief is strongly linked to the quest for a common factor approach (Sprenkle, Davis, & Lebow, 2009). The movement toward a comprehensive and integrative approach heralds the emergence of psychotherapy as a mature clinical science.

The second idea is that the field of psychotherapy has to incorporate the systemic beliefs and practices that drove the creation and growth of the field of family therapy. Over the last 40 years, family (and couple) therapy has become a valued and recognized specialty within the mental health field. Despite this development, the psychotherapy field is still dominated by the concepts of individual psychopathology and individual therapy. It is time for the general field of psychotherapy to recognize that all psychotherapy occurs within a bio-psychosocial context that includes our biology, our selves, our relationships, our families, our community, and even the society in which we live.

The challenge of this imperative is that it complicates things. It is far easier to just think about an individual and his or her problems. It is also far easier to treat an individual than a couple or a family or to include social justice in the mandate of the therapy. Most therapists do not have a framework for simultaneously embracing the individual and his or her context. This book aims to remedy that deficit. The breadth of what we offer in this book extends beyond what is typically called a model of therapy; consequently, we refer to integrative systemic therapy as a perspective rather than a model.

THE HISTORY OF THIS BOOK

This book began over 25 years ago when Doug Breunlin came to work with Bill Pinsof at the newly reorganized Family Institute at Northwestern University (also known as The Family Institute of Chicago). Bill had been working on his *Integrative Problem-Centered Therapy* (1995) since the early 1980s, trying to create a comprehensive framework for integrating family, individual, and biological therapies. Doug had been working on his *Metaframeworks* (Breunlin, Schwartz, & Mac Kune-Karrer, 1992, 1997) perspective for integrating different metatheories or metaframeworks to provide a comprehensive and integrative framework for understanding families and organizing family therapy. Bill's work had been strongly influenced by his long association (since the late 1970s) with Jay Lebow and other colleagues at The Family Institute. Doug's prior work occurred at the Institute for Juvenile Research (IJR) in Chicago, in close collaboration with Dick Schwartz and Betty Mac Kune-Karrer. Not coincidentally, these two institutions were the founding centers for family therapy theory and practice in Chicago.

Bill and Doug came together to integrate their respective problem-centered and metaframeworks models, but more important, to jointly harness their efforts to transform the practice and theory of psychotherapy in line with the core beliefs articulated in the previous section. They began exploring the possibility of integrating their models. At first glance, Doug's metaframeworks perspective provided an elegant and elaborate assessment framework for thinking about family systems. Bill's integrative problem-centered model provided a detailed, integrative, and multisystemic intervention framework that complemented the metaframeworks perspective. Jay Lebow's work on psychotherapy integration elaborated the broader theoretical context of both models, and Cheryl Rampage's work on feminist family therapy laid the groundwork for a modern and nuanced discourse on gender. What has emerged is not yet one more model, but rather a perspective on psychotherapy that transcends the models.

The Family Institute has been a center for psychotherapy training and practice since its inception in the late 1960s. This made it an ideal context for testing and refining the emerging integrative perspective. Specifically, at the same time that Doug came to The Family Institute, Cheryl Rampage arrived to create the Institute's new Master of Science in Marriage and Family Therapy Program (MSMFT Program) at Northwestern University. Under Cheryl's (and a succession of program directors') leadership, the program became an ideal laboratory to explore and refine Doug and Bill's combined perspective.

Bill Russell (hereafter called Bill R.), who had trained with Doug at IJR, joined The Family Institute soon after Doug. Working as a core faculty member of the MSMFT Program, Bill R. taught the combined perspective for many years and progressively got more involved in facilitating its emergence as the core perspective of the MSMFT Program and the clinic at The Family Institute. Eventually, Bill R. began to press Doug and Bill on the need for further articulation and clarification of the key features of the perspective. From that moment in the early 2000s, Bill R. became the absolutely irreplaceable and invaluable shepherd of the project that culminates in this book. Without his supportive and friendly tenacity, his clarity of focus and purpose, and his passion for the emerging perspective, you would not be reading this today. Our debt and gratitude to Bill R. are enormous.

In the last few years, Anthony Chambers joined our team. His youth, and his deep dual understandings of race and couples therapy, energized and expanded the emerging perspective. His passion and commitment to family psychology, building on Bill Pinsof's and Jay's early work in the field, brought the feedback of a new generation of scholars and practitioners to our work. Anthony's feedback drove our decision to change the name of our perspective from *integrative problem-centered metaframeworks* to *integrative systemic therapy*.

WHAT YOU WILL FIND IN THIS BOOK (AND ONLINE)

The mission of this book is to present a comprehensive, unifying, complex, and intricate perspective on the theory and practice of psychotherapy that is accessible to students of psychotherapy as well as informative and useful to seasoned practitioners. It is not a cookbook, nor a primer. It lays out the key concepts of integrative systemic therapy (IST) and details its practice. It is full of transcripts and examples of our work, each an amalgam of the multitude of cases we have all treated and supervised over the last 40 years. Case examples are somewhat simplified to demonstrate in limited space the essential characteristics of IST. We have also disguised details of the case examples to honor individuals' confidentiality.

We begin in Chapter 1 with a case example that includes multiple treatment episodes over a number of years. In Chapters 2 through 4, we then move into the core ideas, the blueprint for therapy, and the essence of IST—the transformation of problem sequences into solution sequences within client systems. In Chapter 5, we present the hypothesizing metaframeworks for thinking about problems and systems, which are followed by the planning metaframeworks in Chapter 6, for intervening into and transforming client systems. After exploring the art of facilitating a transformative and collaborative conversation with clients in Chapter 7, we describe in Chapter 8 how reading the feedback from clients creates and refines our hypothesizing and our planning. In Chapters 9 through 11, we address and illustrate the application of IST to families, couples, and individuals. And we conclude the book in Chapter 12 with a discussion of IST as a framework for therapists' learning and growth over their professional life course.

In addition, we have provided two downloadable chapters online (http://pubs.apa.org/books/supp/pinsof). Online Chapter 1 takes readers through a day in the life of an IST practitioner. It illustrates the comprehensive nature of IST and the diversity of therapeutic pathways that are possible within IST. Online Chapter 2 shows how IST practitioners can use empirical feedback provided by clients to inform decision making. This chapter follows one client system—a couple—through their therapy journey as they provide clinical data via a measurement and feedback system that was developed in concert with IST.

For us and hopefully for you, IST, in its comprehensiveness and richness, will become a challenging, helpful, and evolving framework for your own thinking about and practice of psychotherapy. It will help you find and use a coherent path through the many models of psychotherapy that exist today and that will exist in the coming years. We believe, because it has made us more thoughtful and effective therapists for our clients, IST will expand your thinking and improve your practice. Welcome.

ACKNOWLEDGMENTS

We are grateful to have worked in an environment where thinking systemically has always been valued and encouraged. Even a book with six authors is influenced by many other people. We are grateful for the support we have received from our Institute colleagues, both past and present, especially Jayne Kinsman, Shayna Goldstein, and Liz Jacobson for discussing their IST journeys with us; Janine Jolly, Katrina Sharzinski, Neil Venketramen, and Christine Webster for their careful reviews of an extensive body of literature; and Dick Schwartz and Betty Mac Kune-Karrer for their earlier contributions to metaframeworks, many of which were subsumed into IST. The teaching faculty and supervisors in the MSMFT Program at Northwestern University have helped us test and refine our ideas over the years and have been unfailingly supportive of this endeavor. Our students, who learn IST well, have offered numerous suggestions leading toward valuable refinements.

Jo Ann Casey was devoted, tireless, patient, and obsessive in keeping track of all of our outlines, drafts, and copies. She has literally and figuratively kept us and the book together. Without her passion and care in every phase of the preparation of the manuscript, as well as her extraordinary skills in formatting and proofreading, we would still be working on this manuscript. Diane Russell offered valuable technical assistance with the IST diagrams. Our editors at American Psychological Association Books, Susan Reynolds and Susan Herman, have been patient, supportive, and encouraging from the beginning.

Finally, we pay tribute to the many theorists and model builders whose brilliant concepts and strategies have been incorporated into the integrative systemic therapy perspective.

Integrative Systemic Therapy

1

HOW WE THINK AND
HOW WE WORK: INTEGRATIVE
SYSTEMIC THERAPY IN ACTION

This chapter presents the integrative systemic therapy (IST) perspective in action by describing several treatment episodes with a family over time. The following chapters in the book present, discuss, and illustrate the key concepts and components of the perspective. Many of them are embedded in this chapter and briefly noted within the description of the case. To highlight the unique features of IST we have chosen a fairly complex case. We have thus shortened or skipped many conversations and describe some interventions only briefly.

THE CALL

IST begins with the first conversation between the client making the first contact and the therapist, which usually begins over the phone or with e-mail. In this conversation, the therapist gets an initial picture of the client

http://dx.doi.org/10.1037/0000055-001
Integrative Systemic Therapy: Metaframeworks for Problem Solving With Individuals, Couples, and Families,
by W. M. Pinsof, D. C. Breunlin, W. P. Russell, J. L. Lebow, C. Rampage, and A. L. Chambers

system (the people involved in maintaining and/or resolving the presenting problem), the nature of the presenting problem, and the client's goals and, accordingly, starts to define the direct client system (who will be directly involved in the therapy).

Tom, a 50-year-old husband (to Lena, 48) and father of three (Aiden, 19; Tanya, 16; and Miles, 10) called to set up an appointment to get help with a marital crisis.

> Tom: I am in a ton of trouble and don't know what to do. My wife, Lena, insisted that I get into therapy. I've been drinking a lot recently and got involved with a woman I work with. Lena found out this week and kicked me out of the house. I am living at my brother's place.
>
> Therapist: Tom, where are you with your marriage? Do you want to stay married and work it out or do you want to get out?
>
> Tom: I love my wife and want to work it out. I have been so stupid I can't believe it.
>
> Therapist: Given that you want to work it out, do you think Lena would be willing to come in with you for the first session, and would you be willing to invite her?
>
> Tom: I'd invite her. I've told her about Melinda—the woman at work—and the affair. But she is so hurt and furious that I am not sure if she even could stand to be in the same room with me.
>
> Therapist: If possible, with your goal of repairing the marriage, I think that it would be better if we could start off with both you and Lena in the room. Why don't you give her a call and tell her that I would prefer to start off with both of you? That way we can hear what she thinks, get a fuller picture of your marriage, what's been going on, and what needs to change.

In this vignette, the therapist begins to actively assess the capacities of the client system by stimulating interaction (giving Tom the task of inviting Lena in) between the key client system members. He also avoids defining the therapy as *couples therapy*, which might be offensive at this moment to Lena, and instead defines her involvement as helping Tom and him integrate her perspective into their work. In working to integrate Lena into the therapy, the therapist uses IST's interpersonal guideline that privileges working directly with a relational system whenever feasible and appropriate.

THE FIRST EPISODE

Tom called back the next day to say that Lena had agreed to come in. He shared the concern that Lena, who handled the family finances, was worried about the cost of therapy. The therapist explored health insurance coverage with Tom, and they were both pleased to find that the therapist was a network provider in Tom's insurance plan. The copay would be affordable for them.

To empirically inform their work, the therapist asked that Tom and Lena fill out an online questionnaire to more quickly assess their current situation and track changes over the course of therapy. Tom said he thought that Lena would not mind filling it out and that he would do anything that might help. They scheduled the first session.

The First Session

Prior to the first session, the therapist examined the questionnaires that Lena and Tom had completed. Both spouses reported feeling depressed and anxious, and both acknowledged that Tom abused alcohol frequently, a constraint the therapist thought they would probably have to address. They also reported feeling disconnected in their marriage and unhappy with their sexual relationship. Lena's questionnaire showed her having low trust in Tom and low commitment to the marriage at this point, as well as a great deal of anger. Both partners also were concerned about the social isolation and academic difficulties of their youngest son, Miles. The questionnaires also revealed that Lena was African American, college educated, and employed as an examiner for the state department of employment security and that Tom was Caucasian, high school educated, and employed as a tool and equipment manager at the local power company. Last, they reported that in their families of origin, when they were growing up, both sets of parents divorced. Lena reported feeling connected and safe with her mother, but Tom reported not feeling safe and connected with anyone. The therapist kept this information in mind in case it proved useful in hypothesizing about the case, but the next step was to hear directly from the clients about how they saw the problem(s) and what they wanted to do about it (them).

The therapist began the first session by asking Lena how she felt coming into the session with Tom. One of the therapist's major goals for the session was to clarify what Lena wanted in regard to the marriage at this time and to begin building an alliance with her. Successful therapy depends on building a good alliance with both parties, and an initial key component of the alliance is alignment on goals.

Therapist:	Lena, over the phone Tom was clear that, if possible, he wants to continue with the marriage and work things out with you. What do you want to do about your marriage at this point?
Lena:	I am not sure. I don't know if I can ever trust him again. This affair has shattered my world. If it weren't for the kids, I'd probably be gone.
Therapist:	The affair was devastating. It sounds like you never expected that from Tom.
Lena:	Well, not entirely. He drinks too much, and I worry sometimes about where he is and what he's doing. I never feel fully safe or sure with Tom. But I never expected him to have a serious relationship with another woman—at work no less.
Tom:	I have stopped drinking and that relationship is over. I'm attending AA [Alcoholics Anonymous] meetings and I'm gonna stick with it. I don't know how I could have been so stupid. Lena, give me another chance. I can be the husband you want. [Lena looks away and starts to get tears in her eyes.]
Therapist:	Do you believe what he is saying?
Lena:	I want to, but I am very hurt and angry. I can't believe this happened to me.
Therapist:	Lena, I don't want to pressure you either way, but do you have any conditions, that if Tom could meet, would lead you to explore getting back together and rebuilding your marriage?
Lena:	Stop drinking for sure. I need to know where he is and what he is doing. No more disappearing and lying or getting mad when I ask. He needs to be straight with me and open about everything. [The therapist thinks it is a positive sign that Lena is so quickly able to entertain thoughts about solutions.]
Therapist:	Tom, do you know what Lena means by this?
Tom:	Yeah, I know. Being where I say I am, being accountable, and not avoiding talking about stuff.

Subsequently, the session focused on the revelation of the affair and how each of them reacted to it. It also involved some exploration of the history of their marriage. The therapist believed the presenting problem of the affair was embedded in, and maintained by, a complex set of factors called the *web of constraints*. That web reveals itself through the problem sequence (a patterned set of interactions including associated meanings and emotions). A major goal of the first session was to begin delineating the sequence(s) and exploring what the solution sequence(s) might look like.

Therapist: I'd like to better understand how this came about—what the unraveling looked and felt like.

Tom: A whole bunch of things. I guess it has to do with my drinking and bad judgment.

Therapist: That may be true, but Tom, I'm interested in what goes on with you before you drink. For instance, do you ever feel down or lonely or anxious? [In elaborating the early stages of the problem sequence, the therapist begins exploring the hypothesis that the drinking may function for Tom as a way to avoid difficult feelings.]

Tom: Yeah, lots.

Therapist: Do you ever talk to Lena about those feelings—at those times?

Tom: I've never really been a talker. I think I used to reach out, but now I guess I try to drink them away.

Lena: I think that he used to reach out for sex, but after the kids came along and his drinking got worse, that part of things pretty much went away. I'm not a big fan of having sex on demand with someone who is drunk or close to it.

Therapist: So let me see if I got this right. Tom, it sounds to me like you do feel upset or lonely and at those times you used to reach out for sex with Lena, but that diminished as you drank more and as the kids came along. That led to more drinking and less sex. It also sounds like when you would reach out to Lena for sex, it frequently was preceded by drinking and she was not interested. [Tom's drinking seems to have begun, at least in part, as an attempted solution to the problem of loneliness but has become part of an ongoing problem sequence in which drinking constrains more effective ways of dealing with his emotions, such as sharing them with Lena.]

Tom: Yeah, that's right. And I guess we all know what happened then?

Therapist: You mean the affair?

Tom: Yup. I guess Melinda would take me on any terms—drunk, sober, whatever. [The therapist reflects that the affair may have been an (ill-chosen) attempt at a solution to the problem.]

Lena: So does that mean if I don't have sex with you because you've been drinking or because I am exhausted from all the stuff that goes on with the kids, you're going to go have sex with some 25-year-old who smiles at you at work? [Lena is feeling blamed for the problem. The therapist moves to protect his alliance with her by focusing on Tom's history and responsibility for his maladaptive behavior.]

Therapist: From what I'm hearing, I think that Tom has been dealing with his painful or difficult feelings with alcohol and sex since he was a young adult. That pattern stopped working with the two of you, and he found someone else it worked with. I wonder what would happen if Tom could find some other way to deal with his painful feelings or his emotional needs other than drinking or sex. [The therapist offers a hypothesis about the problem sequence and begins exploring possible solution sequences.]

Tom: Like what?

Therapist: Like first letting yourself know what you're feeling, and then maybe talking to Lena about the feelings, rather than having a few drinks and reaching out to her for sex, getting rejected, and then you know what. [The therapist introduces a specific alternative solution sequence and begins to actively assess the client system's capacity for change.]

Lena: I'm so hurt and pissed off right now that I am not sure I'm going to be very receptive to Tom's feelings. I don't feel very warm and cuddly.

Therapist: Of course, but I think we're talking about what might happen in the future so that Tom can find ways to deal with his feelings other than drinking or getting laid. Maybe sex and alcohol have been a bad, but kind of effective, solution to any emotional pain for Tom for too long. [The therapist reacts to Lena's sense of being pressured and empathically addresses Tom's "bad" behavior.]

Lena: Do you understand what is being suggested, and are you up for this? Sounds like you're going have to find a whole new way of dealing with your feelings.

Tom: I think I understand. I don't know if I can. I don't know much about what I'm feeling or how to talk about it. I just know that I hate what I've done, and I hate being without you and the kids. If this is what I have to learn to do so this never happens again, I will try. I've already stopped drinking.

Therapist: That sounds like a good place to start.

Lena: We'll see if this lasts. I can't really trust it. Maybe with time.

The problem sequence was elaborated with Lena talking about her intense involvement in helping their older son, Aiden, adjust to his first year of college; their 16-year-old, Tanya, deal with her college preparations; and their 10-year-old son, Miles, deal with his social isolation and academic difficulties. Her sense of aloneness in dealing with the children, coupled with Tom's insistence on "sex" as the primary form of connection, made her feel alone and unloved.

Subsequent Sessions

Subsequent sessions focused on Tom and Lena's marriage and, later, on Miles and the rest of the family.

Marital Sessions

As the couple got into working on their core problem sequence, Tom's alcoholism came sharply into view. His parents divorced when he was 10, and he started drinking as a teenager to deal with his sense of social awkwardness and to relieve the tension created by their postdivorce relationship. His drinking worsened over the course of his marriage to Lena, became acute following the birth of each child, and in recent years, took on a life of its own. He was able to keep the drinking from interfering with his work, but it ruined his private life. Melinda was also a heavy drinker, and drinking together was a major component of their relationship.

In contrast, Lena hardly drank alcohol, having come from a divorced family with an alcoholic and inconsistently involved father. Lena said she had always been the "perfect child," a model for her younger siblings and a big help to her mom. Lena and Tom met in high school, where Lena had been at the top of her class. Lena attended college and, on graduation, went to work for the state. Tom began work at the power company within a year or so after graduation from high school. Over the years, Lena bore the brunt of the day-to-day responsibilities for the children and household because Tom often worked overtime. Tom's betrayal cut even more deeply because Melinda was a young Caucasian woman whom Tom met at work. The therapist understands that race, gender, and family role functioning are all important aspects of the couple's context that may constrain the development and/or implementation of solution sequences.

Lena: It really hurt me that Tom ends up having an affair with a young White woman who is free from any major responsibility in life. I have worked day and night to build our family. I raised these kids, and he cheats on me.

Therapist: Lena, you mentioned that Melinda was "White." How is that an issue for you?

Lena: It just makes me wonder whether I should have married him in the first place. My mom was not sure he really loved me, that maybe he was just interested in the exoticness of being involved with a Black woman. Maybe I never should have trusted him in the first place.

Tom: Lena, Melinda being White had nothing to do with why I wanted to be with her. And you being Black was not a reason. I love you and felt like I had lost you. It was you and the kids on one side and me and work and the booze on the other. I was ripe for the picking, and I hate to say it, I probably would have gotten involved with any attractive woman that expressed interest in me—Black or White.

Therapist: Tom, was Lena's being Black a factor for you in marrying her?

Tom: My dad was a real racist, and I always prided myself on not being like him. I had Black friends in high school, and being with Lena felt natural. Also, my mom was really turned off with my dad's racism and was very open to my Black friends, and when Lena came along, she opened her arms and welcomed her into the family.

Lena: I did feel welcomed and accepted by Tom's mom. I worried that maybe I was the "screw you" Tom wanted to aim at his dad.

Tom: If that was the case, which it wasn't, it wouldn't have worked. By the time we got involved, my dad had changed a lot and, as you know, was open to our getting married.

Lena: I guess that's right. He has been pretty accepting. I guess that I just don't like anything about Melinda—White, young, pretty—I hate everything about her.

Tom: I am not defending her, but the truth is that it was me. I responded to Melinda, and I didn't have to. I am the one you should hate. I betrayed you, and she was incidental. [The therapist is impressed with Tom's efforts to draw Lena's anger toward him as the responsible agent in the affair.]

As they dug into the problem sequence, it became clear that Tom's loneliness, disconnection, pain, and general dysphoria predated Lena's rejection of his sexual overtures. His self-presentation as a happy-go-lucky go-getter had begun to wear thin at work and home. His "hardworking and hard drinking" persona was crumbling. He was questioning what his life was about and struggling with feelings of emptiness, general angst, and loneliness. The AA meetings he attended were his only outlet.

Early in these sessions, the therapist considered the possibility of seeing Tom and Lena individually for a session, but he decided that was not necessary because of the surprisingly high degree of self-disclosure and painful honesty that characterized their interaction with each other and with him. Also, their questionnaire data indicated that from the second session on, they both had strong alliances with the therapist and, surprisingly, with each other.

By the end of 5 months of weekly therapy, many things had changed between Tom and Lena. He had moved back into the house and they both decided to tell the children about his affair with Melinda (the older children had been asking all along whether there was someone else in Dad's life). Tom apologized to them as well as Lena for betraying all of them. In sessions, they both talked with remarkable frankness about their disconnected marriage. The therapist helped the couple develop a process for addressing Lena's deep pain and recurrent anger about the affair. This involved Tom responding truthfully to her questions, being empathic to her experience of betrayal, and affirming his commitment. This was reiterative and challenging work that was more complex than can fully be described in this case study. Through this intensive work they were rebuilding trust—no lies about anything for Tom. He had also decided to stop drinking for the foreseeable future and was able to do so with the help of regular attendance at AA. He had come to understand how cut off he had been from himself and Lena and was now communicating about feelings in a new way. He realized that sex had been the only way he knew to connect and feel close and soothed.

Lena welcomed these changes from Tom, although she remained somewhat guarded, concerned that Tom's many changes were motivated by fear and therefore might not last once he felt things were back to normal. She also insisted that he cease all contact with Melinda as a precondition for them continuing their marriage. Fortuitously, shortly after Tom ended his affair with her, Melinda left the power company and found work elsewhere.

However, Melinda's absence from Tom's workplace was not enough to assuage Lena's need for closure. She decided she wanted to have a conversation of her own with Melinda. Tom was worried and reluctant about such a meeting, as was the therapist, but after assessing that Lena's goals were realistic and that safety was not an issue, the therapist supported the idea, believing that taking action on her own would be empowering to Lena and that she had the interpersonal skills and self-control to manage the possible challenges such a meeting would entail. Several weeks after Melinda left the job, Lena called her and arranged a meeting. At that meeting, Lena confronted Melinda about choosing to have an affair with a married man. Melinda burst into tears, apologized, and asked for forgiveness. Lena said she could forgive, but would never forget and would not tolerate Melinda ever reaching out to Tom again. Lena felt strengthened by her meeting with Melinda and felt less like a victim; it significantly reduced her concerns about Melinda trying to reengage Tom in the affair.

As this part of their therapy was winding down, the therapist was impressed with the transformation of their problem sequence. Now, when Tom felt lonely and distraught, he reached out to Lena, not for sex, but for conversation. Lena never rejected these overtures unless she was exhausted, and even then she was able to say "not now; later" in a friendly way. Their connection grew and was affirmed by Lena's commitment and trust scores rising on the weekly questionnaire she completed. More slowly, sexual satisfaction began to improve for both partners.

> *Lena:* What really makes me feel more confident in Tom is that the other night, he told me that he was angry with me about not keeping him in the loop with the kids. He said that he felt excluded, as if we weren't coparents. I apologized and said that I had spent so many years operating as a single parent that I would have lapses and he should just remind me.
>
> *Therapist:* It sounds like you're feeling less alone. For the first time, you really have a partner, but it is taking some getting used to.
>
> *Lena:* That's right, but I still have trouble trusting him. Sometimes I feel he is talking about his feelings just because he wants to get laid. I still feel like I am getting to know this new person I live with. When he can get mad at me for a legitimate reason, ironically it makes me feel more secure. He is not just appeasing me or being a "good boy."
>
> *Therapist:* If he can risk getting mad and making you mad, particularly when the anger is not defending his stonewalling and lies, then you know his new expressiveness is not just manipulation, but real. That's good. Tom, what do you think?
>
> *Tom:* I just want to get laid. [Everyone laughs and the session ends.]

The Miles/Family Sessions

As their marriage began to show substantial recovery, Tom and Lena increasingly talked about their concerns about Miles. In conjunction with the therapist, they defined Miles's problems and their difficulty helping him as a new presenting problem they wanted to address. He was socially isolated in fourth grade and frequently said he hated school. Tom took the position that he was the same as Miles at that age, which was around the time his parents divorced. His position was that Miles would grow out of these problems. Lena was more worried and concerned that they were missing something.

The therapist hypothesized that the emerging focus on Miles might be a way of avoiding certain unresolved marital issues, particularly the slow recovery of their sexual relationship.

> Therapist: I share the concern that both of you are expressing about Miles. I think it is legitimate and appropriate. However, I have another concern, and that is that by shifting our focus to Miles, we are avoiding really digging in to what is going on with you sexually.

> Lena: I don't think that is the case. My sense is that the marital crisis is ending, and we can now give Miles the attention I think he needs. My hunch is that our sexual relationship will take care of itself over time.

> Therapist: Lena, how do you think Tom feels about that?

> Lena: I think he agrees with me, but I am not sure.

> Therapist: Why don't you check it out now with him. [The therapist asks Lena to conduct the exploration of Tom's feelings rather than doing it himself, so he can observe their interaction over this sensitive topic and also assess and facilitate their growing ability to do the work of therapy on their own.]

> Lena: What do you think? Are we avoiding focusing on ourselves and sex by shifting the focus to Miles?

> Tom: I am not sure. Our sexual relationship is not where I would want it to be, but it is getting better. My gut feeling is that we are heading in the right direction and should just trust time. I don't mean to be corny, but this is like the last flower to grow in our new garden and we should not rush it.

> Lena: [To the therapist] He is just saying that, because he knows I love to garden. [To Tom] Do you really mean that, or are you just saying that because that is what you think I want to hear?

> Tom: No. I really mean it. I think we will get there.

> Therapist: Although we are focusing more on Miles at this point, let's not lose this thread. We can loop back to it as well as we go forward.

Toward the end of the session, the therapist suggested that they bring Miles and his siblings in for a family session. He thought it would be worthwhile to talk with all of the kids about what this family crisis had been like for them and to get a sense of Miles without making him out to be the "identified patient" and singular focus of the session. The therapist thought that he would be more likely to open up if the spotlight was not directly on him. A family session was scheduled for the next week.

The family session began with the therapist welcoming the kids and asking them how they felt about meeting him and being part of a family session. Aiden volunteered feeling interested and a little worried. When asked about his worry, he said he was worried that his parents were going to announce in the session that they were getting divorced. Tom and Lena reassured him and the other children they were not getting divorced and their marriage was getting stronger. The therapist asked Tanya how she felt about being there. She said that she did not care and had come because her mom told her she had to. He asked her whether the previous 3 months had been a difficult time and she replied, "Yeah, but I keep to myself and my friends."

Therapist:	How has it been a difficult time for you?
Tanya:	I don't know. I don't like to hear them fight.
Therapist:	When you would hear them fight, what kind of things did they say or do?
Tanya:	She told him to get out of the house and that she never wanted to see him again.
Therapist:	How did you feel when you heard that?
Tanya:	Scared. Scared that I would never see him again. Scared that maybe he loved the other woman more than Mom.
Therapist:	Did you feel mad at either of them?
Tanya:	Yeah. I was mad at him for cheating on my mom and kind of mad at my mom for throwing him out. But I understood. I would have thrown him out too if I was her.
Therapist:	Miles, can I ask you a question?
Miles:	Yeah, OK.
Therapist:	Were you scared too?
Miles:	I hate it when they fight and scream. I was scared when my dad moved out.
Therapist:	Was there anybody that you could talk to about feeling scared? Like Tanya?

Miles:	I would talk to her. I would get in bed with her when I would hear fighting at night.
Therapist:	It's good that you could turn to her and that she could make you feel safer. Could you talk to your dad or mom about your fears about him moving out?
Miles:	Not really. I did not want them to be mad at me.
Therapist:	Miles, do you think you could tell them now how scared you were then, and maybe even sometimes now. [The therapist makes it happen in the room as the first step in implementing a new adaptive sequence.]
Miles:	[To Dad] I thought you would never come back and that I would not be able to see you again. Mom was so mad, and I knew something real bad had happened.
Tom:	I am sorry that I did not talk with you at that time. I was so ashamed about what I had done and upset to be leaving. I wasn't a very good father then.
Miles:	[With tears in his eyes] I know. Why did you do that to Mom and us?
Tom:	[With tears in his eyes] Because I was afraid to deal with our problems and because I was selfish. I wasn't really thinking clearly—like I am now. I am so sorry that I made you feel so bad. But I am glad that you are telling me now.

Miles got up as his dad was talking and went over and sat in his lap. His dad held him and everyone was teary and sad. After a while, the therapist commented that it was a sign of their strength as a family that they could talk about and share their thoughts and feelings about this crisis in their life. The therapist continued exploring Aiden's and Tanya's feelings about the blowup of their parents' marriage and concluded the session by inviting them all to come back for another session a week later.

As the family was leaving, the therapist asked whether Tom and Lena could stay for a couple of minutes while the kids waited in the waiting room. Alone with the parents, the therapist asked whether it was OK with them for him to talk with Miles in the next session about his family, school, and learning issues. He also asked them whether it was OK for him to discuss the possibility of an educational and neuropsychological evaluation with Miles to pinpoint his learning issues. The therapist explained that it would likely be covered by their health insurance, but if not, the evaluation could be done on a sliding scale basis by a well-trained and supervised psychology intern. Tom and Lena wholeheartedly approved of the initiative and said they would assist with the conversation any way they could.

In the next session, after checking in with the kids and Tom and Lena about their reactions to the previous session, the therapist turned to Miles and asked him whether he could talk with him in front of his family about how school had been for him during the past couple of months. (The therapist had used the first session to build an alliance with Miles before moving, in this second family session, into the difficult subject of school and academic performance.) Miles said "OK" and elaborated.

Miles: It was hard. It was hard to remember things. I felt lonely and like crying a lot.

Therapist: Did you ever cry there?

Miles: No. I didn't want to be a crybaby.

Therapist: Yeah. I know how hard that can be. Keeping it all in and trying to pay attention. Miles, why do you think it was or is hard for you to remember things?

Miles: Because I'm stupid. That's what some of the kids call me.

Therapist: How long have you felt that way about yourself?

Miles: Always.

Therapist: You know, I don't think it's hard for you to remember because you're stupid. I think it's something else.

Miles: Like what?

Therapist: I don't know, but I can tell you're not stupid just by talking to you last week and today. In fact, I think you're pretty smart. Would you like to find out why it may be hard for you to remember some things?

Miles: Yeah, I guess so.

Therapist: We have a doctor here who helps kids figure out why they're good at certain things and not good at other things. Would you like to meet with her and see if she can help us figure out and help you with the memory thing?

Miles: Sure. Do you really think she can help me?

Therapist: I do. I will talk to her, then your parents can call her and set up a time for you to meet with her. Would that be OK?

The therapist arranged for Miles to be tested for learning disabilities. It turned out that he had a major auditory learning problem that led to a meeting with the therapist, Miles's parents, Miles, Miles's teacher, a learning disability specialist, and the school psychologist. That meeting led to various interventions that gave Miles the support he needed to be more successful in school. As he met with more success, he started feeling better about himself and started to reach out to other kids at school. As this process unfolded, Tom and Lena started to relax about Miles. They also were able to understand his difficulty following verbal instructions and started either showing him what they wanted him to do or writing things out so he could read them rather than relying primarily on hearing.

Ending the Episode—Termination for Now

After the two family sessions, the therapist met once more with Tom and Lena, who said they were satisfied with the results of the therapy and felt they were ready to stop. They felt their marriage was repaired and things were much better with Miles. They realized their work was not done, but they felt they now had the tools to continue on their own. The therapist asked what they meant by "tools."

Tom: I learned to stop avoiding and started dealing directly with Lena. Now we can talk about the tough stuff we used to avoid. We also learned to talk together as a family about feelings that we were afraid of. This therapy gave us "courage" to face ourselves. Oh yeah, I also learned that sex was not the only way to connect or get comforted and that I don't think I can drink.

Therapist: Lena, how about you? What did you learn or get out of this therapy?

Lena: I got a chance to heal. I felt broken when I found out about the affair. My heart is still healing, but I feel pretty confident that the healing will continue. I also realized how strong I could be when I had to. I realized that I could live without Tom if I had to.

Tom: Oh, boy. I've really got to be careful now.

Lena: You sure do. There will be no second chances. You need to know that.

Tom: I get it.

Therapist: Tom, what did you feel when Lena said "no second chances?"

Tom: I felt scared, I think that I can stay sober and on the right track, but to be honest, I don't feel 100% sure. My not drinking is relatively new, and I am still working on expressing my feelings and staying honest. I also feel a little afraid of not seeing you anymore. You have brought me, and us, back from the brink. I kind of count on you.

Therapist:	Well, Tom, I too am not 100% sure that stopping now is the right thing. Your sobriety is new and you have a new way to deal with your feelings, particularly painful and uncomfortable feelings. And we know that your sexual relationship is not where you want it to be and may reflect some deeper issues we have not gotten to. But I want to respect your mutual sense that this episode of therapy is drawing to a close. What would you do if you felt yourself sliding back? [The therapist shares their ambivalence about stopping now but does not want to undermine their growing sense of competence and strength. He clearly defines their stopping as the end of this episode, implying that there may well be others to come. His last question reflects his desire to be their safety net, while respecting and validating their desire to be on their own.]
Lena:	We'd call you and get our butts back in this office.
Therapist:	Good. I will be here. You both have done very good work.
Tom:	Are we your best patients ever?
Therapist:	[Smiling and chuckling] You sure are. But seriously, when problems come up, which they surely will, use your skills and tools and give them your best shot. If that does not work, come back for another episode of work. Don't wait too long until you're in real trouble.
Lena:	We won't. Thanks so much for helping us and our family.
Therapist:	My pleasure. Goodbye and take care.

THE SECOND EPISODE

The next episode of therapy began 18 months later with a call from Lena.

Lena:	Tom has been acting strangely. He's gotten more secretive and withdrawn. I think he's drinking again. I'm feeling freaked out. Like it's all happening again.
Therapist:	What does he say when you confront him?
Lena:	He says it's nothing—that he's not drinking and that nothing is going on, that I'm paranoid and should not worry. But I feel in my gut that something's not right.
Therapist:	How long has this been going on?
Lena:	I'm not sure. It's been getting worse recently. I started to notice things about 4 months ago.

Therapist:	Let's find a time when you both can come in.
Lena:	He says it's all in my head and that I need you more than he does. I'm not sure he will come in.
Therapist:	Tell him that it's essential that you both come in together. [The therapist feels that his alliance with Lena and Tom was still strong enough, that he could be direct and authoritative about their coming in together.]
Lena:	I'll try.

The First Session

The therapist saw Tom and Lena 2 days later. The session began with the therapist asking Tom what he thought was going on with them. As the session unfolded, Tom stuck to his story that nothing was going on and that Lena was oversensitive and making a mountain out of a molehill. In response, Lena laid out a whole series of "strange" behaviors on Tom's part and added that she had recently found an empty whiskey bottle in their garbage and that 3 days previously somebody texted her, saying Tom was having an affair with a White coworker. She did not recognize the phone number, and the person did not identify him- or herself. Tom was stunned and said that somebody at work was out to destroy him and their marriage and he had an idea who it was. He also said he had no idea how an empty whiskey bottle had ended up in their garbage. Maybe, he suggested, some kids had been drinking in the alley and put it there. Lena said she found it hard to believe that and did not know what she wanted to do.

At that point, feeling that Tom was not being honest in front of Lena, the therapist asked whether he could meet individually with each of them. They consented. Understanding the importance of clarity and consensus with respect to confidentiality and the use of individual sessions in couples therapy, the therapist asked whether they wanted the individual sessions with each of them to be confidential or not. Lena looked at him and said, "Let them be confidential. If he's drinking or having an affair, better you should know than no one." Tom said, "I don't care. I'm not afraid of the truth."

Individual Sessions

Lena

Lena's session began with her bursting into tears and saying to the therapist, "I think my marriage is over." Her pain poured out. She said she felt Tom was "gaslighting" her, making her doubt her own senses. She also said that she felt there was a racial aspect to what was happening, that maybe Tom could not love her or really want her because she was Black. She found it interesting and painful that whoever sent the text said the woman he was involved with was White, as was Melinda. Maybe he had never really loved her.

Lena: Maybe he married me because I was not his mother. I was almost as far as you could get from her. Great student, successful career, but Black. But maybe that isn't what he really needs or wants.

Therapist: Lena, we can and will focus on Tom and why he married you and how much of it had to do with his being White and your being Black, but I think what we need to talk about today is what do you need at this point in your life.

Lena: I don't know. I am not sure who or what to believe. I think he's lying to me, but maybe he's not. Maybe he's relapsed and that's what all this is about. What should I do?

Therapist: I am not sure. The question for me is, what do you need to get both of your feet on the ground and stop spinning? The immediate order of business is for us to figure out what you need to stabilize yourself. You may not be able to figure out the truth at this point, but what do you need to do to get your own equilibrium back?

Lena: The truth for me at this point is that I don't trust Tom. If it comes to a choice between trusting my senses and trusting his words, I have to go with my senses. I think I want him out of the house. I can't live with this and it reopens all the pain from before.

Lena continued to explore her feelings and needs and concluded that she would ask Tom to move out, at least for now. She also said she did not want to work with him in couples therapy because she felt he was not being honest with her. She wanted her own therapist so she could sort out what she needed to do at this point in her life. The therapist agreed to provide a referral but asked that before Lena closed the door on couples therapy, she wait to see what came from Tom's individual session. Lena agreed to wait until the next time all three of them were together to make decisions. In the meantime, Tom could sleep in another room of the house or stay with his brother.

Tom

Arriving for his session, Tom sat down, and sighed. Then he began.

Tom: Boy, have I totally screwed up. I can't believe what is happening. I am drinking and I have started flirting with a woman at work. I am not sleeping with her, but we are definitely talking in ways that I wouldn't want Lena to hear. I know what

Lena said when we stopped seeing you before—"no second chance." If I tell her the truth, we will be done, and that is not what I want.

Therapist: What do you want, Tom?

Tom: I'm not sure. I think I want to be with Lena, but look at my behavior. I think I want to be sober, but I am drinking again. I don't seem to be able to do what I think I want. I am just screwed up and lost.

Therapist: Tom, I am going to be really frank with you. I don't think that you can figure out what you want and why you are getting in your way so long as you are drinking. I know that getting sober and back into some kind of program is not going to solve all your problems, but it is a precondition for figuring out the rest.

Tom: But I can't come out and tell her the truth or it will be over.

Therapist: If you don't tell her the truth, it will be over. If you do, and you take responsibility for what has happened and commit to getting sober and facing your own shit, maybe, just maybe, she will give you another chance. But if you keep stonewalling and denying, you're putting nails in your marital coffin. [The therapist views Tom's drinking as a constraint that prevents him from thinking clearly and being able to integrate his behavior, feelings, and intentions.]

After the individual sessions, Tom and Lena came in several days later together for a follow-up and planning session.

Therapist: How are you both doing, and how did you both feel about the individual sessions?

Lena: I told him that he needed to move out and not just for a couple of days. I need some space, and I am not sure I can go through all of this again.

Tom: Lena, I have some things that I want to tell you that I have been afraid to talk about. I will move out if that is what you want, but I need you to listen to what I have to say. Is that OK?

Lena: Yeah. Go ahead.

Tom: I have been afraid to tell you the truth because I remembered what you said when we stopped therapy before—no second chance. But in coming back to therapy, I came to clearly see that if I am not honest with you, we will be done anyway. So I am going to tell you the truth. I did start drinking, and I have been lying to you about that. The whiskey bottle you found was from me. I now have stopped drinking and have gone back to AA, and I am committed to doing 90 meetings in 90 days. You're also right—I did start flirting with a woman at work, but I have not had any kind of physical relationship with her. I ended that already and told her that I have to get my own head and my marriage sorted out and that we can only be work colleagues. Ironically, she and her husband have gotten into therapy too.

Lena: I knew this was going on. I can't believe you lied to me and tried to make me think I was crazy. If you had been straight with me when you started drinking or about this "flirtation," we could have come back to therapy, and at least there would be no lies. How do I know this won't happen again?

Tom: You can't know. I don't know. I just know that I am not drinking, lying, or doing anything inappropriate with anybody else today. And my plan is to continue that way tomorrow, and I hope forever. I also think that I need some individual therapy to figure out who I really am and what I want.

Lena: That's up to you. I also think that I need some individual therapy to sort out what I want to do. To help me.

Therapist: Tom I am glad that you were honest with Lena. I am also glad that you are pursuing sobriety. I also support and admire your desire to do some individual work and figure out who you really are and what you need. Lena, I admire and support your willingness to listen to Tom and not just walk out. I also totally get your desire to have your own therapist at this time. Let me talk for a little while about some options at this point for going forward. Would that be OK?

Tom and Lena: Yeah, sure.

Therapist: I see three options at this point in terms of therapy. The first is that we stop our couple work and the two of you each see individual therapists. The second is that you both see individual therapists, and we continue our couple work. The third is that we continue working together but bring a greater individual focus to our work—in other words, that we do some individual therapy in the context of our couple work. What are your thoughts about these options? [The therapist, aware of the potential benefits and pitfalls of simultaneous individual and couples therapy, invites Tom and Lena to consider the options and coplan their therapy.]

Lena, I am particularly interested in what you are thinking. [The therapist prioritizes Lena's response to simultaneously support their alliance and acknowledge her autonomy in this decision-making process.]

Lena: I don't know. I feel very shaken and like I need someone in my corner who is just thinking about me and not about the marriage. You're great, but I feel that you are for the marriage and maybe can't be as objective as my own individual therapist could be.

Therapist: Lena, I understand your sense of me being for the marriage. Let me clarify, though. I am for your relationship, not necessarily for your marriage. You two are going to be related to each other until you die. You will have at least a coparental and a cograndparental relationship, if not a marriage. I am for you having the best relationship you can have, whatever form it takes, which, in fact, may not be marriage. I do help couples divorce when they are convinced that is the right thing, or when they are destroying each other and can't stop.

Lena: Are you suggesting that we work with you and not do any individual therapy?

Therapist: I am saying that is a possibility, especially with the particular situation you're in at this point. By that, I mean that neither of you wants to pursue another relationship and the most immediate reasons things have fallen apart now have to do with Tom's drinking and I believe his fear of really turning to you and being your partner. He is taking his drinking very seriously and doing everything in his power to manage it. I also think he is ready to work on his stuff individually and with you. I also think staying separated for a while is not a bad idea. Tom, what do you think about what I just said? [In supporting Lena and the idea of separation, the therapist is sensitive to the potential of Tom experiencing this as a rupture of their alliance.]

Tom: I agree with what you said. I really want to work on myself and my marriage, and if I can do both in this therapy, that would be my choice. I am not thrilled about the separation, but it may be a good thing. It's really up to you, Lena.

Lena: After this all came out, I called an individual therapist and have an appointment set up for later this week. Let me see her and think about it and see what I want to do then.

The session ended with Tom and Lena agreeing to make an appointment for the following week. They both arrived at that session separately, and Lena led off.

Lena: I saw the individual therapist twice since we were here last week and have been doing a lot of thinking. My desire is to work out our marriage if things can really change. I heard what you said about our situation and Tom's commitment to being sober and doing some work, and if we can do that work together and get stronger, that would be the best thing. I think I may be crazy to try again, but I will give it one more chance. Tom, I don't know if you will take me seriously that this is our last chance after what I said last time, but I won't go through this again. I want to continue with the individual therapy for a while, and I want us to stay separated and do couples therapy. If we can rebuild trust and do some serious work, we can talk about you moving back in.

Therapist: Lena, you have been doing a lot of thinking and sorting things out. It sounds like your work with your individual therapist has already been helpful.

Lena: It is very helpful. She gets where I am at. She supports my desire to get stronger in myself and be less dependent on Tom, and at the same time, she understands that I love him and would like to rebuild the marriage if it can be done. She also knows of you and thinks you are very good, and she has also done a lot of work with people with addictions. She seems very level-headed and realistic.

Therapist: Lena, that sounds very good and appropriate. Lena, would it be OK if I made contact with your individual therapist? I regularly do that when people I am working with are in some other kind of therapy. [The therapist is interested in reaching out to, coordinating, and building a therapist system alliance with other therapists working with Tom and Lena.]

Lena: Sure, no problem.

Therapist: Tom, as you listen to Lena reporting on her individual work, what are you feeling and thinking?

Tom: I am not a big believer in all this "higher power" stuff they talk about in AA, but I feel that maybe there is a higher power and he or she or it is watching out for me and us. I feel very grateful to have you, Lena, in my life and open to the possibility of us going forward. I actually feel kind of stunned.

Therapist:	Tom, you look sad. What are you feeling?
Tom:	It's strange, but I feel like crying. I feel very touched by the caring that I feel from both of you and, strangely, from Lena's individual therapist. It's confusing, but I feel kind of taken care of. [Tom quietly weeps. All three sit quietly. After a couple of minutes, Tom resumes talking.] In AA they talk about surrendering to a higher power and letting go, particularly letting go of the fantasy that you are in control and I feel like this is what is happening to me. I cannot control my life on my own, and I am facing that for the first time. To do this, I need AA; I need you, Lena; and in truth, I need this therapy.
Therapist:	Tom, talk to me about letting go. [The therapist wants to support Tom's emerging openness to a spiritual dimension in his life that may facilitate an emotional recovery and spiritual awakening.]
Tom:	I just feel so tired. Like I have been fighting for so long to be a certain kind of person—to look and appear a certain way—and it is not working. And when it doesn't work at home with you, Lena, and with the kids, I run back to work. There they tell me how great I am and I get younger women to respond to me, and I feel powerful and alive, but I have been drinking and lying and pretending all over the place. I can't remember who I have said what to. I am exhausted by my life and my lies.
Therapist:	Lena, what are you feeling about what Tom has been saying and the tears?
Lena:	Lots of feelings. I feel sad, like crying myself. I feel like Tom is being very real and open, maybe for the first time in his life. I feel relieved, like we are taking a big sigh together. I also feel scared that this won't last, that he will close up and shut down, and I will be left alone again.
Tom:	Lena, I pledge to not shut down or run away, no matter how scared or crazy I get. I will bring my shit to AA, to you, and I'll bring it here. If you see me slipping, call me on it. I don't want to go on being the way I have been. I have hurt you and the kids, and I feel ashamed—I have not been a good father or a good husband. I want to run away from that, but I won't. I will just sit here and feel like a shit—present and accounted for.
Lena:	Tom, thank you. I do think you've been a shit, but I don't think that's all you are—you are a lot more, and if you can

continue what you've been talking about today, I think we can have something solid and real. At least that is what I hope right now.

Therapist: I think you are both doing some great work. I think we need to shift before we stop today and talk about what you both want to do with each other and the family this week, between now and our next session.

The therapist helped Tom and Lena talk about what they wanted in the immediate future. Lena said that, on a weekly basis, she would like to see Tom alone for dinner one night and that he should come over and have dinner with her and the kids one night. She said he should also do something, at least once a week, alone with the kids. In fact, she thought he should do something separately with Miles and something with Tanya. Tom agreed, and the therapist ended the session saying that next time he wanted to talk about the roles that Lena and Tom take with each other.

At the next session, Tom and Lena arrived in good spirits. Lena said the week had gone well. Her time alone with Tom and their time with the kids had been good. Tom had gotten together alone with Tanya. When she got home afterward, Tanya told her Mom that Dad had made a nice dinner for her at his apartment. Tom said he had enjoyed making dinner for Tanya and having some time alone with her. He felt they had talked more with each other that night than they had in the previous 6 months. Lena also said Tom was not pressuring her for more time or to get back together, which she appreciated.

Therapist: Lena, I'd like to understand what you appreciated about that?

Lena: He was respecting my space and need to sort things out on my own.

Therapist: Is that different from the way things were between you in the past?

Lena: Yeah, I felt that Tom was always wanting something from me, particularly sex.

Therapist: I have a hunch it was more than sex.

Lena: What do you mean?

Therapist: This was something that I mentioned I wanted to talk about at the end of last week's session—your roles with each other. I think that you have developed certain roles with each other that have kind of burned you out as a couple. Specifically, I think that, Lena, you take care of Tom in lots of ways that are just implicit in your relationship. I was impressed last week by how you took such a decisive and leading role in regard to the terms of the separation and how the two of you would move forward. It led me to think, and I do not mean this at all as a criticism of you, Lena, that you are kind of like the leader and caretaker of your relationship with Tom as well as Tom's relationship with the family. Tom, you seem to respond well, up to a point, when Lena takes leadership in your life. [The therapist begins to explore the way in which Tom and Lena have organized their lives as well as the extent to which that organization constrains their growth and intimacy.]

Tom: I do like it. I like it when Lena takes leadership of things; she is very good at it—just a natural leader. I feel kind of taken care of by her when she does that.

Therapist: Tom, my recollection is that you reported that particularly after your parents divorced, you did not feel connected and safe with anyone in your family. Was your relationship with Lena your first experience of feeling connected and safe with another person? [After stabilizing Tom and Lena's relationship and exploring their current psychosocial organization, the therapist begins to explore some of the more remote and historical constraints impeding their ability to implement and sustain healthier relating.]

Tom: Yes. It definitely was. For some reason, with all of the other women I was involved with before Lena, I was in charge. With Lena, I felt like I could let go and she would be there. She has always been so competent.

Therapist: So when did that change for you?

Tom: It changed with the kids. She was there for them, but not so much for me. I felt they were more important to her than I was. They came first. She is the best mom in the world.

Therapist: And she had been the first person in your life that you could feel connected with, the way you never could with your mom or your dad. She was almost like the mother you never had. [Identifying a constraint to change, the therapist makes the connection between Tom's early experience in his family of origin with his mother and his experience of Lena over the course of their marriage.]

Tom: I never thought of her as my mother, but she definitely was there for me.

Therapist: So when that diminished, how did you feel?

Tom: Alone, kind of lost, I guess a little sad.

Therapist:	What about angry? [The therapist begins exploring the maladaptively and historically denied emotions that have constrained Tom's adaptive functioning.]
Tom:	Yeah, but I did not feel that my anger was legitimate. I hated feeling like I was in competition for her with my kids. Was I that immature and needy?
Therapist:	So you felt ashamed of your feelings. How did they come out? Where did they go?
Tom:	We know where they went. Booze and other women. I guess I ran away from her rather than feel so needy and immature. Like I wasn't a man.
Therapist:	So now, how is it for you to be out of the house and having to organize your own life and your relationship with your kids? Lena still organizes things, but she is not taking care of you very much these days.
Tom:	Sometimes at night, alone in that little apartment, I feel so lonely. Almost a pit in my stomach—an ache. I miss her and the kids—being in my family.
Therapist:	So how are you dealing with that pain? [While illuminating the emotional roots of the problem, the therapist is helping Tom and Lena see the progress he is making in dealing with his feelings more adaptively and appropriately.]
Tom:	I talk about it in AA. A guy in one of my AA groups suggested that I keep a diary, so I've started writing when I feel so bad. It's strange, but it helps.
Therapist:	That's great. Journaling can make a big difference. It's also you taking care of some of your needs in a healthy adaptive way, rather than booze, other women, or demanding sex from Lena. You're tolerating those feelings and not running away from them. That takes a lot of courage. You're also redefining for yourself what it means to be a man—facing yourself and not running away, having the courage to face your pain and write about it. You are growing. [The therapist is also beginning to identify and explore some of Tom's constraining gender beliefs about what it means to be a man.]
Tom:	I also pray for peace and serenity. I don't even know who I am praying to, but when I feel so bad, it helps. I feel like I am sending my pain out into the cosmos and asking for relief. Maybe a higher power is out there that absorbs that stuff that pain and everything else. I don't know.

Therapist: Lena, how are you reacting to what you're hearing?

Lena: It's good. I feel relieved. It's like I don't have to take care of Tom. I am impressed with his courage and honesty. He is letting himself be more vulnerable at the same time that he is getting stronger and that is good. He is also becoming a more real person and less of some kind of cartoon man. It makes me feel hopeful, but I am still feeling very wary.

Therapist: That all makes sense. Your wariness is good too. There is another side to this whole conversation that we haven't touched on. I am talking about your role in this process with Tom. The ease with which you move into that caretaker–mother role and what happens to your needs in that process. I would like to explore that in our next session. [The therapist begins to shift the focus from Tom to Lena and opens the door to explore her role in and contribution to the maladaptive over/under adequate pattern of their relating.]

Tom and Lena came in for their next session, and Tom led off by saying he felt the therapy had been focusing a lot on him and, as the therapist had mentioned last time, they should focus on Lena today.

Tom: I am feeling pretty good and managing well, so I don't need to be the focus today.

Therapist: Lena, shall we pick up where we left off last session?

Lena: Sure. What should I talk about?

Therapist: Have you had any thoughts or feelings about my comment at the end of the last session?

Lena: Yeah, in fact, I talked with my individual therapist about what you said. She said that she thinks I have been the caretaker and little mother in my family growing up and the big mother in this family. I take care of everybody.

Therapist: And does that ring true for you?

Lena: Yes, but I felt that my mom needed me, and I just stepped up.

Therapist: She did need you, as did your siblings. You were kind of your mother's backup and the father in the family as well—the organizer and person that everybody could look up to and respect. I hear that your dad failed the family. You did the opposite. But, I wonder what you missed out on—what needs of yours did not get taken care of—having to grow up so young and having to be so good and competent all the time [The therapist simultaneously validates Lena's early experience in her family of origin and presents the hypothesis that she may have lost out on some things as a result of her family's needs and her innate competence.]

Lena: I'm not sure. I know what you and my therapist are getting at, but I did not have an unhappy childhood. Sure, my dad was a wreck and ultimately not there, but I felt loved and connected with my mom; my grandparents were around. I did not feel alone. And I felt that everybody was proud of what I accomplished.

Therapist: I think you are right. You were very bright and talented and taking the leadership role you took in your family kind of fit who you were, and you definitely felt seen and appreciated. You were not abandoned or unloved. [The therapist moves away from the "lost childhood" hypothesis in the face of Lena's rejection of it, both to preserve their alliance and because it may well be true that there was not a downside for her in what happened.] And when you and Tom got together, the two of you kind of fit together—he had never felt connected or taken care of, and you could connect and care take very well. His need for a mother and to be taken care of got fulfilled and remained kind of invisible or implicit, up until the kids started to come and your caretaking and mothering went more in their direction. Then the pattern you both had created broke down, and he went astray.

Tom: And now I am facing that need and not going astray. Lena, you are still there for me in your heart, I know that, but I am taking care of myself and not doing it in messed-up ways like before.

Therapist: And now the piece that I am wondering about is whether the two of you want to shift the balance of caretaking in your marriage even more?

Lena: Like how?

Therapist: Like maybe Tom taking care of you sometimes instead of you mostly taking care of Tom. Or you putting your needs out there more and asking him to come through more as a partner and as a coparent. For instance, what if you asked him to take care of Tanya and Miles for a long weekend and you went away to see some of your friends or spent some time doing things that you enjoy but may have put on hold. [The therapist proposes a new sequence of interaction to address the imbalance in role functioning that constrains the marital relationship.]

Lena: That would be different. I could use a break. This has been such a hard time, particularly a second time around.

Tom:	You know I made dinner for Tanya at my apartment last week. It was great. I can do more. Why don't you leave them with me and take some time for yourself? I'd like that and feel less like such a selfish jerk.
Lena:	Yeah, I would like that.

After this session, Tom and Lena planned for her to go away for 3 days while the two younger kids stayed with Tom at his apartment. They talked about him moving into the house for the weekend, but Tom said he knew Lena would then make sure everything was perfect in the house and taken care of. If they came over to his place, they'd gripe about it, but Lena would have less to take care of and worry about. Also, Lena felt she was not ready for Tom to move back in, even for a weekend when she was not there.

WINDING DOWN THERAPY

Tom and Lena continued in couples therapy for another 6 months, cutting down to every other week during the last 2 months. During this time, they worked intensively on building trust, communicating openly, and finding new patterns of mutuality and interdependence. Insights gained during the early sessions of the second episode of therapy provided direction for much of the rest of the therapy but required repeated interpretation and application to the actual patterns of their marital and family life. There were challenges and complications in this successful process that are beyond the scope of this discussion. Lena continued her individual therapy and felt it was helping her express her needs and desires with greater clarity and strength. Tom continued AA attendance (recommended by a formal evaluation for addiction) and moved back in at the end of the third month. Several weeks after Tom moved back in, the following conversation took place.

Therapist:	How is it going with Tom back in the house?
Tom:	[Smiling shyly] Pretty good.
Therapist:	What does that mean?
Tom:	It means that lots of things are better and different. For me a huge difference is that we are not only talking with each other so much more, we are making love in a different way.
Therapist:	How do you mean?
Lena:	We are connecting more in all ways. We are making love and not just having sex. It is slower and closer and warmer.
Tom:	I did not know that this kind of thing was possible.

Therapist: I think that the work you have done, particularly the physical and psychological separation, has allowed you to be together in a new way. That's great. [The therapist validates the differentiation work they have done and the way it lets them be together in a new way.]

Toward the end of the sixth month, the therapist brought up the idea of termination.

Therapist: You two are doing so well these days and have shifted things in your marriage and family, I feel like I am almost superfluous [For the therapist, a visceral feedback signal that termination is happening.] You come in and I don't have much to say because you are saying and doing it all so well. When this happens, those feelings are usually a signal to me that we are approaching the end of our work. What do you think about that?

Tom: I really don't feel ready to stop completely. What do you feel about stopping, Lena?

Lena: I think he's right. We are doing well and lots has changed. But I agree with you, Tom, that I am not ready to say good-bye yet.

Tom: Maybe we should slow it down, but not cut the cord.

Therapist: What about we meet every month for a while, say 2 or 3 months, and if things continue as they are now, maybe go to every couple or 3 months. If you wanted, we could even move to booster sessions every 6 months. I am open to however you would like to do it.

Lena: I think that would be good. I would feel safer not cutting the cord, just lengthening it—at least for a while.

Therapist: After the relapse, it is hard to fully trust all the changes you have made. I understand that. So keeping me in the picture, but more and more remotely, sounds like a good idea, a plan in fact.

Tom and Lena continued in therapy, meeting less and less frequently for another year and a half. The last two sessions were 6 months apart. At the last session, they all agreed that Tom and Lena were ready to stop but could and would come back if things started to slip and they could not get back on a good track. At the last session, all three of them were teary at the end, and Tom and Lena each embraced the therapist. They gave him a gift of a beautiful frosted glass egg that had clear cracks in it, but was whole. Their therapist graciously accepted it.

2

THE FOUNDATION OF INTEGRATIVE SYSTEMIC THERAPY: FUNDAMENTAL ASSUMPTIONS ABOUT PEOPLE AND THERAPY

Integrative systemic therapy (IST), formerly known as integrative problem-centered metaframeworks, is, as its title suggests, an integrative therapy (Breunlin, Pinsof, Russell, & Lebow, 2011; Pinsof, Breunlin, Chambers, Solomon, & Russell, 2015; Pinsof, Breunlin, Russell, & Lebow, 2011; Russell, Pinsof, Breunlin, & Lebow, 2016). It can be contrasted with early psychotherapies that were based on a monochromatic theoretical model that focused exclusively on one aspect of human systems and a set of methods that flowed from that aspect. Each of those models hypothesizes a set of crucial concepts, a set of strategies for conducting therapy based on these concepts, and a set of specific interventions designed to carry out the strategies. For example, psychoanalytic therapies emphasize the concept of internal conflicts, the strategy of allowing feelings to emerge in therapy, and the intervention of providing insight (Freud, 2003). Similarly, behavioral therapies focus on the concept of learning, leading to strategies such as shaping behavior with interventions

http://dx.doi.org/10.1037/0000055-002
Integrative Systemic Therapy: Metaframeworks for Problem Solving With Individuals, Couples, and Families,
by W. M. Pinsof, D. C. Breunlin, W. P. Russell, J. L. Lebow, C. Rampage, and A. L. Chambers

such as exposure (Wolpe & Lazarus, 1966). Structural family therapy emphasizes the concept of family structure, leading to strategies aimed at changing family structure using interventions such as enactment (Minuchin, 1974).

In contrast, integrative therapies draw their concepts, strategies, and interventions from multiple theoretical frameworks. From an integrative vantage point, best practice extends beyond considering a case through the lens of a single theory and using a similar set of strategies and interventions applicable to all situations. Instead, clinical decision making is viewed as being most usefully grounded in the concepts and intervention strategies that have particular relevance to a particular case or problem and in how to collaborate in creating the most coherent, effective, and acceptable pathways to change for specific clients (Fraenkel, 2009; Lebow, 2014; Pinsof et al., 2011; Sprenkle, Davis, & Lebow, 2009).

On the basis of this integrative vantage point, IST therapists mix elements of different theories, strategies of change, and interventions. IST provides both an integrative way of thinking about people and problems and a set of specific paths for intervention. It builds on the best evidence-informed knowledge available about the resolution of human problems. IST has its foundation in a number of diverse metaframeworks, described in Chapter 5 of this volume. Whereas in some approaches, one lens and one tool derived from that lens are viewed as the cure-all for all problems, IST gives coequal attention to such diverse domains as mind, culture, and biology, building a coherent way of incorporating such a diverse range of evidence-based concepts and methods into practice. It draws from the rich array of theories, concepts, strategies of change, and interventions that are the major achievements of 100 years of development and testing in the practice of psychotherapy. At its foundation, IST moves away from simplistic either–or formulations of difficulties to a vision that considers a particular problem in the context of a particular social system with all its complexity.

IST also tries to find the simplest path to change. Consequently, the breadth of the perspective is viewed not as an invitation simply to do more things but as an opportunity for better planning and collaboration with clients to arrive at the best therapeutic decisions.

As an integrative therapy, IST is structured in marked contrast to the earlier stereotypes of seemingly haphazard eclectic therapies. IST emphasizes creating a structure for case formulation and intervention that suggests under what situations which intervention strategies are likely to be most valuable. It aims to allow for both complexity of understanding and simplicity of action. In this book, we provide a set of core guidelines so that the relevant options are clearly understood, and an ever-evolving plan for intervention is created.

IST can readily be used by the beginning therapist, who may have a more limited repertoire of intervention strategies. It is also relevant for the practice of experienced therapists because it leaves much room for them to add to their range of intervention as they gain experience and master more interventions. IST also accentuates a core conceptual framework that can be embellished and tailored by the therapist over time.

COMMON FACTORS

Like most integrative psychotherapies, IST draws heavily on common factors that are present in and underlie all successful models of therapy (Norcross & Lambert, 2011b). Common factors associated with the therapist include therapist empathy, positive regard, and genuineness. Although these conditions identified long ago by Carl Rogers (1965) have something to do with personality (and thus come more naturally to some therapists than others), all therapists most certainly should cultivate these characteristics, which are also learned skills in the context of psychotherapy. Other common factors associated with the therapist are a strong belief in the efficacy of one's approach, collecting and providing client feedback about progress, and managing therapist countertransference (Norcross & Lambert, 2011b). Other common factors reside principally within clients—for example, clients' belief that therapy will be helpful and clients' readiness to change. Clients who are open to the change process, being in what is called the *action* stage of change, are far easier to engage in an alliance in therapy and have better treatment outcomes than those who do not believe they have a problem (the *precontemplation* stage of change; Norcross, 2011; Norcross, Krebs, & Prochaska, 2011). The third set of common factors is associated with the relationship between clients and the therapist; these include the therapeutic alliance, repairing alliance ruptures, and achieving goal consensus and collaboration. Again, strong evidence is available that each of these factors enhances the probability of client change (Norcross, 2011). IST views common factors not just as phenomena that happen in successful therapy but also as aspects of therapy that therapists can consciously emphasize and build on as the foundation of treatment.

Clinicians and researchers have debated whether "common factors," themselves, or the specific strategies and interventions of particular treatments account for more of the outcome in therapy. Meta-analyses have suggested that the shared common factors are more important than specific treatment interventions (Norcross & Lambert, 2011a). This finding has led some to contend that therapists need only attend to common factors and nothing else. A moderate common factors position, however, contends that the therapist's methods remain important, both in providing effective pathways to change and in constituting part of what makes for the generation of the common factor. There is a circular process between doing something effective and generating common factors toward change in which each mutually enhances the other (Sprenkle, Davis, & Lebow, 2009). It also is striking that almost all evidence-based treatments (which typically emphasize intervention strategies) include both strategies and interventions to create change and strategies to maximize the presence of common factors such as the therapeutic alliance (Lebow, 2014). IST adopts the moderate view of common factors believing that it is indisputable that common factors are of great importance in achieving successful outcomes but that specific treatment methods also contribute to good outcome.

The Therapeutic Alliance

Of all common factors, a strong therapeutic alliance between those involved in the treatment is the most highly correlated with successful outcome (Norcross & Lambert, 2011b). Evidence strongly supports this conclusion for individual (Horvath & Bedi, 2002), couple, and family therapy (Friedlander, Escudero, Heatherington, & Diamond, 2011).

Alliances consist of multiple components: tasks, bonds, and goals (Pinsof, 1994a; Pinsof & Catherall, 1986). The *task* component of the alliance represents agreement about the value of the specific activities involved. The *bonds* focuses on the quality of the human connection between clients and therapist. The *goal* component is about what clients want to accomplish in therapy. When therapist and client are aligned regarding tasks, bonds, and goals, the alliance is stronger than when they are not. Alliance building and maintenance, therefore, is far more than a therapist's being likable, grounded, and gregarious; it is interwoven with effective goal setting and intervention. IST views a positive alliance as an essential ingredient of effective intervention and positive intervention as a contributor to the alliance.

Following Pinsof (1994a), because IST is a systemic and relational form of therapy, it envisions not one but several alliances that contribute to good outcome. The most obvious alliance is the self–therapist alliance that exists between each client and the therapist. In couples therapy, for example, the therapist has alliances with each partner. However, other more subtle forms of alliance also play a role. The other–therapist alliance represents the connection between significant others (either participating directly in therapy or not part of it) and the therapist. To the client in couples and family therapy, the other–therapist alliance is the alliance between the individual's partner or family and the therapist. In therapy with only one individual therapist and one client, the other–therapist alliance is the alliance of the others in the client's life (who are not in therapy) in support of the therapy.

A third alliance relevant to couple and family formats is the shared alliance between the clients as a unit and the therapist. Surprisingly, the shared alliance sometimes substantially differs from each party's self–therapist alliance. For example, in couples therapy, individuals may each feel a positive connection on their own with the therapist, but each may not feel a shared sense of connection as a couple with the therapist about the therapy.

The fourth variation of the alliance is distinct from the others in that it does not involve the therapist. This "within" alliance is the alliance between the family members themselves with one another. It is a particularly challenging circumstance when family members begin therapy with a poor within alliance because it will almost inevitably imperil accomplishing therapeutic goals. An example of this would be couples therapy in which there is little connection between the couple.

The components of the alliance (content dimensions) along with the systemic levels of the alliance (interpersonal dimensions) are represented in Figure 2.1. This model, the theoretical structure of the therapeutic alliance (Pinsof, Zinbarg, & Knobloch-Fedders, 2008), facilitates a systemic understanding of the alliances that influence therapy. Specifically, it helps therapists go beyond the conventional way of thinking about the alliance as

Interpersonal dimensions	Content dimensions		
	Tasks	Goals	Bonds
Self–therapist			
Other–therapist			
Group–therapist			
Within-system			

Figure 2.1. Theoretical structure of the therapeutic alliance. From "Factorial and Construct Validity of the Revised Short Form Integrative Psychotherapy Alliance Scales for Family, Couple, and Individual Therapy," by W. M. Pinsof, R. Zinbarg, and L. M. Knobloch-Fedders, 2008, *Family Process, 47*, p. 282. Copyright 2008 by John Wiley & Sons. Adapted with permission.

something that only exists between the client and therapist, to thinking about and addressing the alliance as something that exists within the multiple and distinct clinical subsystems and relationships that compose the client system.

IST views these alliances as evolving with inevitable ebbs and flows in which the alliances may get stronger and then weaken sometimes to the point where there is a rupture in one of the alliances. There is considerable evidence that the repair of a ruptured alliance, if such a repair can occur, strengthens the alliance. This can accelerate the pace of change and thus accelerate and improve the outcome of therapy (Norcross, 2002; Norcross & Wampold, 2011). Of course, ruptures can also lead to the end of therapy and poor outcome if handled poorly.

Establishing a Therapeutic Alliance in Integrative Systemic Therapy

There is no one simple way to establish a therapeutic alliance. By definition, alliances are interactional. A client who does not initially want to be challenged will likely connect better with a therapist who is less intrusive, whereas one who wants to be challenged will engage better with someone who is more active and challenging (Beutler, Consoli, & Lane, 2005). Ultimately, being skillful at alliance formation lies in tailoring the alliance to the clients.

There are several key ingredients to establishing and maintaining a therapeutic alliance. An alliance begins when the therapist listens so clients feel heard (Nichols, 2009). Privileging and understanding the client's experience is vital, as is respecting and adapting to the client's cultural context. Creating a sense of collaboration helps, as does enlisting and promoting client strengths. Alliance has a foundation in a therapist's social and emotional intelligence; therefore, therapists should cultivate and develop these skills.

Consider Leanne and Josie, a lesbian couple. They entered therapy demoralized, with Josie, in particular, feeling they had tried therapy several times and that their relationship was just not what it used to be. They began therapy with Ruth, wondering whether they had the right therapist and whether this therapy would help. In the first meeting, Ruth listened to and understood their concerns. She reached out to each of them and directly addressed the issues of their collective despair and their concern about her comfort and familiarity with a lesbian couple. Thus, she began to build a connection. When Ruth revealed that she frequently works with lesbian couples and had seen many couples begin with little hope and reach a good resolution, this offer of hope further created the alliance.

IST therapists also work to establish balanced alliances—that is, alliances in which each member of the client system has a similar positive level of alliance. A major problem in conjoint therapies is the split alliance that occurs when one client has a good alliance with the therapist and the alliance for another client is poor. Outcomes tend to be notoriously poor and early termination frequent in the wake of split alliances, especially in conjoint therapies (Knobloch-Fedders, Pinsof, & Mann, 2007). Keeping alliances in balance can be a considerable task, particularly when one client is much more sympathetic than another. Directly dealing with whatever underlying issue is interfering with the alliance is the ultimate solution to such an alliance problem.

When Stefan and Marietta came for their first couples therapy session, Marietta lit into Stefan, berating him for being unemployed and lazy and being a bad lover. Stefan, in turn, was hurt, passive, and withdrawn. Midway through the second session, Marietta turned her anger toward the therapist, who she experienced as siding with Stefan when the therapist tried to slow down her attacks long enough to get a better sense of the problem. The challenge was how to keep an alliance with each when they had at present almost no alliance with each other and when Marietta derived some level of temporary relief by engaging in cathartic but destructive sorts of behaviors that are associated with marriages ending in divorce (Gottman & Levenson, 2002). The therapist, noting that a major alliance problem was emerging, found a way to improve the alliance with Marietta while continuing to join with Stefan. With Marietta, the therapist focused on validating her level of frustration and the difficulties she had encountered, while also challenging her form of expressing her feeling, which in turn led to an exploration of her underlying feeling of helplessness. With Stefan, the therapist empathized with how he felt attacked and blamed, while making certain not to support the dysfunctional behaviors that were so troubling to Marietta. Although in this process Marietta and Stefan continued to feel a level of frustration, their alliances became more balanced.

Alliance is also served by finding effective and acceptable ways of approaching client problems, the reasons clients engage in treatment. And, as already noted, it is essential for the therapist to attend to tears in the alliance. Ruptures that go unattended almost always lead to trouble in therapy and often to client dropout. In addition, as we discuss in Chapter 8, tracking alliances can help enhance the alliance by quickly identifying difficulties in connection before they result in problems in treatment.

ADVANTAGES OF INTEGRATIVE THERAPY

Integrative therapies have a number of distinct advantages over other therapies that are based on one theory and set of strategies (Lebow, 2014).

- In drawing from a broad theoretical base, integrative therapies can offer a more sophisticated explanation for human experience than monochromatic explanations based on a single theory and, therefore, can better account for a larger range of human behavior. When you have only one view, you are limited to what that view can envision and account for, whereas multiple views broaden possibilities.

- Integrative therapies allow for greater flexibility in the treatment of any given case and thus offer the opportunity for increased efficacy and acceptability of care. When therapists have more options, they are more likely to find interventions that are both effective and embraced by them.

- Integrative approaches apply to a broader range of clients. Some clients are more verbal, others less so. Some come from highly communal cultures and others from those that are individual focused. Furthermore, clients present with a wide range of specific problems and family contexts. There are, in fact, an almost endless series of client factors that affect treatment. Integrative methods can extend to different client populations.

- Integrative therapists are better able to match the treatment they offer to their personal conception of problem development and change as well as to their personality characteristics. Therapy differs from many other professional activities in that the person-of-the-therapist matters a great deal (Kramer, 1980). What may be comfortable and flowing for one therapist may feel awkward and off-putting for another. An integrative framework provides a set of methods readily adapted to each therapist. This is not to suggest that integrative therapists do not have to stretch themselves; they do if they want to capture the spectrum of opportunities offered by integration.

- Integrative approaches combine the major benefits of the specific approaches. For example, some approaches are rich in providing ways of approaching emotion, whereas others focus on evidence-based ways of altering cognition and behavior.

- Integrative therapists can bring a greater objectivity to case formulation and treatment planning. Although no one is perfectly objective, having an array of choices increases the possibility of viewing the case with less distortion engendered by the lens of the therapist's preferred theory.

- Integrative frameworks provide the scaffolding essential to include new interventions and concepts that enable therapists to stay current with the evolving field of psychotherapy and thus to continue to feel vital in practice. In particular, this scaffolding allows both concepts and interventions to be modified and expanded as evidence accrues about their utility and impact.

For example, integrative practice a generation ago might have considered incorporating into practice ideas from the double-bind theory of schizophrenia. The substantial evidence that has accrued showing there is no validity to this theory, coupled with the considerable evidence showing the importance of reducing expressed emotion (the presence of criticism coupled with high affect) in the management of schizophrenia, makes it infinitely more likely that today the effective treatment of a family of a person with schizophrenia will not attend to a double-bind formulation but will provide much more impactful psychoeducational information and other help toward reducing expressed emotion (Hooley, 2007).

Because of these considerable strengths, it is no surprise that the majority of therapists already see themselves as working in an integrative way. For example, Norcross, Hedges, and Castle (2002) found that 36% of psychologists describe themselves as integrative, whereas Thoma and Cecero (2009) found that the majority of psychologists use interventions beyond those in their preferred theory. In the largest study of therapists worldwide (Orlinsky & Rønnestad, 2005), the majority of psychotherapists labeled themselves as integrative (Orlinsky & Rønnestad, 2005).

HOW WE SEE HUMAN PROBLEMS

IST goes beyond eclectic practice by providing a set of conceptual pillars that explain why certain theories, strategies, or interventions are being adopted at various points during the course of therapy. These pillars point to understandings about the nature of reality, human beings, and their processes, including the nature of problem formation and how change occurs. The pillars create the conceptual foundation of IST and pervade its frameworks and guidelines. Each pillar represents what we believe is the best synthesis of some of the vexing issues that underlie clinical practice.

The Epistemological Pillar

At the foundation of every psychotherapy model is the question of how objective or subjective reality is. Watzlawick (1977) posed the question with the title to one of his books: *How Real Is Real?* Philosophers from antiquity onward have debated whether the world around us has a reality of its own or whether it is a product of our subjective construction. Therapists have followed their lead, creating therapies based on different views about this question.

Some, such as poststructural therapies (Tarragona, 2008), view the world as a completely social construction, whereas others, such as behavioral therapies (O'Donohue, Henderson, Hayes, Fisher, & Hayes, 2001), envision a world of real objective behaviors that are the ultimate targets of change. Such issues particularly fascinated early family therapists, who devoted many articles and book chapters to ascertaining the most appropriate epistemological position (Bateson, 1972; Dell, 1984; Keeney, 1982).

In the early era of family therapy, this debate about epistemology was for some a fascinating and necessary plunge into the origins and nature of human knowledge, whereas for others it was labeled an arcane conversation of little practical value (Gurman, 1983; Keeney, 1982). IST's take on this complex question is that therapists cannot not have an epistemology; therefore, it is helpful to be clear about what it is. Moreover, IST takes a simple and straightforward position, targeted not at the aesthetics of philosophy but at the pragmatics of which position on this question best informs treatment. We believe this position represents the best synthesis of the crucial elements from this dialectic.

IST purports that there is an objective reality in which real behaviors do occur. When Charles hits his partner, Jordan, this is not the stuff of interpreting reality. Similarly, sequences occur in which a first behavior leads to a second, and IST holds that such behaviors, whether the expression of emotion or doing something, do exist. However, IST also holds that human knowledge of any observed reality is by definition imperfect and evolving. Each behavior is thus also subjectively experienced and people bring their own lens to events that occur.

The ramifications of this synthesis are crucially important for psychotherapy. First, various people involved in a problem, whether they are participating in therapy or not, will subjectively experience the same events in different ways; therefore, an action that has one meaning to one person may have a different meaning to another. Through the process of therapy, an IST practitioner believes it is possible to achieve a better approximation of reality by synthesizing the subjective experiences of various family members. For example, an often-unstated goal of conjoint therapies lies in constructing such a shared but also more objective reality.

A second ramification of the IST view is that over time and with more experience our knowledge about a family becomes more accurate but never complete. Knowledge and truth are seen as human constructions produced by the available cognitive and emotional constructs of each party and the state of objective reality at distinct points in time. So therapists must embrace the idea that they deal with what is an ever-evolving subjective reality.

Science, the systematic knowledge of the physical or material world gained through observation and experimentation, matters. IST does not view

science as a perfect representation of reality but as a set of rules and procedures that help maximize the likelihood of people telling the truth to each
other about the extent to which their methods approximate reality (Pinsof
& Lebow, 2005). It is still subjective (from a limited human perspective), but
it is systematic and rigorously intersubjective.

We view science as an antidote to a drift toward too much anchoring in
subjective reality. As the reader will see, IST often invokes scientific information as an important source of knowledge that is more credible than subjective conjecture. Everyone has their own experience, and they are the best
experts about that experience, but there are truths that transcend individual
experience. One hundred years of scientific investigation about individuals,
couples, and families have articulated many such widely applicable truths
that apply to most, if not all, people. For example, Gottman's research established the toxic impact of contempt on relationships (Gottman & Levenson,
2002). If a therapist observes a contemptuous interaction in a session, it is
essential to find some way to alter this process. If when the therapist points out
the contempt and its toxic effect, the contemptuous husband responds that he
was just "kidding," the therapist may accept that this may well be his experience
of his words, but nonetheless, the couple must reckon with its toxic impact on
their relationship and decide what to do about it.

Although the scientific method creates knowledge applicable to therapy in general, it can also be applied locally to the treatment of each particular clinical case. In this way, therapists become what Stricker and Trierweiler
(1995) called "local clinical scientists," who can track the relationship
between processes that occur in clients and in therapy in relation to an evolving set of outcomes (see Chapter 8). From such a perspective, each event in
the life of the clients or each intervention can be viewed as an experiment—
an opportunity to use the data that emerges (either from observation or the
collection of measures) to determine the effect of a particular pattern or
test whether an intervention is helpful. The IST therapist is a local clinical scientist. The last powerful implication of our epistemic position, which
we call "partial and progressive knowing," is that assessment (what we call
"hypothesizing") and intervention are two co-occurring processes that span
the course of therapy. In IST, there is no assessment or intervention phase.
Both are ongoing from the first phone call to the last goodbye.

The Ontological Pillar

Ontology is the study of the nature of things. In the realm of therapy,
ontology explains how humans interact and how problems emerge from this
interaction. The ontological pillar for IST is grounded in a 21st-century understanding of systems theory and cybernetics. Systems theory has a long history

as the principal foundation of family therapy. The systems theory that serves as a pillar of IST, however, is not the systems theory that fascinated early family therapists. That early systems theory likened humans to inanimate objects and featured notions that humans were like "black boxes" within which the content (cognitions and emotions) was of no importance or that everything is explained by current interaction, signifying that history does not matter.

Over the years, systems theory has evolved from its origins in the work of Ludwig von Bertalanffy (1975). It has been expanded and interwoven with cybernetics by Wiener (1961); Bateson (1972); Maturana and Varela (1980); von Foerster (1984); Poerksen, Koeck, and Koeck (2004); Bronfenbrenner (2005); and numerous others. Hence, the ontological foundation of IST is 21st-century systems theory informed by this evolution over the years.

The core concepts of systems theory that apply to human systems and underlie IST are simple yet vital. First, human systems are composed of a nested hierarchy of subsystems that include society, community, family, relationships, individuals, and the biology of individuals. Each subsystem has parts. A marriage is a subsystem of a family that has two spouses. Individuals can also be conceptualized as having different parts, as they were by Freud (1994) when he envisioned id, ego, and superego.

Second, systems are organized, such that boundaries (who is in what operation), alliances (who sides with whom), and power (who has what control) matter.

Third, as Bronfenbrenner (2005) highlighted in his ecological systems theory, humans are influenced by their interactions with multiple systems, such as family, school, peers, community, and the larger culture. That is, there are multiple systems that influence any family or individual. Part of the task of the therapist lies in locating which systems are most crucial to the problem in focus and its solution.

Fourth, the whole is greater than the sum of its parts. People together in a system are more than their individual characteristics; they blend and interact in ways that extend beyond their individual personalities.

Fifth, all behavior can only be understood in context, most especially in the context of the various systems for which that behavior has relevance (Watzlawick, Bavelas, & Jackson, 1967). Focusing on behavior alone can be deceiving because the behavior has to be understood in the context in which it occurs. For example, to see a person shouting in the street only provides some information. That information is understood quite differently if the observer sees that the shouting is in response to the person's spouse being hit by a car. Perspectives of human functioning that are fully based in biology and individual psychology often ignore such contextual factors.

Sixth, all behavior generates important consequences for social systems, and behavior sometimes serves a function for the system. Behaviors have meaning in the social context. IST holds that some early family systems formulations took this notion of the function of behavior too far, assuming the behavior had to have a purpose for the system. For example, now outdated and debunked notions argued that a person in a family who had schizophrenia or bipolar disorder would inevitably serve the function of distracting other members of the family from other concerns.

Seventh, feedback provides essential information for regulating the operations between people. Formally, feedback is the furnishing of data concerning operation or output, so that subsequent or ongoing operations can be altered or corrected. Information passed on through various channels (e.g., verbal, nonverbal) in reaction to behavior is important in influencing that behavior. Feedback, as the term is used in cybernetics, is referred to as "positive" when the information leads to more of the behavior that is occurring or "negative" when the information leads to a diminishing of that behavior. The implication here is that it is important to focus not only on behavior that occurs but also on the sequences of feedback that occur between people. The primacy of sequences will be discussed as a separate pillar of IST.

Eighth, there are forces within systems that transcend the particular individuals that move both toward change (termed *morphogenesis*) and toward remaining the same and minimizing change (termed *homeostasis*). Early systems theory and early family therapy could only see systems as homeostatic; that is, systems were viewed as moving back toward the steady state before the change occurred. More recent developments in systems theory accentuate the forces toward change that can occur when change is initiated (Maturana & Varela, 1980). The message for therapists is that we have to attend to both of these forces that affect those working to change in therapy—to build on the forces moving toward constructive morphogenesis and to anticipate and work with the forces diluting constructive change.

The ontological pillar and its grounding in systemic thinking have important ramifications for the practice of IST, which envisions therapy as an encounter of client and therapist systems (Pinsof, 1983, 1995, 2002). The two systems form the therapy system that is represented in Figure 2.2. As is seen in this diagram, each system consists of multiple subsystems. The client system consists of all people in any way connected to the problem. The client system is in turn composed of two subsystems, termed the direct client subsystem and the indirect client subsystem. The *direct client subsystem* is composed of the people who attend any given session; this may be an individual, a married or unmarried couple, a nuclear family, or any other combination of people (e.g. several members of different families in a multifamily group). The *indirect client subsystem* is composed of people who have a stake in the problem and are affected by the treatment but are not present for the sessions.

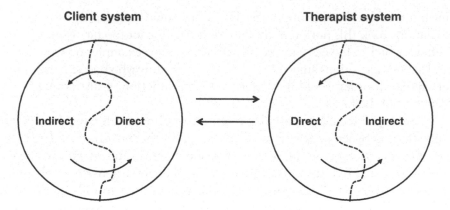

Client system   Therapist system

Indirect   Direct   Direct   Indirect

Figure 2.2. The therapy system. From *Integrative Problem-Centered Therapy: A Synthesis of Family, Individual, and Biological Therapies* (p. 6), by W. M. Pinsof, 1995, New York, NY: Basic Books. Copyright 1995 by Basic Books, an imprint of Perseus Books, LLC, a subsidiary of Hachette Book Group, Inc. Adapted with permission.

As illustrated by Tom and Lena in Chapter 1, an important decision point within IST lies in deciding which clients to include in the direct client system for any given session or set of sessions. For example, consider a client with generalized anxiety disorder who has a partner. Although therapy may involve using cognitive behavior therapy (CBT) interventions for the anxiety disorder, the IST therapist would prefer to meet initially with the client and partner to lay out the trajectory of treatment and secure the partner's cooperation. After this, several CBT sessions may be offered to the anxious client alone, and the partner may attend intermittently. The boundary between the direct and indirect client subsystems is fluid. The therapy is always "systemic"; consequently, who is in the direct client system for any given session is not a function of a therapy modality but rather what is likely to be most useful and pragmatic for the moment.

The therapist system consists of all the treatment providers involved in the problem. These may include supervisors, other therapists, psychiatrists or physicians prescribing medicine, school personnel, probation officers, and so forth. Returning to the example given previously, were the IST therapist in training, he or she would have a supervisor and possibly a supervision group. These professionals would influence the course of therapy. Unaddressed or intractable conflicts in the supervisory relationship or team, as well as conflicts with consultants, potentially affect the therapy as much as conflicts within the client system. The client might have a psychiatrist who prescribes medication for anxiety, and the spouse may have a therapist. Typically, IST therapists reach out and try to build an alliance with other therapists involved in the case. This is especially essential when problems in coordination emerge between therapists. For example, a couples therapist arrived at a mutually agreed-on plan with a couple to work toward increased intimacy only to have one partner relate that in individual therapy he was receiving support for "going slow" and avoiding intimacy. A coordinating phone call (after appropriate consent forms were signed) was immeasurably helpful in working toward mutually agreed-on treatment goals. IST therapists consult directly with other therapists, even at times collaborating by hosting a phone consult and/or face-to-face meeting among therapists and treatment providers.

Psychotherapy, therefore, becomes the mutual and directed interaction of client and therapist systems. IST is systemic in its focus, always remaining cognizant of the people who are affected by and who affect the treatment. The pragmatic questions of how to make decisions about who to invite into treatment in a specific case are discussed in detail in Chapter 3.

The Sequences Pillar

The ontological pillar of IST dictates that therapists paint on a large canvas; that is, the course of any given therapy can be multifaceted. To break therapy down into the actual brushstrokes of practice, IST focuses on the specific sequences played out by clients (Breunlin & Schwartz, 1986; Breunlin, Schwartz, & Mac Kune-Karrer, 1997). A *sequence* is nothing more than a cycle of actions, meanings, and emotions that is patterned and repetitious. Sequences provide the most concrete, accessible, and ultimately changeable route to working with a problem. If we attend to "what follows what," we can help assess and create alternative sequences that work better for clients.

The primary task of the therapist, therefore, is to facilitate the replacement of key problem sequences with solution sequences that eliminate or reduce the problem (this is called the *sequence replacement guideline*). IST therapists collaborate with clients to identify these solution sequences, believing clients possess the strengths to implement the solution. The specifics of the solution come from the recognition of client strengths, failed attempted solutions, collaborative analysis, common sense, therapist expertise, and cultural fit. In Chapter 3, we highlight how IST emphasizes the tracking and alteration of sequences.

The Constraint Pillar

Every model of therapy has a theory of how change takes place. Because most therapy models posit that problems are the result of some deficit in the client system (usually an individual), for these models change takes place when this deficit is addressed in therapy. For example, if a client labeled with borderline personality disorder repeatedly fails in life because of emotional dysregulation, a therapist might work to enhance emotional regulation for the client using object relations therapy and mood stabilizing medication. Such an approach, like many therapies, is grounded in ameliorating the underlying sources of emotional dysregulation. IST is grounded in a different question: What keeps the person from being emotionally regulated? For IST, the answer to this question best defines what has to be addressed in therapy. IST argues that the clients we treat cannot, themselves, solve the problems they present in therapy because they are caught in a web of constraints that keeps them from doing so.

The difference between the two questions (what causes the problem? vs. what keeps the problem from being solved?) is grounded in Bateson's (1972) distinction between positive and negative explanation. *Positive explanation* maintains that something happens because some force propels it to happen, whereas *negative explanation* maintains that what happens occurs because other things are prevented from happening. Labels are often used to capture positive explanations. For example, Joe lies because he is a pathological liar. The corresponding negative explanation question about Joe's lying is, what keeps him from telling the truth? Bateson argued that all explanation of human behavior is ultimately grounded in negative explanation. What presents as a positive explanation, therefore, always has a corresponding negative explanation. The mood disorder of a client may contain a biological constraint that interferes with mood regulation, a constraint that can be at least partially lifted with medication. The client, however, may also live in a high-conflict family where repeated provocations keep her from learning how to regulate her feelings.

An IST therapist was referred a court-ordered case involving the Thierry family, consisting of divorced parents John and Marcia, and their son, George. John Thierry came from a family of origin in which severe corporal punishment, which today would be labeled as child abuse, has been passed on from generation to generation. In his postdivorce home, he continued to use these methods with his son, George. When George told his mother, Marcia, about his dad's form of punishment, she reported him to the state's child welfare department, which launched a child abuse investigation and a legal process by Marcia to severely limit John's time with his son. A therapy grounded in positive explanation would ask why John engages in this abusive behavior and perhaps conclude that he has an explosive personality disorder. Conversely, once safety concerns have been addressed, an IST therapist would focus on what was preventing John from changing his abusive style of discipline despite abundant information about child abuse, various admonishments by others about it, and even punishments for engaging in this behavior. As the therapist explored this question of constraints with John, it became clear that not only was this behavior familiar and ego syntonic for John given the many generations during which family members essentially taught that child abuse was acceptable, but also that John had a catastrophic fear that his son would become out of control if he were not properly disciplined. This fear was also associated with John's concern that Marcia was too lenient.

The therapist worked with John to lift these constraints by directly addressing his fears through psychoeducation about parenting, strategies from cognitive therapy for challenging beliefs, and interactional work between John and George when they discussed John's fears and George's adolescent behavior. The therapist also met with Marcia to help her trust that a different relationship between John and George was possible. These interventions ultimately lifted the constraints by creating a father–son and coparental subsystem that was better able to set limits and monitor George's behavior.

A constraint is anything in the client system that keeps the problem from being solved. In IST, therapist and clients begin searching for constraints when the clients are unable to solve the presenting problem in a straightforward manner. The search involves two questions: Where are the constraints located in the client system, and what are they? The "where" question flows from biopsychosocial systems theory; constraints can exist at the biological, psychological, relational, family, community, and societal levels. For example, a person of color presenting with depression may be constrained from getting over the depression by any or all of the following constraints: a biochemical imbalance, internalized racism, a relationship marked by domestic violence, caretaking demands of an elderly parent, repeated stops by police, or a sense of insecurity bred by repeated events of violence against persons of color that dominate the media.

The IST therapist must also ascertain what the constraints are. This "what" question is answered by using the hypothesizing metaframeworks to understand and evaluate clients' answers to what prevented them from solving the problem. The hypothesizing metaframeworks gather together relevant theories about domains of human functioning. They are described in detail in subsequent chapters. For example, the development metaframework encompasses the vast conceptual territory of biological, psychological, relational, and family development.

The IST therapist's confidence that clients can lift constraints is grounded in a basic premise of health that assumes individuals and systems function well until there has been a clear demonstration that some other process is at work. Whether people are innately healthy or troubled is another long debated question for those in mental health disciplines and philosophy long before that. Some have accentuated pathological processes (Freud, 1920), whereas others have accentuated resilience (Walsh, 2006). IST emphasizes resilience while remaining cognizant of the possibilities that problems may be deeply rooted and at times difficult to change. Even when this proves to be the case, the so-called deficit is still treated as a constraint that can be lifted or at least managed.

IST begins by evoking the strength guideline that suggests that until proven otherwise the client system can use its strengths and resources to lift constraints and implement adaptive solutions with minimal direct input from the therapist system. Chapters 3 and 4 explicate in more detail how IST therapists proceed toward these ends. For our purposes here, the essential thought is that people and systems are mostly healthy and that most therapy should consist of a parsimonious process of lifting constraints to resolve problems.

The Causality Pillar

Causality, the relationship between cause and effect in human systems, has been a much-debated entity both in philosophy and the mental health field. Early on, linear causality dominated mental health. Linear causality purports that something happening at Time B is caused by something that happened earlier at Time A; that is, A causes B. Linear causality focuses change on the theorized causes of problems such as early childhood experience and the effects of that experience on the individual with the problem. This led to an emphasis in therapies for a search for how to alter individual behavior, either by locating what was occurring inside the person or simply changing the behavior itself.

Early systems theory and family therapy substituted the equally simple notion of circular causality purporting that A and B mutually influence each other in an endless bidirectional and recursive feedback loop (Watzlawick, Weakland, & Fisch, 1974). From this vantage point, causality lies in the system rather than in the person where the system is embodied by circular patterns or sequences of interaction. The emphasis, therefore, is on changing the circular pattern and thus the system. Change the system and the individuals constituting the system can change.

IST emphasizes patterns of interaction (sequences) and the mutual effects people have on one another in recursive cycles. However, consistent with more recent systems theory, there is also considerable emphasis on the arcs of linear causality that are part of a recursive cycle (Dell, 1986). Within these arcs, one person's behavior can be the primary determinant of what happens in that arc. In an extreme example, most relational violence is the product of one person's behavior inflicted on a partner (Goldner, Penn, Sheinberg, & Walker, 1990). The recipient of the violence may also play some role in the cycle of violence, but that aspect of the relational dynamic is dwarfed by the impact of the linear arc of causality from perpetrator to recipient of the actual violence.

IST, therefore, adopts the position that causality is circular but often differential (Pinsof, 1995). The people in a system and different subsystems contribute differentially to what occurs within a system. Sometimes their contributions should be taken as equal, but sometimes they should not.

A corollary of differential causality is that individual personality and psychopathology matter. In IST, far from the view of radical systems therapies of early family therapy, there is ample room to consider what is occurring within people and how this affects their behavior. IST is fully informed by evidence-based views of personality (McAdams, 2001). IST views problems as typically having multiple causes at multiple systems levels; what is the ultimate "one" cause is in the eye of the beholder. As is discussed further in Chapter 4, we see a web of mutual influence in which various people contribute differentially to the variance in any process or outcome. The total set of contributions may be quite complex; nonetheless, IST tries to find the most parsimonious way of approaching problem resolution even as it acknowledges complexity.

IST also takes a position with regard to the issue of psychiatric diagnosis. IST uses an evolving case formulation anchored in the salient problems clients first bring to therapy and that emerge during the course of therapy. We contrast this approach with treatments tailored only to client diagnosis. The latter approach is at the foundation of much of biological psychiatry and of evidence-based psychological treatments for specific disorders (Barlow, 2008; Nathan & Gorman, 2007). In such treatments, specific methods are mandated simply because a client has a particular diagnosis. IST respects that these treatments often do produce positive outcomes for most clients who have the disorders for which these treatments were developed. Although often effective, such treatments are tailored to only one aspect of the client system: changing specific psychopathology and symptoms. Other salient clinical issues of the case, therefore, are not addressed, sometimes leading to poor overall client outcome and satisfaction with the therapy. Furthermore, there is no alternative when following the manual of prescribed ingredients is not working. Because these treatments are organized around a single diagnosis and have a one-size-fits-all approach, they are less effective for some clients, and for others they are unacceptable, leading to client dropout. Even the best evidence-based treatments organized this way leave at least a third of people unresponsive to treatment (Kazdin, 2011).

When placed in the context of the blueprint that organizes how IST therapists make decisions about which interventions to use, the strategies of evidence-based treatments can serve as important resources for the selection of interventions. For example, using self-monitoring, thought records, and exposure, principal aspects of CBT treatments for anxiety, would be likely early interventions with a client with panic and anxiety.

In the next chapter, we segue from the conceptual foundation of IST explored in this chapter to delineate how IST therapists begin therapy through the process of identifying and solving client problems. This process includes the identification of sequences in which the problem is embedded, efforts to solve the problem by introducing solution sequences, and initiating the search for constraints when this process fails, as it often does.

3

THE ESSENCE OF INTEGRATIVE SYSTEMIC THERAPY: BEGINNING THERAPY

In Chapter 2, we introduced the pillars of integrative systemic therapy (IST), each of which addresses important practice considerations. But just as the pillars of a building are designed to blend in and not dominate its appearance, so the pillars of IST are not at the forefront of an IST therapist's mind when starting a new case. Rather, the focus is on how to engage the clients about their concerns, create hope, and intimate initial direction for the therapy. In this way, the practice of IST is quite simple. The moment-to-moment unfolding of events in a session is understood and driven by a simple process we call the *essence of IST*.

In this chapter, we explain the components of this process and their logical connections. To illustrate, consider the following vignette involving the Cook family, consisting of a mother, Ann; father, George; and 16-year-old daughter, Kim.

http://dx.doi.org/10.1037/0000055-003
Integrative Systemic Therapy: Metaframeworks for Problem Solving With Individuals, Couples, and Families,
by W. M. Pinsof, D. C. Breunlin, W. P. Russell, J. L. Lebow, C. Rampage, and A. L. Chambers

Following introductions and establishment of therapy ground rules, the therapist sought a definition of the presenting problem.

Therapist: I am interested in what brings you here today.

Father: My wife thinks our daughter isn't eating enough and is losing weight.

Therapist: Between you and your wife, who is more worried about this issue of eating?

The therapist wanted to focus the conversation on eating rather than weight as the problem because eating is part of the family dynamic, whereas weight is a characteristic of Kim.

Father: I know Kim has lost weight, but I sometimes think my wife sees it as a bigger problem than it is.

Therapist: OK, so maybe you and your wife aren't completely on the same page?

Father: Yes.

Therapist: [To daughter] How do you see this issue of what you eat, and how it is related to your body?

Daughter: They are making too big a deal out of how I eat. I am a gymnast, and I have to be a certain weight to perform well. I am doing what my coach tells me to do and what every other girl on the team is doing.

Therapist: I see. So one problem may be eating, but another problem is that the three of you aren't in agreement about what the eating should look like?

Parents: [Together] That's right. [The problem is not just eating; it is how the family cannot agree on it.]

Therapist: There are some activities for young women such as gymnastics, swimming, dance, cheerleading, where weight is involved. Unfortunately, this can be expressed as weighing less is better. Research has shown that weighing less can be a slippery slope and that some young women take their weight so seriously that they begin to have symptoms of an eating disorder. Are any of you worried that this might be the case here?

Mother: You named my fear.

Father: I don't know.

Daughter: My mom's a fanatical worrier. I do not have an eating disorder, period.

Therapist:	So is it correct to say that a related problem is that you all can't agree on whether or not weight is a problem?
Mother:	That's correct.
Therapist:	Have you gotten an opinion from Kim's pediatrician?
Mother:	Yes, she says that Kim's weight does not put her at risk yet, but she should maintain her current weight. [The therapist prefers not to label the problem as an eating disorder at this time.]
Therapist:	Would you give me permission to check with your pediatrician so we can all be in agreement on whether we should consider this problem to be a disorder?
All:	Sure.
Therapist:	For the moment, then, can we agree the problem is you aren't able to agree on how Kim's eating can allow her to maintain a healthy weight and still be a competitive gymnast?

When all family members agreed, for the moment there was consensus on at least one presenting problem: eating.

The therapist next asked the family to describe how they interact regarding food—that is, to articulate the typical sequence of interaction in which the problem is embedded. IST calls this a *problem sequence*. Patient and nonjudgmental interviewing by the therapist helped the family describe a sequence wherein the mother prepared the food she believed Kim should eat, and Kim either rejected it or ate sparingly, complaining it was not the food she needed. The mother replied that she was not going to prepare a separate meal for Kim. Because George was frequently not home for breakfast or dinner, the battle over food primarily involved Ann and Kim, but Ann engaged George late at night by revealing her fears that Kim would develop a serious eating disorder and die. She begged George to talk to Kim, which he did in a half-hearted way. These conversations made Kim feel guilty but also angry that Ann involved George. This fueled her tendency to be oppositional. In the end, Ann was never satisfied that Kim was eating enough; therefore, her constant worry was perpetuated by the sequence, and she interacted with Kim concerning food in a predictable way.

As the family described this problem sequence, the therapist wondered whether there was a way to change it such that it would contribute to solving the eating problem. This change would have introduced a *solution sequence* that replaced the problem sequence. The therapist mused to the family: "What would happen if Kim were given more responsibility for managing her food intake?" At first, the mother flat out said no, but when the father said it was not a bad idea and Kim enthusiastically embraced it, the mother showed some interest. The family worked together to define how this solution sequence would work. The therapist was cautious to include monitoring behaviors during the trial period when Kim first took responsibility for managing her food. This monitoring addressed the mother's fear that only she could prevent Kim from developing a full-blown eating disorder. By the end of the session, the family agreed to a plan that incorporated the solution sequence.

There are myriad ways the Cooks could approach the solution sequence, ranging from complete compliance to complete disregard. If they fell short, the therapist evoked the constraint pillar and asked what kept them from succeeding. In this example, the family had initial success, but after several weeks, Ann and Kim resumed their battle over food because Ann sharply disagreed with Kim's choices. When asked what kept her from being able to support Kim's choices, Ann revealed that her sister committed suicide shortly after Ann left for college. Ann believed her parents failed to see the signs of the sister's distress and had Ann been there she might have prevented the suicide. This news revealed a major constraint to Ann's ability to back off and allow Kim to manage her food intake.

In what follows, for heuristic purposes, we first present the textbook application of the essence diagram (see Figure 3.1), acknowledging at the

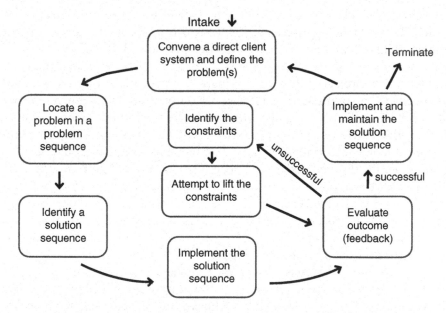

Figure 3.1. Essence of integrative systemic therapy. From "Integrative Problem Centered Metaframeworks (IPCM) Therapy," by W. P. Russell, W. Pinsof, D. C. Breunlin, and J. Lebow, in T. L. Sexton and J. Lebow (Eds.), *Handbook of Family Therapy* (p. 531), 2016, New York, NY: Routledge. Copyright 2016 by Routledge. Reprinted with permission.

beginning that nothing in the practice of therapy is ever a textbook case. Following this textbook analysis, we introduce a set of clinical issues that often necessitate some modification to this textbook approach. Moreover, in this chapter, we focus primarily on the problem-solving tasks of the essence diagram while acknowledging that conducting therapy involves the use of a broad set of clinical strategies.

THE PRESENTING PROBLEM

IST is premised on the problem-centered contract: that clients seek therapy to solve problems and hire therapists to help them do so. The first problem-solving task, therefore, is to define the presenting problem, the problem the clients want to solve. The problem is like a signpost pointing the direction to be taken. For the Cook family, the problem was Kim's food intake (which affected her weight and potentially put her at risk of having an eating disorder). The problem reflects clients' goals for therapy and enables the therapist to discuss how they interact concerning it (how they engage in a problem sequence).

Having a problem as the focus for therapy has several other advantages. First, by addressing the concerns of the clients, the therapist strengthens the alliance (Pinsof, 1995). Agreement on the problem means goal consensus. Second, only those sequences in which the problem is embedded are of interest; hence, the problem focuses therapy. The problem functions like the anchor of a fishing boat. When fishing on a lake, the fisher rows the boat to the spot on the lake where she or he believes there are fish. She or he drops the anchor at that spot, so the boat does not drift. Without the anchor, the boat would begin drifting, and before long, the fisher would be fishing where there are no fish. So it is that therapists can find themselves adrift in a sea of irrelevant details by listening to the clients without the focus of a problem. Third, the problem points to a way to measure progress. When it is solved to the satisfaction of the clients, they feel a sense of success. Fourth, a focus on the problems provides a way of determining that therapy has served its purpose. When all the problems of concern have been addressed, it is time to end therapy. Fifth, clients are encouraged to return to therapy should they encounter another problem for which they cannot find a solution.

Arriving at an agreement on the presenting problem may seem straightforward and, therefore, a task to be dispatched without much labor. Sometimes this is the case. For example, a family might seek therapy to mourn the death of a member or to cope with a medical diagnosis such as cancer. A couple might seek therapy in an attempt to repair the damage caused by an affair. An individual might seek therapy for treatment of anxiety or depression. Often, however, the source of clients' distress might be clear, but an operational definition of the problem associated with that distress is much less clear. In these cases, considerable effort must be devoted to extracting the problem from the narrative offered by the clients. Clients can make vague statements about the presenting problem: "We just aren't close anymore," "We don't know how to communicate." Such statements must be molded into operational definitions of that problem. The acid test of a problem definition is whether we know what it will look like when the problem is solved. For the first problem, the definition might become, "We do not spend time together because when we do, we do not enjoy each other's company." The problem could be solved once the couple knows how to plan time together and looks forward to the activities they have chosen. For the second problem of communication, the definition might be that the clients cannot talk about important and potentially controversial topics. The problem would be solved when the clients agree there is a topic needing discussion, make time to discuss it, have the discussion, and reach a decision that does not leave the relationship fractured.

Some clients do not enter therapy viewing it as a problem-solving exercise. They might say, "I am upset in my life, and I just need a place to talk." This is particularly true for clients who previously had been in "supportive" therapy. In such cases, the IST therapist is initially in a bind. The therapist knows the therapeutic alliance is, in part, determined by goal consensus with the client, but good outcome requires progress be made, and this requires having operationalized goals. The IST therapist can openly discuss this with the client and see whether the client is open to viewing therapy as a problem-solving exercise. Sometimes more patience is needed, and the therapist has to wait for an opportunity to operationalize one of the client's concerns: "So the fact that you too often find yourself at home on a Friday or Saturday night is something that upsets you? If that changed, would your life look different to you?"

Because IST therapists prefer to have sessions with more than one client, it raises the issue of how to handle multiple perspectives about the problem. For example, a child might be referred for treatment of attention-deficit/hyperactivity disorder (ADHD). An IST therapist would recommend that the whole family attend the first session. A discussion of why they are seeking therapy would reveal a set of interconnected problems. The parents might say they have conflict over how to parent the child with ADHD. The siblings might say that ADHD so dominates family life that they feel like the parents pay little attention to them. The child with ADHD might say his parents overly restrict what he can do, fearing ADHD will lead to some catastrophe. The therapist would hear each perspective and acknowledge it as a concern. One strategy for dealing with multiple perspectives is to place them under an umbrella problem. For instance, the therapist might externalize ADHD and say, "ADHD is certainly tyrannizing your family, and all of you are affected. Would it be helpful if we could find a way for ADHD not to have such power over the family?"

In still other cases, the clients offer a disparate list of problems that cannot be subsumed under an umbrella problem. In these cases, the IST therapist acknowledges that there are a number of problems and guides the clients through a discussion of how to prioritize the problems such that one is selected to start therapy, with a recognition that the others will be addressed in due time.

Therapy begins with the presenting problem. Other problems may be revealed during the course of therapy. These problems are targeted for solution only when clients themselves declare a need to solve them. For example, couples often reveal they have less-than-satisfactory sex lives. When asked whether they want to focus on improving sex, one couple may say yes, whereas another might say that sex is not that important to them. The sexual problems would merit attention for the first couple but not the second.

THE PROBLEM SEQUENCE

Because IST seeks a systemic understanding of the presenting problem, obtaining a problem definition is just the first step of beginning IST. The second step is to contextualize the problem by understanding how it is embedded within the client system—that is, how the system maintains the problem. Myriad explanations have been posited to explain how problem maintenance occurs. Although the full articulation of problem maintenance may be quite complex, IST asserts that it is important not to get lost in the labyrinth of the entire system at the outset of therapy. Rather, IST posits that it is sufficient to obtain a "good enough" systemic explanation and to use this explanation as the starting point for solving the problem. The need to seek a more complex explanation of the client system arises when the "good enough" explanation proves to be inadequate.

This balance between systemic complexity and systemic pragmatism is a hallmark of IST and distinguishes it from most systemic therapies that lean in one direction or the other. Milan systemic therapy (Selvini Palazzoli, Boscolo, Cecchin, & Prata, 1978), for example, elegantly constructs a complex hypothesis about the system, whereas solution-focused therapy (de Shazer et al., 1986) is pragmatic in its view that problem maintenance need not be understood beyond the acquisition of an understanding of exceptions to when the problem is occurring.

Although at the beginning of therapy IST aspires to use a parsimonious understanding of the client system, there are cases in which issues emerge early in therapy that necessitate a more complex understanding and handling. Examples of this are the revelation that a client has a complex trauma history or that the former spouse of the mother in a blended family constantly takes her back to court over issues pertaining to the divorce settlement. How IST approaches these situations will be elaborated later in this chapter.

In IST the parsimonious and pragmatic path to systemic understanding of the client system is the problem sequence. A *problem sequence* is a predictable, patterned, and recursive set of actions, meanings, and emotions in which the presenting problem is embedded. The problem sequence represents the client's first explanation of what is going on when the problem occurs. It reveals at least one important way the client system maintains the problem. The problem sequence has to be constructed with sufficient detail to show how it contributes to the maintenance of the presenting problem. For the Cook family, the problem sequence included how Ann pushes certain foods on Kim, how Kim reacts, and how George is triangulated in Ann's attempts to regulate what Kim eats.

Although the exercise of collaborating with clients to articulate the problem sequence may seem straightforward, it can, in fact, be quite challenging. In part, this is because clients often do not see that they participate in a problem sequence. As they begin therapy, they expect to complain about the problem, and they often project the blame for the problem onto other family members. They can become quite uncomfortable when asked to describe how they participate in the problem sequence. The therapist must be persistent and persuasive in bringing the focus back to the problem sequence. For example:

Therapist: I know that what you just said is important, and at some point it needs to be discussed, but for the moment, can I go back to my question of what happens when he gives you that look?

Wife: It just crushes me inside because I know that he is disgusted with me.

Therapist: [To husband] Did you know that your wife interprets the look as disgust?

Husband: I had no idea.

The task of defining a problem sequence proceeds in a spirit of curiosity and acceptance so as to avoid making the clients feel judged. The therapist might begin by asking, "So, I am curious, can you tell me what is going on when the problem happens?" This question encourages clients to supply the antecedent and consequent actions, meanings, and emotions associated with the problem. Some clients are readily able to see how their respective interactions are connected, whereas others have great difficulty grasping the stimulus–response nature of their interaction. It is unlikely that a clear articulation of a problem sequence will emerge if the therapist listens passively to the clients describe their problem. Rather, the therapist must actively engage them in the search for the problem sequence. Gregory Bateson's mantra "What is the pattern that connects?" must be ever present in the therapist's mind (Bateson, 1972). Persistence must be measured with tact, so the clients stretch to define their problem sequence without feeling badgered by the therapist: "This might seem like nitpicking to you, but I still don't quite understand what happens for each of you when your son is disrespectful to one of you. Can we go over that moment one more time?"

An IST therapist participates in the construction of the problem sequence in several ways. First, the therapist uses questions that help contextualize the problem within a sequence of interactions: "So when he acts that way, what do you do?" or "What happens after that?" Tomm (1987a, 1987b) demonstrated how questions are used to establish the temporal relationship among action, meaning, and emotion in a problem sequence. For example, "When she turns away from you, what do you think it means?" or "When she turns away from you, how do you feel?"

Glimpses of the problem sequence also appear in the interaction during the session itself. The therapist must decide whether simply to file the observation or to comment on it to further define the problem sequence. At stake here could be the budding alliance between client and therapist. If pointing out an interaction to clients is going to shame and/or make one of them defensive, it is better to hold off. There are times, however, when calling attention to an interaction has the effect of unlocking a part of the problem sequence outside the client's awareness.

> *Therapist:* Tom, I just noticed that you shifted your posture away from Sally when she said you don't spend enough time with the kids. Does that shift convey any meaning?
>
> *Husband:* She's always on my case about what I do or don't do with the kids. She thinks I'm a lousy father, and she makes the kids feel that way too.
>
> *Therapist:* I can see how you can feel pretty bad about your wife's views of your parenting. Are you able to talk to her about this?
>
> *Husband:* What's the use? Nothing will change.

A problem sequence consists not only of clients' actions but also their internal experiences. Clients' internal experiences consist of the meaning and emotions they have about the problem sequence. These internal experiences occur both during the problem sequence itself and at other times when clients are thinking about it. Meaning derives from the cognitions clients have about the actions and emotions of the sequence. This includes cognitions about their actions and the actions of others and the cognitions they have about their emotions and the emotions of others in the sequence. Emotions occur as immediate reactions to events and interactions or in response to meanings that are created.

Because problem sequences occur in a context, clients' internal experiences can relate to any of the following: (a) a moment in the sequence ("That's just like him to say that"), (b) the sequence as a whole ("I hate it when this happens"), (c) how the sequence is part of a current situation ("I knew this would happen"), (d) how the same sequence has occurred over and over ("Here we go again"), and (e) how the sequence relates to the respective narratives of clients' lives ("I can never catch a break").

Although problem sequences are always made up of elements of action, meaning, and emotion, at the outset of therapy IST privileges action as the preferred pathway for change. It is hoped that any relevant meaning and/or emotion will shift if the action shifts. Of course, this assumption is often not borne out, but failure in the realm of action provides an opportunity to explore important constraints related to meanings and emotions.

Although every problem sequence has many components, it is not necessary to know them all to initiate a solutions sequence. Rather, the rule of thumb is that the problem sequence has been defined adequately when the description feels accurate to the therapist and clients and when it contains enough detail to begin to suggest a solution sequence.

THE SOLUTION SEQUENCE

IST fosters change through a systemic focus on changing sequences. IST calls this the *sequence replacement guideline*; that is, IST solves problems by introducing a solution sequence that replaces part or all of the problem sequence. If the clients understand how the problem sequence maintains the problem and a solution sequence can be envisioned, it is time to suggest it. Initially, this can be done in the spirit of curiosity: "So this sequence seems to be a problem for all of you. I wonder what would happen if you did X instead of Y?" By being tentative, the therapist allows the clients to agree or to express reservations (we will see later that such reservations often signal the presence of a constraint). If they say the change makes sense, the therapist invites them to try it. For the Cook family, the solution sequence involved a shift toward giving Kim more autonomy over decisions that would enable her to make good choices about food so she could be both healthy and a competitive gymnast. The solution sequence also required Ann to be less central in Kim's food consumption and for the triangulation of George to stop.

The conviction that clients can and do solve problems in therapy is grounded in IST's *strength guideline*, which states, until proven otherwise, that clients possess the resources to solve their problems (see the Appendix to this volume for a summary of all the guidelines). The therapist identifies these strengths and uses them to introduce the *solution sequence*. The solution sequence will contain new action, meaning, or emotion that will eliminate and/or replace the dysfunctional aspects of the problem sequence and, therefore, partially or completely eliminate the presenting problem.

An experienced IST therapist can frequently define the problem, articulate the problem sequence, and introduce a solution sequence all in the first session. Beginning therapists may take several sessions to do the same thing. The length of time required to execute the solution sequence only becomes an issue when multiple sessions fail to produce a presenting problem, a problem sequence, or a solution sequence. When this occurs, the therapist should ask whether the focus of therapy has been lost.

The solution sequence can be implemented in the session and/or as a between-session exercise. When implemented in session, the therapist constructs some form of an enactment (Minuchin, 1974) wherein the clients practice the solution sequence. Rarely do clients get it right the first time. Successive approximation is more the norm. They will make and attempt and then revert to all or part of the problem sequence. The therapist must urge them to try again. When they succeed, validation is in order. The therapist asks what feels easy for them, what is challenging, and what gets in the way of implementation. All these issues must be addressed for successful implementation of the solution sequence.

The practice of creating change by altering the problem sequence is conceptually sound but raises several important questions. First, are clients not entitled to be who they are? If so, what right does a therapist have to suggest that they act, believe, or feel differently? In a society grounded in individualism, in principle this may be true; however, it must be remembered that the clients have sought therapy for distress that they themselves cannot resolve. By doing so, they invite the therapist's involvement. Furthermore, IST therapists offer (vs. impose) solutions and invite client feedback about them. Second, if IST is a collaborative therapy, should the clients not come up with their own solution sequence? In IST, therapy must be collaborative, and, in the course of therapy, clients generate or contribute to solutions; however, IST would not suggest that the therapist can never serve as an expert in the process of creating the solution sequence. In IST it is incumbent on the therapist to possess expert knowledge that informs the selection of solution sequences.

The *education guideline* dictates the therapist's role in the creation of the solution sequence. This guideline states that therapy is an educational process in which therapists give away their skills, knowledge, and expertise as quickly as clients can integrate them. In short, IST therapists freely offer suggestions for solution sequences. The therapist offers suggestions, however, in a collaborative spirit that includes clients' input, including the right to decline the suggestion.

The solution sequence can emerge from several sources. The first is knowledge of best practices about how to handle difficult situations. For example, in a blended family together for a year, the presenting problem was the acting out of a 9-year-old boy. The adults reported that the stepfather disciplines his stepson. Best practice for blending families recommends that the stepparent not participate in discipline until the stepchildren have developed an attachment to him or her. The solution sequence, therefore, would recommend that the biological parent, the mother, be the one to provide discipline, with the mother and stepfather having time alone to discuss the stepfather's point of view about parenting.

Second, solution sequences can be drawn from empirically supported findings from models of therapy that address particular problems or situations. For example, the psychoeducational model for the family treatment of major mental disorders (Anderson, Hogarty, Bayer, & Needleman, 1984) has shown that high levels of expressed emotion exacerbate the disorder of the diagnosed family member. The solution sequence suggested by this research would be to educate the family on expressed emotion and work to reduce it.

A third source of solution sequences is the therapist's experience with similar difficult situations. Although this experience is not always empirically supported, all experienced therapists have accumulated templates that fit a variety of common presenting problems and problem sequences. Their ability to catalog and recall solution sequences they applied in the past enables them to apply them in similar circumstances.

Fourth, everyone possesses common-sense knowledge about how to solve problems. This common sense is often obvious when the problem sequence includes components that would lead the average person to say, "That's just not right." For example, if a client has an extreme or unrealistic point of view related to the presenting problem, the solution sequence may include replacing it with a more considered view. Finally, therapists' intuition and feelings about the clients and their problem can suggest a solution sequence. For example, if one client professes not to be bothered by something another client is doing but the therapist senses that client's anger or sadness, the therapist can point this out and make recognition and expression of that feeling part of the solution sequence.

This is not to suggest that the solution sequences simply boil down to the correct way to approach problem sequences. Therapists must also incorporate the idiosyncratic nature of the client system into the solution. This includes characteristics of the clients and the unique fit among the clients and their cultural context. For example, a wife kept asking for emotional closeness with her husband, who often reacted to such bids with anger. When the therapist recognized that the husband's behavior seemed to place him somewhere on the autism spectrum and confirmed this through testing, his failure to respond to emotional needs was reframed from "He doesn't care about you" to "He doesn't recognize what you are looking for in those moments." This enabled the wife to be less frustrated with the husband and the husband to respond without anger when she made bids for affection.

The nature of the relationships among clients must also be accounted for when understanding the problem sequence and developing a solution sequence. Gottman (1993), for example, identified types of couples that can have healthy interaction. One is the validator couple, and another is the volatile couple. It would be easy to assume that validation is good for all couples; hence, a problem sequence of high conflict should always be modified to include validation. However, volatile couples not wounded by the harsh words they exchange in conflict would not thrive if they were encouraged to replace their conflict style with validation.

Likewise, clients' culture must also be accounted for in the creation of the solution sequence. It is incumbent on IST therapists to be culturally literate and to inquire respectfully whether some component of a problem sequence is, perhaps, normative within a given cultural group. For example, although Americans value directness, in some cultures it is offensive to be direct. The indirectness of the client's communication, therefore, should not be automatically interpreted as passive–aggressive behavior needing to be changed.

Successful implementation of the solution sequence in a session does not guarantee that it will be generalized to clients' lives at home—hence, the importance of prescribing the solution sequence between sessions. To do so, the therapist must be certain that all clients understand the solution and know their role in it. Troubleshooting the client's context at home anticipates obstacles to implementation. For example, the demanding routine of a couple could keep them from finding the time to talk, let alone practice the solution sequence.

The following example illustrates the first four problem-solving tasks of IST: (a) define the problem, (b) construct the problem sequence, (c) identify a solution sequence, and then (d) implement it. A wife complained that her husband believed she is not competent. The husband countered that it was not so much that she was not competent but seemed so indecisive that he had to decide what should be done in most situations. They agreed that she was underactive and he was overactive in deciding how to live their lives. They then articulated the problem sequence as follows. The husband stated that his wife had to rehash something over and over and could never get to the problem-solving part of the conversation. The wife stated that the husband was impatient. Not long after the conversation started, he butted in to say, "This is what you should do." This made the wife feel incompetent, and she deferred to the husband's suggestion because otherwise, he would get frustrated and walk away.

To introduce the solution sequence, the therapist wondered what would happen if the husband agreed to be more patient and listen to several iterations of the wife's point of view. The wife agreed to signal that she had thoughts about how to deal with the situation, so the husband did not erroneously conclude that she was just "spinning her wheels." They each agreed, therefore, to do one thing differently. In the session, they practiced successfully and agreed to do their best to keep these changes during the ensuing week.

WHEN THE SOLUTION SEQUENCE DOES NOT WORK: IDENTIFYING CONSTRAINTS

When clients cannot implement the solution sequence, the therapist adopts a spirit of curiosity in an effort to determine what went wrong. The first line of inquiry establishes whether something was wrong with the process of setting up and implementing the solution sequence. Did the clients understand what they had agreed to do? Did some pragmatic obstacle keep the solution sequence from being successful? For example, did one of the clients get sick, or did a change in the routine preclude trying the solution sequence? Sometimes a key component of the problem sequence has yet to be revealed that would necessitate tweaking the solution. Whatever is learned, the therapist must decide whether there is value in rebooting the solution sequence and trying it again.

If the process of implementing a solution sequence seemed sound and the clients simply could not perform it, an IST therapist's response would be guided by the constraint pillar—something is keeping the clients from implementing it. Accordingly, rather than ask, "Why didn't you do it?" the therapist would ask, "What kept you from doing it?" Clients' responses to this question contain feedback that reveals one or more constraints. A *constraint* is anything in the client system that keeps the problem from being solved. Further, a constraint keeps the solution sequence from being able to alter the problem sequence. For the solution sequence to be successful, therefore, the constraint must be lifted.

Consider the following example. A family's problem sequence included emotional escalation that inevitably led to all family members screaming at each other. The therapist suggested that better emotional regulation would facilitate less volatile conversations. The therapist suggested that each family member takes stock of his or her emotions before engaging in the conversation and that they refrain from engaging if they were close to becoming emotionally flooded. They all agreed to try this and had some success in the session. When they returned for the next session, however, they reported that conflicts during the week had been just as volatile. When the therapist asked what kept them from checking their emotions as they had agreed to do, the father responded,

> I thought more about it and decided I'm not sure it's the right thing for me. I think there are times when a father should raise his voice and say essentially, "Now I mean business." The problem isn't my emotions. It's that I have gone to the mat with them too often and now they don't pay any attention. Hell, I'm the father.

The ensuing conversation revealed that the father's patriarchal beliefs kept him from embracing the solution sequence; also, by not doing so, he engaged in a subtle gender war with the female members of the household, who constantly challenged his leadership through the high emotion conflict of the family.

IST therapists begin therapy hoping a single solution sequence targeted at a single problem sequence will result in a resolution of the presenting problem. Every therapist has a few stories about how such parsimonious successes occur. They are, however, the exception to the rule. More often, the situation is more complex and, often, far more complex. The degree of complexity is directly correlated with the number of constraints that have kept the clients from solving the problem. The win–win of working with a solution sequence is that it is either effective in solving a problem or provides a gateway to the constraints that must be lifted to solve the problem.

When clients answer the constraint question, the therapist frames their feedback in constraint language. There are several variations of constraint talk: "So it seems like X is stopping you from doing Y," "So this X is keeping you from doing Y," "So do you agree that X is an obstacle for doing Y?" All of these speculations about a constraint invite the clients to explore the nature and impact of the constraint on the presenting problem, the problem sequence, and the solution sequence. Sometimes the discussion focuses on an isolated constraint that alone is blocking the solution. In this case, the conversation moves quickly to strategies for lifting the constraint. The implementation of this strategy represents the next step in the early stages of IST when the clients and therapist collaborate on finding ways to lift the constraint. If the clients lift the constraint, they can then implement the solution sequence and thus solve the problem. In many other clinical situations, however, the discussion of one constraint leads to the identification of still more constraints. In these situations, the initial constraint is like the loose end of a knotted ball of string: pull on it, and rather than loosening the knot, it tightens, signaling more constraints. In Chapter 4 we present the IST framework for identifying and cataloging constraints, the *web of human experience*.

This description of IST is captured in the essence of IST diagram, Figure 3.1. The essence diagram is not the totality of IST but rather represents a core set of processes that are repeated throughout the course of IST. In summary, those steps are as follows:

1. Convene a direct client system and define the problem.
2. Locate the problem in the problem sequence.
3. Identify a solution sequence.
4. Implement the solution sequence.
5. Evaluate the outcome (successful or unsuccessful).
6. If successful, go to Step 9, maintain the solution sequence, and if unsuccessful, identify the constraints preventing the solution sequence from working.
7. Use strategies to lift the constraints.
8. Implement the solution sequence.
9. Maintain the solution sequence.
10. Terminate therapy or repeat the steps with additional constraints and/or new problems.

WHEN PROBLEM RESOLUTION REQUIRES MORE COMPLEXITY

Thus far we have presented the textbook case for using the essence diagram. In many therapies, however, the application of the essence diagram is not as straightforward and requires attention to additional factors that render the case more complex. Additional factors include the complexity of sequences, the complexity of client systems, and the readiness of the client system to change.

The Complexity of Sequences

Sometimes the problem sequence consists of a nested collection of sequences that must all be changed if the presenting problem is to be addressed successfully. It is vital, therefore, that IST therapists possess a framework for recognizing and working with the nested property of sequences. Breunlin and Schwartz (1986) proposed a framework for classifying sequences based on *periodicity* (the length of time it takes the sequence to go through one cycle). They identified four classes of sequences: (a) face-to-face sequences that occur in seconds or minutes, (b) sequences involving clients' routines with periodicity that ranges from 1 day to a week, (c) ebb-and-flow sequences that occur anywhere from several weeks to a year or so, and finally, (d) transgenerational sequences that play out across generations. Ebb-and-flow sequences typically have one of two properties: the ebb and flow of a key variable such as sadness or intimacy over time or the involvement of an intermittent event such as violence, binge drinking, or an anniversary reaction.

In this framework, sequences of shorter duration are nested in longer sequences; hence, face-to-face sequences occur at some point during the daily and weekly routine. For example, parents often report that conflict with their children is the worst in the morning when they are trying to get out the door for school and work or in the evening when the routine includes events such as homework, monitoring the various screens in the household, and getting to bed. Likewise, a parent's struggle with an adolescent's weekend curfew can be affected by the adolescent's monthly visit with an out-of-state biological parent whose views about curfew are quite different. Transgenerational sequences occur when a process is replicated from generation to generation. For example, a couple had a long-term stable relationship until the husband contracted an illness that put the wife in the role of caregiver. Initially, the couple seemed to adapt to the new roles, but eventually, the wife experienced episodic hostility toward the husband. One constraint was the impact of caregiver fatigue, but this did not seem to account for the strength of her feelings. With further exploration, the wife revealed that growing up her brother had a debilitating illness that preoccupied her parents. She was expected to be the "good" child, so they could focus their limited resources on her brother. She had never appreciated how much she resented being in this role and made the connection that caring for her husband made her feel the same way.

Sometimes it is obvious from the outset that multiple sequences are involved, so they are all reviewed as part of the problem sequence. An example is sexual problems. The sexual problem may involve sequences of sexual practices taking place in the bedroom—how a couple is making love. A sexual encounter also takes place at some point in a day and week that includes issues of routine. One partner may prefer having sex in the morning and the other at night. Some routinely problematic ebb-and-flow sequences involve the couple's pattern of initiation, the respective ebb and flow of desire for each partner, and the biology and decisions they make about a female partner's menstrual cycle. Finally, sexual beliefs or practices may be passed from generation to generation. A couple may describe a particular sequence as the primary problem sequence, but constructing a solution sequence for it often reveals that other sequences are involved.

There are other situations in which the therapist initially believes an adequate problem sequence has been revealed only to learn that the problem is embedded in other sequences. In these situations, the therapist must step back and gather additional information about the problem sequences before formulating a solution sequence. For example, in a first session, parents discussed their conflict about discipline. As they articulated a face-to-face problem sequence, one of them revealed that the conflict was most intense when the mother returned from business trips that occurred several times a month. The father said he had no problem with discipline while she was away. It was only when she returned and questioned the decisions he made in her absence that the conflict emerged. The face-to-face interaction, therefore, was embedded in the intermittent event of travel. The solution sequence for this case may include better communication about discipline, but it may also include an agreement that when the mother is away on a business trip, the father's discipline operates, and the mother agrees not to call it into question when she returns.

The Client System and Sequences

The clients attending the session provide the information about the problem and the problem sequence. Per our discussion of the ontological (systems theory) pillar in Chapter 2, these clients are in the direct-client system. All other clients in the client system not attending the session are in the indirect-client system. These clients may participate in the problem sequence, but their role in it can only be described from the perspective of the clients who are in the session. For example, if a woman enters individual therapy, her description of spousal conflict comes from her perspective and will inevitably have substantial blind spots. The husband's description is likely to be somewhat different. Further, the two perspectives provide the most complete description of the problem sequence.

The best approximation of a problem sequence, therefore, is one provided by all the clients who participate in that sequence. Mindful of this, IST therapists invite all relevant clients to the initial session. Both partners of that couple, therefore, would be invited to the initial session. If the caller initially requests to be seen individually, an IST therapist would explain why it is better to include the spouse, but if the caller is adamant about wanting to be seen alone, the therapist will apply the alliance guideline and grant her wish to be seen alone. Likewise, the parents of an adolescent may prefer to place their adolescent in individual therapy. Again, mindful that the richness of the problem sequence will come from hearing all perspectives, an IST therapist would invite both parents and the adolescent to attend the session. The therapist might also request that other siblings attend some sessions because their perspective can shed light on the client system. For example, when one child has a problem, the other children are often described as perfect. These children are burdened by the problem sequence because they resent having to be perfect so the parents have the energy to focus on the problem child.

Sometimes in the course of gathering information about the problem sequence, the function of another family member, not present, is revealed. This information creates choice for the therapist: to stay with the problem sequence as articulated by the clients in the direct system or to expand the focus by including other family members. For example, a single parent raising an oppositional child described the problem sequence of getting homework completed. How the parent made requests and how the child responded seemed to constitute the problem sequence until the parent revealed her mother is home after school and is supposed to monitor homework. When the grandmother allowed the homework to slide and an exhausted mother had to deal with it, the mother–child conflict was embedded in the larger sequence of the grandmother's inability to get the homework done. At this point, the therapist could work with the mother and child or invite the grandmother to attend the next session. If the latter happened and the grandmother was helped to insist that homework was done right after school, the mother–child conflict would also be resolved.

Readiness and Ability to Change

IST seeks to initiate the process of change as quickly as possible. Therapists know well, however, that when clients enter therapy, they are sometimes not yet ready to change. The therapist's enthusiasm for change, therefore, must be tempered by recognition that some clients will be hesitant to engage in a change process early in therapy. IST therapists must, therefore, simultaneously work with the essence diagram while also listening for client ambivalence about change. If the therapist fails to read feedback about ambivalence to change, a struggle between the client and therapist can result that can damage the alliance and lead to early termination.

Reluctance to or ambivalence about change can manifest for an individual client, a couple, or the whole family. For a specific client, the following are often markers of ambivalence: addiction, trauma, risk of suicide, or a psychiatric disorder. Violence, commitment, and trust issues predict ambivalence for a couple. When the presenting problem serves a function for the whole family, reluctance to change will be present because the family will resist giving up the problem to preserve their homeostasis.

Because IST does not use formal assessment at the outset of therapy, the therapist must detect ambivalence to change by listening carefully to what clients say, observing clients' behavior and interactions, and noticing client reactions to the therapist's attempt to define a problem, a problem sequence, and a solution sequence. We recognize there are trade-offs in taking this approach and prefer the benefits accrued to alliance formation achieved through an active and direct engagement with the presenting problem.

Because readiness to change is a common factor, IST therapists are sensitive to the stage of change each client presents at the outset of therapy. The stages are precontemplation, contemplation, preparation, action, and maintenance (Norcross, 2011; Norcross, Krebs, & Prochaska, 2011). For clients to implement their part of a solution sequence, they must be in the action stage of change. Sometimes therapy must pass through each of the stages of change before IST can be fully implemented. Feedback enables the therapist to recognize ambivalence. For example, a client may present with flat affect or burst into tears with little provocation, thus revealing a possible depressed state. Or a client might appear to become triggered when a particular circumstance and/or issue is being discussed, thus raising the question of a trauma history. On occasion, clients arrive for their session under the influence of alcohol. Sometimes one client will call attention to another client's psychiatric condition, trauma history, or chemical dependency. If the other client denies the issue or becomes defensive, it often signals that the issue is part of the problem sequence that cannot yet be discussed. When the issue broached involves danger to self or others, however, it must be addressed regardless of its impact on the alliance.

When ambivalence is encountered at the outset of therapy, the therapist plans whether to slow down the pace of therapy. One strategy is to name, acknowledge, and discuss the ambivalence. Another strategy is to conduct a cost–benefit analysis of not changing. Another strategy is to study the problem by assigning a monitoring task. For example, clients can be asked to monitor the frequency, intensity, and duration of a target variable such as conflict episodes. Although monitoring tasks do not ask for change, their use can trigger change or induce contemplation of change because it is hard for clients to observe their behavior without thinking and/or changing some aspect of it. Clients can then be asked to discuss their thoughts and feelings about the task.

For example, Marlene, a 29-year-old heterosexual woman, was referred to Elizabeth by Marlene's family therapist because she was unable to tolerate being in therapy with her family. In this therapy, Marlene paralyzed the family therapy sessions by exhibiting anger and defensiveness that the family's therapist could not modify. In the first individual session, Elizabeth found her to be similarly reactive to questions about the presenting problem. Elizabeth hypothesized that Marlene felt unsafe in therapy because the very process of defining the problem was threatening to her. Reading this feedback, Elizabeth departed from the more typical IST path and deferred the problem-solving process until a sense of safety could be established. She did so by inviting Marlene to discuss what might be comfortable for her, and she assured her that she had a say in what would be discussed. Further, Elizabeth described the process of therapy in IST so Marlene would know what to expect, adding that things would proceed at Elizabeth's preferred pace. She added that she would invite Marlene to explore the pros and cons of any in-session activities or proposed solutions. In the third session, Marlene began to define her presenting problem as feeling emotionally out of control and having frequent conflict with family members. As therapy became safe for her, she began to work on the sexual abuse she had experienced as a child. In that work, Elizabeth used a diverse set of strategies and interventions that had originally been developed within dialectical behavior therapy, cognitive behavior therapy, trauma therapy models, and self-psychology.

SPECIAL CIRCUMSTANCES INFLUENCING PATHWAYS WITHIN INTEGRATIVE SYSTEMIC THERAPY

In IST there is no one correct way to approach a type of problem and no one correct way to work with a particular system. Some circumstances alter the path that IST takes, such that the work varies somewhat from what otherwise might be expected. These circumstances include dangerous situations requiring a social control function, mandated therapy, alternative contexts of therapy (secondary treatment settings, outreach programs), and cases in which a client experiences the process of beginning therapy, including defining a problem sequence or solution sequence, as a threat. Although an extensive discussion of these factors is beyond the scope of this book, we address each of them briefly here.

Dangerous Situations

The presence of danger to self or others alters the path of IST. Such circumstances as suicidality, homicidal threats, child endangerment or abuse, and elder abuse require the therapist to focus carefully on these risk factors whether or not they are presented by the client as a problem. The therapist may be able to establish with the clients a mutual concern about the issue (e.g., agreeing that suicidality is a presenting problem), but the therapist is required by law and professional ethics to address such risk-management issues as effectively as possible to prevent harm from occurring. In a sense, under such circumstances, the therapist represents the community, society, and our professions, which define the "presenting problem" as a danger that has to be addressed. The normal path of IST is supplanted with a social control function to ensure safety. This may mean calling the state child protection agency or hospitalizing a client (hopefully voluntarily; if necessary, involuntarily). Strategies and procedures for such situations are important for every therapist to know but are not substantively covered here. The point is that danger to self or others and child or elder abuse are situations that will likely require the therapist to suspend the ordinary IST practice of focusing on clients' presenting concerns.

Mandated Therapy

Mandated therapy is another circumstance that requires modification of the IST approach. Examples of mandates include a referral from child protective services for work toward family reunification, divorce court referral for resolution of parental conflict, juvenile court referral of an adolescent, and court referral of an individual adult offender. The literature on mandated clients addresses strategies of intervention within a task-centered casework approach (Rooney, 2010), the importance of cultural sensitivity and therapist self-awareness (Baker, 1999), social work ethics and values pertaining to involuntary clients (Barsky, 2010), alliance issues with high-conflict divorcing families dealing with custody and visitation disputes (Lebow & Newcomb Rekart, 2007), and the use of group motivational interviewing with substance abusers (Lincourt, Kuettel, & Bombardier, 2002). If you work with mandated clients, we refer you to this literature as well as to the policies of the agency context in which the therapy takes place. The discussion here is meant to clarify in a general way how IST can be adapted to work with involuntary clients.

Essentially, mandated therapy requires an accommodation to a triangular arrangement involving the client, the mandating agent, and the therapist. Specifically, the mandating agent is defining a presenting problem (at least in general terms), and the client is reacting to the mandate. Although the IST process of establishing an alliance through a focus on the client's presenting problem is skewed from the start, the IST approach will apply once this skew is addressed. We strongly recommend that the therapist establishes a clear understanding with both the mandating agent and the client about the requirements of therapy and the type of reporting, if any, that will be done. The next task is to discuss with the clients how they feel about the mandate and whether they want to work on what the mandating agent specifies. Solution-focused interviewing (De Jong & Berg, 2001) and motivational interviewing (Miller & Rollnick, 2012; Miller & Rose, 2009) provide helpful guides to the type of conversation that can enhance cooperation. The goal is to bridge the mandated requirements to something the client wants to accomplish. If this can be established, then IST's problem-solving tasks (essence diagram, Figure 3.1), the decision-making process of the blueprint, and the planning strategies apply.

Alternative Contexts of Therapy

IST is most typically practiced in mental health agencies, group practices, and private practice. It is, however, also practiced in alternative settings such as schools, medical settings, social service agencies, and community-based social service programs. The course of therapy in these settings is affected by such variables as the mission of the agency, whether the therapy is mandated, and how clients are referred to the therapist. These settings may present very different points of entry for therapy than mental health centers or private or group practices. First, therapy may not be the primary mission in these alternative settings. Because the nontherapist staff may or may not fully understand the therapy process or value it for a particular family, the IST therapist has to establish and maintain an alliance with these staff members. Ideally, a team approach will apply, and the teacher, nurse, social worker, child care worker, or outreach worker will collaborate with the therapist and family. Clear boundaries for confidentiality and the release of information are essential. Second, the presenting problem may well be defined by the agency staff member who referred the case. In some cases, the problem and solution sequence may be at least partially defined by an organization outside the family. For example, a school may refer a child to a school-based therapist for anger management. Or a family in a community outreach program that focuses on job readiness may refer a person for what the worker sees as depression.

Because the point of entry to these cases is often a statement of a concern by a third party, the IST therapist has to acknowledge in session the referring agent's definition of the problem. If the therapy is mandated, the considerations regarding mandates discussed earlier apply. If not, the referral is still the starting point, and the therapist will have to determine whether the family wants to accept the problem or goal of the referrer and consider any consequences of not doing so. For example, a referral for a child's disruptive behavior in day care may not be explicitly mandated, but it may carry the implicit message that if the child's behavior does not improve significantly, she or he may be excluded from the program. Once the therapist and client system have decided what to do about the referral agent's concerns and whether they can agree on a goal of therapy, the therapist begins to explore the problem sequence and continues with the normal course of IST. Boyd-Franklin (2012) provided many practical guidelines for home-based, school, and community interventions that can be incorporated into IST. Discussions of therapy in medical settings are provided by Edwards and Patterson (2006); Heru (2014); McDaniel, Doherty, and Hepworth (2013); Pisani and McDaniel (2005); and Ruddy and McDaniel (2016).

Case Management and Support Services

In some community-based programs, case management or support services are offered by means of outreach to an economically disadvantaged or vulnerable population. IST therapists working in such contexts understand that these clients may be much more concerned about meeting basic needs for food, shelter, clothing, and physical safety than they are with the hope of solving a psychological or relational concern. In such programs, it is important to meet the family at their level of need. Kilpatrick and Holland (2005) proposed a model for family assessment and intervention that is based on level of need and suggested that in some cases more basic human needs may require attention before the family can focus on the issues traditionally associated with family therapy (e.g., boundaries) or individual therapy (e.g., inner conflict). These basic needs are the equivalent of a presenting problem and, in turn, are the entry point for the IST-trained caseworker or therapist to assist the family and form a therapeutic alliance. This involves assessing need and locating resources for the family. The therapist works to access strengths and support problem-solving skills, but when the adult family members are constrained from navigating the community and societal systems that can be of assistance, the caseworker or therapist will have to advocate on their behalf. The alliance that develops from meeting the family where they are and responding to their needs may lead the family to feel more comfortable presenting other issues such as child-focused problems, relational concerns, substance abuse, or depression.

Although the special circumstances we have discussed may alter the path therapy takes, IST, with the modifications discussed, can be used in each of these circumstances. The versatility and adaptability of IST make it applicable in a wide variety of circumstances and contexts.

THE ESSENCE DIAGRAM AND OTHER TOOLS OF INTEGRATIVE SYSTEMIC THERAPY

To describe how to use the essence diagram, in this chapter we have focused almost exclusively on it. Although the essence diagram is the anchoring tool that enables the therapist to stay focused, it is just one of several tools that make up IST. To fully engage, understand, and work with a client system, therapists must also understand the intricacies of how the client system works in both the context of the client system and also in the broader context of community. Therapists must also develop and maintain alliances with all clients. Hence, in addition to working the essence diagram, the IST therapist is also attending to myriad other tasks. Finally, sessions are both a whole experience and a microcosm of the entire course of therapy, so the therapist must track the therapy over time and anticipate and make decisions about what might be up ahead. In short, IST is thoughtful therapy at each point along the way.

In Chapter 4 we introduce another tool for managing thoughtfulness in the sessions. We call it the *blueprint for therapy*. With its four recursive components of hypothesizing, planning, conversing, and feedback, the blueprint grounds therapy in the moment by enabling therapists to both attend to the unfolding process and reflect on what has to happen next. Chapters 5 to 8, in turn, expand on each of the blueprint components, with Chapter 6 adding an additional tool, the *IST planning matrix*. This tool is designed to assist the IST therapist in choosing the best methods for lifting the constraints that emerge through the efforts to solve the problem. Moreover, the matrix is designed to help therapists decide what to do next when what they are doing is not working.

4

A BLUEPRINT FOR THERAPY: TESTING AND REVISING HYPOTHESES

The processes of developing and maintaining a therapeutic alliance and leading a collaborative exploration of the tasks specified in the integrative systemic therapy (IST) essence diagram (see Figure 3.1) require many decisions that are conditional on what the therapist thinks would be helpful at a given point and what the key clients agree to discuss and do. The IST therapist takes primary responsibility for formulating and addressing the many decisions the therapy system will have to undertake. This is an ongoing and continually evolving process that invites client participation and welcomes course correction as therapist and clients address the various tasks of therapy. In this chapter, we present a schema, the IST blueprint for therapy, that guides our decision making, facilitates evaluation of the effects of our work, and provides the basis for the clinical–scientific method of our integrative approach to therapy. Further, we discuss the first of its four components in

http://dx.doi.org/10.1037/0000055-004
Integrative Systemic Therapy: Metaframeworks for Problem Solving With Individuals, Couples, and Families,
by W. M. Pinsof, D. C. Breunlin, W. P. Russell, J. L. Lebow, C. Rampage, and A. L. Chambers

somewhat greater detail and establish the operational significance of the body of knowledge associated with it.

Therapists face innumerable decisions with each case they see. Whom should they invite to therapy? Should they contact a family member's therapist or a child's school? What would they want to learn or communicate in such a call? Which problem should they prioritize? What can they suggest to help solve the problems brought to therapy? What do they do when the family does not follow their suggestions? What do they do when clients follow the suggestions and things do not improve? How do they know when therapy should end? What would they like to accomplish in the last session? Each of these larger questions may involve many "real time" decisions about what to say or do at particular moments within a session. What language should they use to describe the problem sequence? What should they do about the fact that the husband turned away when the wife was describing her concerns? How long should they let him talk about a particular issue? What should they do when a teenage boy refuses to answer their questions? How long should they wait before interrupting a conflict in session? It seems that there are about as many decisions as there are moments in therapy. A therapist has to have a knowledge base and a schema for making these many decisions. The blueprint is both our decision-making schema and our means for organizing the bodies of knowledge required for conducting our systemic, integrative, and empirically informed approach to therapy.

A BLUEPRINT FOR THERAPY

IST provides guidelines, discussed in Chapters 2, 3, 4, and 6 of this volume and listed together in the Appendix, that address many of the questions that arise in therapy, but the specific course of therapy at any point is also determined by a recursive decision-making and decision-evaluating process we call the *blueprint for therapy* (Breunlin, Pinsof, Russell, & Lebow, 2011; Breunlin, Schwartz, & Mac Kune-Karrer, 1992; Pinsof, Breunlin, Russell, & Lebow, 2011). The blueprint, shown in Figure 4.1, has four key components: hypothesizing, planning, conversing, and giving feedback. It describes a process in which hypotheses about the therapeutic relationship and the problem-solving tasks of the IST essence are generated, tested, and progressively refined until the clients solve the presenting problems. The blueprint serves as an organizing tool for managing the moment-to-moment events in a session and planning therapy between sessions.

In *hypothesizing*, the therapist and clients consider descriptions and explanations for a wide variety of events and processes that occur within the therapy and in the clients' lives. They study the problem and consider formulations

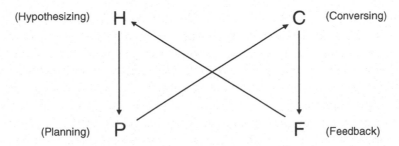

Figure 4.1. Integrative systemic therapy blueprint for therapy. From "Integrative Problem-Centered Metaframeworks Therapy I: Core Concepts and Hypothesizing," by D. C. Breunlin, W. Pinsof, W. P. Russell, and J. Lebow, 2011, *Family Process, 50,* p. 300. Copyright 2011 by John Wiley & Sons. Reprinted with permission.

(hypotheses) of the problem sequences and solution sequences. When clients have difficulty implementing a solution sequence, further collaborative hypothesizing progressively reveals the factors (constraints) that prevent its enactment. In the course of formulating such hypotheses, the therapist pays careful attention to the therapeutic alliance and formulates hypotheses about it as well.

Planning involves the development of strategies to implement the solution sequences and, when necessary, to lift the constraints identified in hypothesizing. Planning also involves developing strategies the therapist uses to promote adaptive sequences between her- or himself and the client system that create and maintain the therapeutic alliance.

Conversing refers to the conversation through which plans are explored, developed, and initiated. Conversation is a collaborative process in which the therapist gathers information, learns about client concerns and viewpoints, educates, formulates descriptions of sequences, and suggests courses of action.

Last, *feedback* involves reading feedback—that is, paying careful attention to any information, response, or reaction that seems to make a difference to the relational and problem-solving tasks of therapy. Are they with me? Did this intervention work? What can we learn from it? The therapist tracks the content and themes of conversation, observable behavior and interaction, reports of actions and interactions, empirical data regarding progress in therapy, and her or his internal (emotional) reactions. Reading the feedback provides the information the therapist needs to confirm or revise hypotheses and modify plans or specific conversational elements as needed. Considering client feedback about progress is one of the common factors that underlies all successful therapy (Norcross & Lambert, 2011b).

Recursively, in each session, between sessions, and over the course of therapy, the therapist, in concert with the client system, hypothesizes, plans, converses, and reads the feedback. The process of the blueprint applies to any and all of the relational and problem-solving tasks of therapy. Further, it has utility on a moment-to-moment basis within sessions (micro level of therapy) and between sessions as a means of planning therapy (macro level of therapy). The therapist uses the blueprint as a guide in leading the therapy while knowing that there will be many minor course corrections, as well as major shifts as the therapy progresses. In a sense, each therapy is a single case study in which the blueprint is continuously used to intervene and correct the course until the presenting problems are solved. Significantly, the blueprint logic is the tool for integrating intervention strategies from a variety of models and the basis for the incorporation of feedback, including empirical feedback, into the work. It, along with IST pillars and guidelines, guides therapists seeking to work in both an integrative and empirically informed manner.

A brief case example illustrates the nature of the blueprint in operation. A father called with concerns about an escalating family conflict over his son's school achievement. The family consisted of heterosexual parents married 15 years and their son, Josh, a 12-year-old sixth grader in a suburban public middle school. This was a middle class, second-generation, Polish American, Catholic family. In the first session, the mother, who worked full-time as a nurse at a local hospital, expressed concern about the ongoing high level of conflict between the father and Josh concerning homework. The father, a former software developer and stay-at-home dad, expressed his strong concern that Josh is successful in school. Josh, reticent at first, stated that he wanted to do his work on his own and that his father was "making me crazy" with his pressure and close monitoring of the assignments. All members agreed that the father had always worked closely with Josh on his schoolwork and that this had always been a source of tension in the household, but that the tension and conflict had escalated significantly this year. A recent incident in which Josh shoved his father during a conflict brought the family to therapy. Josh stated that he was sorry for this incident but that his father was putting too much pressure on him.

In the first session, the family agreed that the presenting problem was the ongoing conflict between father and son. The son asked his father directly to let him do his work independently, and all agreed this would be a reasonable thing to try, though the father stated his reservations. The hypothesis at this point was that, given greater independence and a personal commitment to being responsible for his homework, Josh might well be able to complete his assignments on a daily basis (a solution sequence). The plan was developed for Josh to do his homework each night after dinner. The parents agreed to let him do so without interruption but to ask him later in the evening whether he had completed his work. The therapist supported the plan and framed it as an experiment. This all occurred in the medium of the therapeutic conversation in which the therapist facilitated the process and attended to clients' concerns and reactions. The therapist felt that the feedback within and from the conversation in session was positive overall, though it was clear that the father had some concerns.

More significant feedback came when the family returned for the second session. They seemed tense. Josh appeared sullen. They reported that the week had been peaceful until that day. The father had stayed out of Josh's homework, but he had been worried about whether Josh was doing all of it. The morning of the session, the father had gone on the school assignment website to see whether Josh was keeping up with his work and discovered that Josh had a number of missing assignments. He confronted Josh with this in the afternoon. There was an angry exchange, and the father said they would talk about it in therapy. The therapist supported the father for having performed the experiment and asked the mother to share her perspective. She stated her appreciation for the father's efforts and asked Josh why he did not do all of his work. Josh said he did not know and then added that middle school grades do not matter for college admission. The conversation came to a halt. The therapist viewed (hypothesis) Josh's remark about college admission as a sign of his discomfort and an attempt to save face. Further, the therapist assumed that Josh had good intentions and was constrained in some way from doing his work. At that moment the therapist decided to reach out (the plan) in a positive, accepting way; acknowledge Josh's likely good intentions; and ask about the constraints. This would be initiated immediately in the therapeutic conversation.

> *Therapist:* Josh, this is probably an uncomfortable conversation for you. I don't know you that well yet, but I would guess that you really want to complete your homework, but that something is getting in the way of that. Would you agree?
>
> *Josh:* Yes. [His tone is quiet and respectful, which the therapist takes as feedback that Josh appreciated the positive view of his intentions.]
>
> *Therapist:* What do you think might be getting in the way?
>
> *Josh:* I don't know. I don't like homework, but I want to get it done. I sometimes get sidetracked with things.
>
> *Therapist:* Like what?
>
> *Josh:* Computer games or texts from friends. I keep thinking I will get to it, but then the night goes by, and I sometimes don't.
>
> *Father:* You often don't.
>
> *Josh:* [With a bit of a scowl] Pfft.

At that moment the therapist wondered (hypothesis), given the challenge Josh described and given the history of the father's close monitoring of homework, whether Josh had had the opportunity to learn progressively over time how to take responsibility for his homework. The therapist decided to bypass the father's interjection and the son's reaction to introduce the hypothesis.

Therapist: I understand that you want to do your homework on your own. Have you ever put your homework completely on your shoulders? You know, taking full responsibility for it?

Josh: Not so much.

Therapist: [To the parents] Would you agree with Josh on this?

Mother: Yes, I would.

Father: I try to get him to be responsible for the work, but no, he does not assume it.

The therapist felt this feedback supported the hypothesis that Josh had not progressively learned how to assume responsibility for his homework. This led immediately to the decision to develop that theme in the conversation.

Therapist: I think that responsibility is a skill that needs to be learned— and learned in a progressive, step-by-step manner. Does that make sense? That as we grow and develop and are given more responsibility, a bit at a time, we learn to accept it—put it on our shoulders?

Parents: Yes. [Nodding]

Therapist: Then maybe it would make sense for us to approach the homework like that. Josh, would you be willing to work with your parents so that you get to do parts of your homework on your own and, step by step, move toward accepting more and more responsibility for it until you have it all on your shoulders?

Josh: Sure.

With discussion, the family agreed with this idea, and the therapist and family designed a new plan that involved a structure within which Josh would more independently perform portions of his work under his parents' supervision. The mother would work in tandem with the father as cosupervisor. The couple would support each other in managing their worries and sticking to the plan. Josh would ask for help as needed, but otherwise complete bits of work on his own and report periodically throughout the evening on his progress. The understanding was that, over time and with success, more autonomy with schoolwork would be extended to Josh. The therapist and family felt good about this plan that had been developed on the basis of the failure of the initial plan. More feedback would be observed in the coming sessions, and the therapist would be prepared to revise the hypothesis, plan, and/or conversation as the family continued in therapy.

From the first moments of this therapy, the therapist communicated—directly and indirectly—that the family had significant strengths and abilities, that therapy would involve a set of experiments, and that struggles and even failure in the course of the work would be important sources of information and opportunity. At the end of the second session, the therapist was hopeful that the family would make progress with the plan and was prepared for the many twists and turns the work might take. Would the son respond to this structure with better performance? Were there any other factors that constrained his school performance? Would the parents work well together as cosupervisors? Would the father be able to calm his fears and anxieties about his son's schoolwork? Would a contact with the school provide information that would require modification of the plan? Rather than basing therapy on a comprehensive initial assessment, the blueprint, in the spirit of parsimony and with respect for IST's epistemology pillar, facilitates recursive and progressive discovery of what the therapist has to know to help the client system resolve their problems.

It can be argued that the blueprint, in its most basic form, is a universal process that underlies every form of therapy. IST's approach to the blueprint, however, is distinguished in four ways. First, we elevate its importance by placing it at the center of our work and encouraging a conscious use of it. Second, we organize the knowledge, theories, and skills required for the practice of therapy with the blueprint, using it as the means of bringing the entire field of therapy to our practice. Third, we use it as a guide for integrating concepts, strategies, and interventions from specific models of therapy, common factors that underlie successful therapy, and accepted clinical competencies and practices. Last, as local clinical scientists (Stricker & Trierweiler, 1995), we use it as the logical basis for the clinical–experimental process that empirically informs (through observation and/or formal measures) each case we see. In Chapter 8 we discuss formal empirical measures that can be incorporated into this therapist-as-local-scientist approach.

We have discussed the blueprint as a decision-making and decision-evaluating process, but as noted before, IST is also a tool for containing and organizing the knowledge, theories, and skills required for the practice of therapy. In this sense, the blueprint is used to carry all of the details and operations of the IST approach and, to a great extent, the information and strategies of the field of psychotherapy. Each component of the blueprint carries a framework (or frameworks) and knowledge base for understanding the variables a therapist has to consider within that component of the process. Hypothesizing uses a set of frameworks (hypothesizing metaframeworks) that facilitate the description and assessment of the complex, multileveled functioning of the client system with a particular focus on the identification of alternative adaptive patterns (solution sequences), client strengths, factors that constrain problem solving (constraints), and the state of the therapeutic alliance. Planning organizes strategies for enacting solution sequences and removing constraints into a set of frameworks (planning metaframeworks) that are applied according to the IST guidelines and in concert with evolving hypotheses. Each of the planning metaframeworks includes extensive lists of strategies and interventions that have a common mechanism of change. Organized within conversing is a body of knowledge about the linguistic choices and communication skills that are used to build alliances, understand the client system, and execute interventions. Last, feedback contains a body of knowledge about various types of client responses and how they inform the therapy. Associated with feedback are empirical approaches to measuring change in therapy, including a multisystemic instrument—the STIC (see Chapter 8).

Chapters 5 through 8 delineate the factors associated with the blueprint components. Full comprehension of IST requires an understanding of the blueprint that is "loaded" with all of the information provided in these chapters; however, we believe it is important to have an initial grasp of the blueprint prior to learning in depth about each of its components. Einstein's observation, "The only reason for time is so that everything doesn't happen at once," may provide some encouragement for our dilemma of understanding the whole of the blueprint before fully comprehending the complexity of its various parts. Following the chapters on each of the blueprint components, we present three case studies that comprehensively illustrate the use of the blueprint in IST. Further, a bonus chapter, available online, provides a summary and synthesis of IST targeted for those who have an understanding of its components. For now, we proceed with a more general discussion of the blueprint that focuses somewhat less on all the information it contains and more on how it facilitates the development and testing of hypotheses. For this, we have to put forth a brief, initial discussion of the hypothesizing metaframeworks and introduce a case-formulating tool, the IST web of human experience.

THE INTEGRATIVE SYSTEMIC THERAPY WEB OF HUMAN EXPERIENCE

The blueprint prescribes a continuous and collaborative process of case formulation and intervention. Although this is a recursive process that does not have an identifiable starting point, hypothesizing is a reasonable place to begin the discussion in that the hypotheses are what we test and revise as we work our way through the blueprint. Any discussion of hypothesizing must acknowledge the range and complexity of the factors that may come into play when learning about how a family, couple, or individual functions, struggles, and solves problems. Although IST privileges parsimonious case formulations at the outset of therapy, it acknowledges the complexity of human systems and, as necessary, progressively explores it by considering two fundamental questions: What are the factors governing the system's functioning, and where in the multilevel system are they located? The "where" question draws on the concept of inclusive organization, suggesting that we can understand a system by looking at the various levels of it, including the levels of person, relationship, family, community, society, and civilization. The "what" question is considered in relation to seven hypothesizing metaframeworks (organization, development, culture, mind, gender, biology, and spirituality), each of which distills and organizes empirical findings and ideas from various models of therapy into domains that can be drawn on to describe and understand human systems.

The "what" and "where" questions generate a heuristic device called the *IST web of human experience*, shown in Figure 4.2. The concentric circles

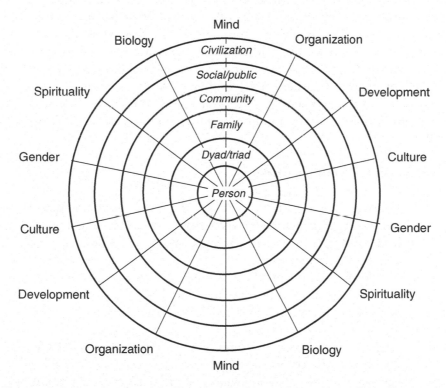

Figure 4.2. Integrative systemic therapy web of human experience. From "Integrative Problem-Centered Metaframeworks Therapy I: Core Concepts and Hypothesizing," by D. C. Breunlin, W. Pinsof, W. P. Russell, and J. Lebow, 2011, *Family Process, 50,* p. 301. Copyright 2011 by John Wiley & Sons. Reprinted with permission.

represent the psychosocial system levels, and the axes represent the hypothesizing metaframeworks. The web facilitates an integrative approach to hypothesizing and the identification of pattern and context in the lives of clients. It suggests where to look and what to look for. Of particular importance is the use of the web as a tool for understanding ways in which the tasks specified in the essence diagram (Figure 3.1; defining the problem, describing a problem sequence, identifying and enacting a solution sequence, identifying and removing constraints) can be formulated with a particular client system. Beginning therapists appreciate the web's structure that enables them to manage large amounts of clinical information. Experienced therapists internalize the web and readily connect their clients' patterns of behavior and experience to the web's levels and the hypothesizing metaframeworks.

In IST, hypothesizing metaframeworks transcend and replace the specific theories of human functioning, problem formation, and problem maintenance that underlie most models of psychotherapy. Hypothesizing metaframeworks are IST's case formulating factors. Each hypothesizing metaframework organizes a domain of human functioning and provides a multisystemic concept that applies isomorphically at each level of the system. These frameworks embody ideas (many of which are derived from empirical research) about what constitutes adaptive functioning within that domain. Metaframeworks are fluid bodies of knowledge that incorporate emerging information and ideas as new research emerges and the field of psychotherapy develops. A detailed description of each of the hypothesizing metaframeworks is provided in Chapter 5; to facilitate an initial understanding, we provide a listing and brief definition of them next.

Hypothesizing Metaframeworks

- *Organization*: a set of concepts that describes how the components of a system fit together and function as a whole (boundaries, leadership patterns, and the levels of harmony and balance among members and subsystems).
- *Development*: concepts and information concerning developmental stages and competencies of families, relationships, and individuals; fit of developmental demands among members and across levels of the system.
- *Culture*: a framework for examining the impact of membership in contexts of race, ethnicity, religion, class, geographic region, economic status, education, sexual orientation, and age; cultural fit across levels of the system.
- *Mind*: concepts and information that facilitate understanding of patterns of cognition, emotion, and intentionality.

- *Gender*: gender-based analysis of power and role functioning; gender identity; fit of gendered expectations and preferences across levels of the system.
- *Biology*: medical and neurobiological factors (e.g., brain chemistry, physiology of emotional arousal, patterns of health and illness, disability).
- *Spirituality*: spiritual resources such as faith, hope, prayer, transcendence, letting go and acceptance, religious beliefs; fit of religious beliefs and/or spiritual practices across levels of the system.

Hypothesizing metaframeworks carry the information therapists need to understand biological, psychological, and interactional aspects of human functioning in a multilevel system. They can be used to construct a simple and straightforward understanding of the problems clients bring to therapy, and they can support the most complex formulations of challenging cases. Hypothesizing metaframeworks inform any and all aspects of the therapeutic process but are particularly useful in helping us understand four tasks of therapy. First, they inform us about factors related to developing and maintaining a therapeutic alliance with the client system. Second, hypothesizing metaframeworks carry information that can suggest possible solution sequences. Third, they facilitate the identification of constraints to change. Fourth, they help us identify strengths that can be used to enact solution sequences or remove constraints. Next, we discuss how the blueprint is used to formulate, test, and revise hypotheses regarding each of these therapy tasks.

Testing and Revising Hypotheses About the Alliance

Developing and maintaining a therapeutic alliance, the most acknowledged common factor in psychotherapy (Sprenkle, Davis, & Lebow, 2009), is fundamental to the practice of IST. Because the presenting problem is the focus of therapy, the alliance is the vehicle by which therapist and clients collaborate to solve the problem(s). The integrative psychotherapy alliance model (Knobloch-Fedders, Pinsof, & Mann, 2007; Pinsof, 1983, 1994b), discussed in Chapters 2 and 3, supports the importance of tracking the development and maintenance of the alliance with careful attention to whether the therapist and clients are aligned in terms of the goals and tasks of therapy. The therapist leads a conversation that addresses clients' concerns and carefully monitors the dimensions of the alliance (tasks, goals, and bonds) as hypotheses and plans develop and evolve. He or she uses the decision-making schema of the blueprint to test hypotheses about whether the clients are on board with the direction (tasks and goals) of therapy and are developing an alliance with the therapist. Specifically, the therapist solicits feedback (ideally including empirical feedback) at many steps along the way and is prepared to notice signs of alliance issues and ruptures.

The hypothesizing metaframeworks inform and enrich this process by providing information about patterns of organization, development, culture, mind, gender, (human) biology, and spirituality that provide possible explanations for alliance issues and point toward ways to make a better connection with particular clients. Therapists deal with such questions as: Do the clients think I understand and respect how their religious views affect the problem and the therapy? What effect is my gender having on this couple's discussion of power in their relationship? As I ask about what brings this family in, are they feeling emotionally safe? Hypotheses about the alliance are tested and revised as plans to strengthen the alliance are made and implemented, and the therapist reads the feedback that results.

For example, a first-generation Mexican American widowed mother presented for therapy with her two children (Alejandro, age 13, and Gabriela, age 11). In the first session, the therapist joined with the family and began to define the problem, which involved conflict between the mother and son over his bids for greater freedom and independence. He had never been allowed to leave the immediate vicinity of their apartment building on his own, but now that he had begun high school, he thought it was time for him to do so. He was engaging and animated in the session and cited several specific examples to make his point. The mother was polite and rather formal. Although she was fluent in English, she presented a somewhat less well-formulated case. She verbalized concern about Alejandro being successful in school and not becoming involved with the boys who get in trouble in the neighborhood. The therapist asked Alejandro and his mother to talk directly to each other about their concerns, and the conversation became conflictual. The therapist was inclined to think, but did not directly say, that an adolescent boy should have more freedom than Alejandro was being allowed. At the conclusion of the session, the therapist indicated that it would be important to talk further about these issues and set a goal for the therapy. The family agreed to return the next week. As the session ended, the therapist felt a little uncomfortable about the look on the mother's face (feedback), but time was up, and the next client was in the waiting room.

The mom called to cancel the next session and did not request to reschedule (feedback). The therapist hypothesized that the alliance was damaged by something in the session, perhaps by the son's success in presenting a winning argument for more freedom that frightened the mother. She also wondered whether there was a difference in level of acculturation between mother and son that disadvantaged the mother in the therapy. This hypothesizing led to a plan to reach out to the mom to discuss her response to the therapy.

The therapist contacted the mother by phone, acknowledged the cancellation, and asked whether she had any concerns. The mother denied she had concerns, but the therapist pushed gently further and said that she was worried that the mom was concerned the therapist might support the son's bid for greater freedom. The mother then acknowledged (feedback) that she was concerned about her son's safety in a neighborhood, given the level of gang activity. She further said that in her family of origin there was a tradition of keeping children with family or friends of family and close to home. The therapist realized there was a need to better understand issues of culture and community in the life of this family to establish a working alliance with the mother. The therapist apologized for alarming the mother and expressed understanding and support for her concerns and promised to factor these issues into the process of therapy. The mother scheduled another appointment, and the family returned to therapy.

In IST, a positive alliance is viewed as an essential ingredient of effective intervention and, conversely, interventions that are effective and well received by the clients contribute positively to the alliance.

Testing and Revising Hypotheses About Solution Sequences

In IST, problems are viewed as being embedded in sequences of interaction. IST's sequence replacement guideline states that the primary task of the IST therapist is facilitating the replacement of key problem sequences with solution sequences that eliminate or reduce the problem. IST therapists strongly believe that clients, unless otherwise constrained, have the ability to identify and enact solution sequences. The solutions developed in therapy emerge from a collaborative exploration that considers such variables as prior and current attempted solutions, common sense approaches, client resources, cultural fit, and therapist expertise. In Chapter 3 we discussed areas of therapist expertise, including knowledge of best practices, empirically supported findings, therapist experience with similar situations, and therapist intuition. Although respecting the ideas about solutions presented by clients, the IST therapist does not hesitate to propose general ideas or specific suggestions for alternative sequences. Whether generated in the therapeutic conversation or specifically proposed by the therapist, the solutions may target the implementation of a new course of action, a shift in beliefs about the problem, and/or better expression or management of emotion. IST privileges action-oriented solutions, particularly at the outset of therapy, but the evolving hypotheses often reveal the need to focus on the meaning and emotional aspects of the sequence as well.

The therapist works to establish a consensus: "So, do we agree that this might be a good way to work on this problem?" The road to that consensus requires therapist curiosity, empathy, encouragement, persistence, and sometimes persuasion. The therapist takes into account clients' readiness to change, both in the initial conversation about the solution and in the subsequent discussion of its enactment. The blueprint provides a moment-to-moment decision-making schema as client feedback (both informational report and behavioral response) in the course of the therapeutic conversations continuously allows the therapist to revise hypotheses about solution sequences that would be worth a try.

The hypothesizing metaframeworks, briefly discussed earlier and covered in detail in Chapter 5 (and the planning metaframeworks discussed in Chapter 6), provide extensive information that informs the search for solution sequences. In some cases, the solution sequence is directly drawn from the metaframework. For example, the organization metaframework articulates the importance of coherent and effective leadership within a parent subsystem. This knowledge suggests that a therapist working with a family that presents with behavioral issues of a 10-year-old boy should be interested in tracking how leadership functions in the parental subsystem. If the therapist discovers the parents usually respond to their son's protests and demands by giving him his way (problem sequence), one solution sequence might involve the parents establishing and enforcing expectations and limits.

In other cases, the hypothesizing metaframework provides information that suggests the therapist modify the solution sequence or take particular care to see whether it fits for the client. For example, in the case of Alejandro and his family described earlier, there were issues of family culture and realities at the community level of the system that would have to be considered when deciding what the family would do about Alejandro's bid for greater freedom.

The hypothesis that a particular solution sequence may improve the presenting problem can lead to a change in who is involved in the direct system. For example, Rose, a 71-year-old widow, presented with depressed mood. During the first session, the therapist learned that she was somewhat isolated, had periodic contact with her two adult children, and did not tend to reach out to them because of a belief that they were busy and should not be bothered. The therapist began to hypothesize that Rose's mood might benefit from increased contact with her family. This led to a discussion of involving her adult children in the therapy, and she agreed to invite them to attend the second session.

Given the plethora of psychotherapeutic approaches, the traditions for problem solving in various cultures, family oral histories of growth and development, and human ingenuity, there may well be an infinite number of possible solution sequences. Our task in this chapter is not to provide an extensive list of solution sequences but to describe and illustrate in a general sense how the blueprint is used to identify and enact them. In later chapters, more extensive exploration of the hypothesizing and planning metaframeworks provides further detail about the kinds of solution sequences IST incorporates into therapy.

A hypothesis about a solution sequence is tested as the client system agrees to a plan to enact the sequence and attempts to enact it. The feedback that results from the enactment of the problem sequence informs the process. Did the clients enact the sequence? Did it affect the problem? Is it a basis for further experimentation? If they did not enact the sequence, what kept them from doing it? The feedback opens new territory for conversation and for the modification of the hypothesis about what would be an adaptive approach to the problem and problem sequence. For example, in the case of a relatively disengaged couple that spent little time together, the therapist hypothesized that a starting place for them would be to spend more time together. On the basis of a collaborative conversation in therapy, the couple agreed to be more disciplined about putting their young children to bed each evening and spending 20 minutes or a half hour together. At the next session the therapist "read" the feedback from this experiment. The couple reported that they did spend the time together but felt too tired to make much of it. A discussion at that point led to a plan for a revised sequence that involved getting childcare twice a week for 2 hours so they could begin to have time they could count on and be prepared to use. Enacting this solution sequence would provide more feedback to the process of therapy. Did they make it happen? If not, what kept them from doing it? If they did it the first week, would they maintain it? What was the time like (connecting, enjoyable, conflictual)? The feedback and subsequent conversation led to revised hypotheses about what will make a difference for this couple.

IST therapists work diligently to identify problem sequences and solution sequences and to encourage clients to enact new patterns. Careful follow-up on client efforts is essential to focus their motivation, guide them to successful patterns, and/or identify what gets in the way. Failure to enact the solution sequence presents the opportunity to understand further how the system works and what has to happen to move toward resolution of the problems that are of concern to the client.

Testing and Revising Hypotheses About Constraints

As discussed in Chapter 3, the IST therapist typically begins with the idea that a particular solution sequence, if implemented, may result in the resolution or improvement of the problem. This often does not prove to be quite so straightforward, but the plan to implement an alternative sequence is both a way of initiating change and a means of identifying what constrains the system from solving the problem. Struggle or failure with the solution sequence opens an examination of the system that leads to more complex hypotheses about what limits problem solving. To understand more about this, we turn to constraint theory.

The constraint theory pillar of IST (Breunlin, 1999; Breunlin et al., 2011) states that therapy involves the identification and removal of constraints that prevent problem solving. It addresses the age-old question of why people are often unable to resolve their personal and relational problems by suggesting that some factor or factors (constraints) are keeping them from doing so. Although positive explanation explores why human systems have problems (causes), negative explanation and constraint theory describe the factors that prevent problem solving. Both of these inquiries can lead to useful hypotheses about human problems, but we have found the concept of negative explanation as formulated in the theory of constraints particularly useful for the following reasons (Breunlin, 1999). First, removal of obstacles to problem solving is the most direct and efficient approach to problem resolution. Second, negative explanation supports the search for strengths because it assumes clients are constrained, not unable or unwilling or unskilled. Third, negative explanation leads to less resistance and more cooperation from clients.

The practical clinical expression of constraint theory is found in the study of what prevents people from solving their problems. When clients perform solution sequences and therapy improves their lives, we highlight their success and continue to support their efforts with this and other solution sequences. When they struggle with enacting the solutions, we ask them what keeps them from doing so. The questions "What keeps you from . . ." and "What prevents you from . . ." are signature questions in IST. We find that these questions are more productive and client friendly than "Why didn't you . . . ," which can come off as critical or judgmental to clients.

As depicted in the essence diagram (Figure 3.1), a central focus of IST is to identify and modify constraints sufficiently to allow clients to use their strengths to solve their problems. A broad range of factors can constrain problem resolution. A family can be kept from solving problems by such factors as patterns of leadership, boundaries of relationships, developmental challenges, gender beliefs, economic circumstances, religious conflicts, health issues, catastrophic fears, or internal conflicts. The hypothesizing metaframeworks provide information that helps the therapist understand all these types of constraints.

Addressing constraints begins with the creation of a hypothesis about what prevents the clients from implementing the solution sequence. Consistent with IST's epistemology pillar (partial and progressive knowing), there is no perfect or definitive hypothesis. Rather, the therapist and clients search for hypotheses they can agree on and that are good enough to facilitate the resolution of the presenting problem. To achieve this, we seek to understand as fully as necessary the clients, their problems, and the context in which they exist. Each client system presents with its own unique constraints. In some cases, these appear to be relatively simple, whereas in others there seems to be a complex set of multiple, interacting constraints that make the consistent enactment of the solution sequence difficult. The web of human experience (see Figure 4.2), composed of the hypothesizing metaframeworks and the levels of the system, is a heuristic device well suited to identifying simple as well as more complex patterns of constraint. It helps us address two fundamental questions: What factors constrain the system, and where in the multilevel system are they located? The web of human experience in this context is conceptualized as a web of constraints (Breunlin et al., 2011; Breunlin, Schwartz, & Mac Kune-Karrer, 1997) that, due to its multilevel nature and the breadth and depth of its hypothesizing metaframeworks, is comprehensive enough to facilitate the identification of virtually any constraints that influence problem solving in human systems.

The following case of a couple illustrates how hypotheses about constraints are formulated and tested. A White, heterosexual couple (John and Nicole), married for 10 years with a 6-year-old son, presented after John's 8-month affair with a coworker. At the first appointment, it was established that the affair had been discontinued immediately when Nicole confronted John about text messages she had discovered on his phone. This was traumatic for Nicole, but she wanted to save the marriage. She demanded, and John agreed, that he would discontinue contact with the other woman and begin the process of looking for a job with a different company. She demanded, and again he agreed, that she have access to his phone and e-mail as proof that the relationship had ended. John stated he was desperate and would do anything to save the marriage. There were a number of problem sequences that would have to be modified if the couple was to make the marriage work, but they had established that the sequence involving an affair and lying about it would end.

Nicole reported that she was pleased with John's willingness to demonstrate that he had ended the affair (and that she tended to trust that this was the case), but she was angry that he continually resisted talking about it. She stated that when she tried to talk about what it was like for her—feeling lost and betrayed—or ask questions to try to understand the relationship with the other woman, he would state that the affair was over, that he could not change what was in the past, and that he wanted to move on. This would typically lead to Nicole's feeling and expressing anger ("Why don't you move in with that bitch? You obviously don't want to be here") because she felt in those moments that John did not care about her pain. The therapist identified this as a problem sequence. Seeing both Nicole's pain and John's significant discomfort, the therapist provided some information about recovery from affairs and shared the view that recovery would involve, among other things, the husband demonstrating that he sees the damage done and is sorry for it. This would involve a solution sequence of his listening and responding to her feelings, concerns, and questions. Nicole strongly agreed with this suggestion, and John seemed to understand and stated he would do all he could.

In the second session, the therapist followed up with the couple on their communication during the week. Nicole reported that the problem sequence continued with John trying to shut down her questions and expression of emotion (sadness, betrayal, anger). In a curious and accepting manner, the therapist asked John what kept him from hearing and responding in a supportive manner. John shared his belief that it was best to put these things behind them. The therapist then asked what he thought would happen if they did not put it behind them quickly. John seemed to struggle with his reasoning on this. The therapist asked whether perhaps John did not fully understand what kept him from being able to hear Nicole out. Was it something he felt when she began to talk about it? "Maybe." The therapist, having studied the process couples go through to recover from an affair, hypothesized that Nicole's strong emotions and quest to make sense of what had happened stimulated within John profound feelings of guilt and shame, and he sought to prevent these feelings by stopping the conversations. The way he managed the difficult emotions seemed to constrain the solution sequence. The therapist shared this idea with John and Nicole and wondered whether it was difficult for John to accept that he had, indeed, had an affair. John stated that he would never have imagined that he could have an affair and that he had always been highly disapproving of those who did. Nicole shared that he had always been a moral person and she would never have guessed this could have happened. The therapist acknowledged how painful this was for both of them and suggested that the next step would be to work in session with the process of Nicole expressing herself and John tolerating his emotion to hear what was on her mind and in her heart.

In the third session, the therapist structured a conversation that involved close monitoring of the communication process. Nicole began to share her anguish. The therapist made space for her expression and worked with John to help him tolerate his emotion and stay in the conversation with Nicole. At one point, Nicole asked John how he could have been unfaithful and hurt her so deeply. John fairly exploded in grief, and when his crying subsided, he began to talk about how horrible he felt about himself and how sorry he was for hurting Nicole. Moved, Nicole told him she wanted to be with him and thought she could trust and forgive him in time. The therapist and couple agreed that the way John had been dealing with his emotions had indeed been a constraint to the solution sequence. In addition to confirming the constraint, the couple had begun to remove it and had taken the healing solution sequence further than they or the therapist had expected. The therapist congratulated the couple on taking this important step and stated there would be more work to do to keep the constraint from derailing future conversations.

After the session, the therapist wondered how the work would progress. Perhaps the work with the constraint of John's avoidance of his feelings of shame and guilt would require some exploration of his family-of-origin issues. That would remain to be seen because the therapist would let the ongoing feedback from work on the solution sequence guide the hypothesizing. There was significant work ahead for this couple regarding forgiveness, trust building, and modification of the patterns that had become problematic over their years together. The therapist would be prepared to draw on any or all of the hypothesizing metaframeworks in the ongoing formulation of the case and would have the opportunity to use strategies of intervention drawn from the planning metaframeworks and planning guidelines explicated in Chapter 6.

Testing and Revising Hypotheses About Strengths and Resources

IST's problem focus and emphasis on identifying constraints should not be confused with a deficit-based approach to therapy. IST is strongly committed to recognizing and drawing on client strengths while attending carefully to the concerns clients bring to therapy. The IST strength guideline asserts that, until proven otherwise, the client system can use its strengths and resources to lift constraints and implement adaptive solutions to its problems with minimal and direct input from the therapist. Whether developing solution sequences or removing constraints, therapists have to mobilize clients' strengths and resources to do so. Commitment to the search for strengths, however, does not suggest naïveté on the part of IST therapists, who also understand that some client systems are severely and multiply constrained.

When it comes to IST's approach to identifying client system strengths, believing is seeing, and seeing is believing. A passionate conviction that every person (and every system) is able and adaptable supports the search for strengths. This is an article of faith, yet it is operationalized within the blueprint, which provides the clinical–experimental tool for testing hypotheses about client strengths. Considering the multilevel system as depicted by the web of human experience, strengths and resources exist on the individual level (e.g., inner resolve, willingness to try something new, openness to feedback, will and determination, courage, awareness of emotions, good judgment, self-care, spiritual beliefs and practices), the relational level (e.g., nurturance, communication skills, commitment), the family level (e.g., shared views, role flexibility, clear boundaries, support, cohesiveness, shared spiritual beliefs and practices), and the community level (e.g., social support, social services, educational institutions, job opportunities). The hypothesizing metaframeworks as depicted on the web of human experience (and explained in detail in Chapter 5) facilitate understanding of strengths and adaptive functioning in systems. Operationally, the question the therapist ponders is, Which strengths at which levels of the system as described by which hypothesizing metaframeworks can be brought to bear on the enactment of solution sequences or the removal of constraints? As we identify and then draw on those strengths, the feedback we receive will confirm their utility, invite us to explore what keeps clients from using them, or mobilize the search for other strengths.

In the case of the John and Nicole, the therapist believed that Nicole could recover from the affair with time and, more important, within a healing process in which John faced and responded to her pain. The therapist also believed that John had the strength to tolerate his sense of shame and guilt about the affair (the constraint) and communicate with Nicole in a way that would be helpful to her and their relationship (the solution sequence). A plan was developed to help John access and stay with his pain. The conversation and feedback in session and the following session confirmed that he had the ability to experience and tolerate her pain and his. Although the emotion was initially overwhelming, he would learn to manage it well enough to participate in healing the relationship. The therapist hypothesized that this would pay a dividend in John's personal growth and in his ability to contribute more to the relationship in the future.

FURTHER EXAMINATION OF THE BLUEPRINT COMPONENTS

Although the blueprint as a whole provides the clinical–experimental process for the conduct of therapy, its components contain the bodies of knowledge needed for the conduct of therapy. In Chapters 5 through 8 we discuss in detail the frameworks and bodies of knowledge associated with one of the components. We begin this exploration in the next chapter with an in-depth discussion of each of the seven hypothesizing metaframeworks, IST's case-formulating factors.

5

THE HYPOTHESIZING
METAFRAMEWORKS

In the course of an episode of psychotherapy, clients reveal fragments of their experience. For example, Bill complained that Sarah, his wife, was completely unreliable.

> Bill: The taxes are due on Tuesday, and all you had to do was get a donation receipt from the thrift shop.

> Sarah: I was on the phone five times with my mom yesterday. I just didn't have the time.

Here the therapist wondered whether the five phone calls (or the five with her mother) are a relevant fragment of Sarah's experience that might be part of the problem sequence and decided to ask about them.

http://dx.doi.org/10.1037/0000055-005
Integrative Systemic Therapy: Metaframeworks for Problem Solving With Individuals, Couples, and Families, by W. M. Pinsof, D. C. Breunlin, W. P. Russell, J. L. Lebow, C. Rampage, and A. L. Chambers

Therapist:	Is that a typical day where you talk that much with your mom?
Sarah:	Ha, that's a light day. My dad died last year, and my mom isn't doing well. In fact, she has never done well and has always leaned on me.
Bill:	And so we have no life.

Although there may be many legitimate reasons why Sarah talks to her mom frequently, the boundary around the couple seems weak with regard to the mother. Opening the organization metaframework, the therapist could, therefore, hypothesize that a weak boundary between the couple and Sarah's mom is part of the problem sequence. Is this weak boundary keeping Sarah from being reliable in the marriage? Integrative systemic therapists must balance when to work with a hypothesis based on known fragments and when to recognize that a new fragment modifies and/or expands the hypothesis. Can the problem of sharing responsibilities in the marriage be solved without addressing the boundary issue? Here the therapist decided to follow up.

Therapist:	No life. That's big. Have you two talked about the time commitment Sarah makes to her mom?
Sarah:	We have, but we always end up fighting, so it's sort of the pink elephant in the room.

The multisystemic nature of integrative systemic therapy (IST) encourages therapists to be open and curious to all reports of clients' experiences related to the presenting problem. When clients provide feedback on those experiences, IST therapists choose whether the experience is an additional part of the problem sequence and/or a constraint to implementing the solution sequence. To be successful, they efficiently recognize the relevance of experience and integrate it while still conducting therapy in a parsimonious way.

In this way, IST differs from most models of psychotherapy that circumvent this conundrum by excluding large swaths of human experience from the purview of the therapy. For example, some therapies exclusively focus on the couple interaction and would not explore boundaries as part of the therapy. Such therapies create focus but also huge blind spots that can render therapy ineffective. An IST therapist might begin with the hypothesis that Sarah is caught in a loyalty dilemma between her marriage and her mother, viewing her as doing the best she can to balance her commitment to both and that, no doubt, both her husband and her mother feel shortchanged.

A SHORTCUT TO UNDERSTANDING
HUMAN EXPERIENCE IN THERAPY

When IST therapists open their hypothesizing lens to encompass a wide range of human experience, they mitigate the risk of losing focus by grounding their understanding in seven hypothesizing metaframeworks: organization, development, culture, mind, gender, biology, and spirituality. Each metaframework organizes a domain of human experience. This greatly simplifies the task of reading feedback about clients' experiences. In the earlier example, the therapist read the feedback of multiple phone calls as a lot of contact time between Sarah and her mother. Knowing that contact time is a marker of interpersonal boundaries and that too much contact time can signify a weak boundary, the therapist decided to ask about it. This efficiency is made possible because knowledge about boundaries exists as part of the organization metaframework.

All seven metaframeworks are relevant at each of the levels of the biopsychosocial system. Hence, we can talk about constraints of organization at the level of the family or development at the level of relationship. Although the knowledge evoked for a given metaframework at each level may differ, the isomorphic nature of the web of human experience suggests that the principles of organization and development exist across levels (Breunlin, Schwartz, & Mac Kune-Karrei, 1997).

Not only are there adaptive and constraining alternatives within each metaframework but the metaframeworks also interact with each other, sometimes for better or worse. More often, several are relevant, and the therapist must decide how to privilege them. A further challenge of hypothesizing is determining which are most important to a particular web of constraints for a particular presenting problem within a specific case. In essence, using IST's causality pillar, the therapist generates hypotheses about the relative contributions of the constraints from the different metaframeworks to each problem's web of constraints.

Each of the seven hypothesizing metaframeworks addresses a domain of human functioning. They embody ideas (many of which are derived from empirical research) about what constitutes adaptive and maladaptive functioning within that domain. In IST, adaptive functioning does not suggest an ideal, but rather functioning that is "good enough" to solve the problems.

THE SEVEN HYPOTHESIZING METAFRAMEWORKS

The following is a brief synopsis of what we consider some of the most relevant knowledge about human experience in each of the hypothesizing metaframeworks. The knowledge is by no means intended to be exhaustive; hence, the reader is encouraged to add to it. Moreover, the knowledge in the hypothesizing metaframeworks is always changing and expanding as scientific discoveries are made and shifts in societal norms prescribe what is important. For example, functional magnetic resonance imaging technology is revolutionizing constructs of the mind, the utility of a binary concept of gender has been called into question, and the way families are organized is not the same today as it was two generations ago.

IST therapists are students of the human experience and draw their understanding of this experience from related fields of knowledge such as sociology, anthropology, gender studies, and medicine, to name just a few. Every new case represents both the opportunity to help clients solve their problems and a journey through the lives of a unique system.

Organization

Two college-age sisters sought family therapy to address issues they had with their father. The therapist invited the parents and daughters to the initial session. As the family entered the office, the two daughters sat on the ends of a sofa, and the mother sat between them rather than take one of the vacant chairs. The father entered last, glanced at the seating arrangement, and glumly sat alone in one of the chairs. The therapist noted this spatial arrangement of family members and formed an initial hypothesis that the daughters and mother might be aligned in some way, perhaps against the father.

At that moment, the therapist read the feedback, opened the organization metaframework, and formed a hypothesis based on observations of the interaction in the session. Readers familiar with structural family therapy (Minuchin, 1974) will recognize the structural concept of a cross-generation coalition. The organization metaframework borrows Minuchin's (1974) concept, and thus it can be accessed without working fully within the logic of structural family therapy.

Why is an organization metaframework essential to IST? For decades, the abstract concepts of systems theory have been operationalized through the construct of organization. In general systems theory, von Bertalanffy (1968) suggested that living organisms possess an organizing force that establishes and preserves relationships among their component parts and gives them integrity. The essence of a living system (a digestive system, a person, a marriage, a family, a corporation) is not its components but its organization—how it fits together as a whole. A system's organization defines how its various parts are structured, as well as the function that each part serves for the whole. Organization reveals how "the whole is greater than the sum of its parts." The client system is a network of relationships that possesses the properties of an organization and can, therefore, be understood through the constructs of the organization metaframework.

Organization can be thought of as a spatial depiction of relationships captured at one moment in time. Minuchin (1974) emphasized these spatial metaphors with structural diagramming. The seating arrangement of the family described earlier is an example of a spatial depiction containing organizational information. The same information is captured as part of the problem sequence: who speaks and how others respond. Organization uses the metaphor of space, and sequences use the metaphor of time. IST's emphasis on sequences means that our understanding of organization grows directly out of understanding the problem sequences.

Applied to therapy, organization has two primary constructs: boundaries and leadership. The first, boundaries, regulate the type and quality of connections among clients and the various subsystems (relationships) in which they participate. The second is leadership, which regulates how power, influence, and the distribution of resources are regulated in the client system.

Boundaries

Boundaries exist at all levels of the biopsychosocial system: individual, relationship, family, and community. Boundaries regulate the connection among the various subsystems of the client system. Minuchin (1974) defined a boundary as "the rules defining who participates and how" (p. 53). The "who" is an issue of membership. The membership of a subsystem is defined by a characteristic of the members or by the functions they have. Obvious subsystems are the parental, sibling, and grandparental. In a single-parent household with several children, the parenting subsystem might include the parent, an older child, and a grandparent. The variables of gender and age can define subsystems. For example, in a family of four children, the siblings' four-person subsystem might also include two further subsystems of brothers and sisters or subsystems of older siblings and younger siblings. Subsystems are also created for interests and beliefs. In a family of four, the parents and one child might be musicians, whereas the second child is not. Every time the musicians practice, listen, perform, or attend a musical event, boundaries are created that can exclude the nonmusician child.

Therapy can create subsystems when one child is presented as the problem and others are not. Parents are often concerned about not disrupting the lives of the so-called "well" children by having them attend family sessions. Exclusion creates a rigid boundary around the parents and problem child that often causes the other children to be resentful. IST therapists invite all children to at least some of the sessions. Their attendance allows the therapist to observe the problem sequence of the whole family and to recruit the other children as resources for the solution sequence.

Minuchin (1974) conceptualized boundaries on a continuum. The ends of the continuum are diffuse and rigid boundaries, and in the middle are clear boundaries. Dysfunctions arise when boundaries are too rigid and/or diffuse. The solution sequence incorporates a plan to make boundaries clearer. First, boundary dysfunction must be recognized, named, and acknowledged, at which point clients can decide how to make the boundaries clearer. In the earlier case example, Sarah has to recognize that giving her mother so much attention puts her marriage at risk. Parts of the solution sequence include Sarah talking to her siblings and finding ways to share meeting the mother's needs. Sarah may have to explore why having this exclusive role was satisfying to her and what it means to her to share it.

The quality of the connection among the members of any given subsystem or between subsystems is regulated by a boundary. Wood (1985) proposed six process dimensions that can be used to assess interpersonal boundaries. The common denominator of these processes is proximity, whereby an optimum proximity creates the best connection and too much or too little proximity adversely affects connection. The six dimensions are (a) time members spend together, (b) physical closeness, (c) emotional separation, (d) shared general information, (e) confided personal information, and (f) decision making. These six dimensions can be tracked as the therapist seeks to define the problem sequence. For example, the physical proximity of the mother and daughters sitting on the sofa together suggested an enmeshed boundary. Further, as the daughters began to express their issues with the father, they seemed distressed, and the mother began to weep, suggesting an enmeshed boundary. They were not emotionally differentiated. Later in the interview, the daughters stated that they called the mother several times a day and frequently complained to her about the father, indicating a high level of shared information. The problem sequence, therefore, included an important boundary component. Moreover, the solution sequence may well contain a new behavior that involves the daughters dealing directly with the father without the intercession of the mother.

The language of boundary creation, maintenance, and expression is both verbal and nonverbal. The corresponding communication is both verbal and nonverbal. Eye contact, tone of voice, body posture, and other nonverbal messages indicate who is part of a subsystem and how it operates. Interventions aimed at changing boundaries are often nonverbal as well as verbal. For instance, in the case of the two-sister family, the therapist may suggest the mother move into a chair next to her husband.

Technology has revolutionized how people communicate. Today, cell phones and texting and e-mail have replaced much if not most of the communication that once took place face-to-face or at least voice-to-voice via the telephone. The ubiquitous presence of technology has a profound impact on relationships and particularly on how boundaries are managed (Turkle, 2011).

Cell phones now make it virtually impossible for a rigid boundary to exist in a relationship. The connection between two people, therefore, is always mediated through the imposition of many other relationships that seek connection with the people in the relationship through the ubiquitous cell phone. Many families have battles over the presence and use of cell phones during dinner conversation.

Texting also creates on-demand communication that was unthinkable before cell phones. Parents expect to reach their children at all times and become fearful or irate when a teenager does not respond to a text. With global positioning systems capability, some parents are even keeping track of their adolescents' whereabouts. Gone are the days when an adolescent could get beyond the reach of parents and experience autonomy for a brief time. Many a marital conflict has been stoked by the failure of one spouse to acknowledge the text of another. This is often notwithstanding the vicissitudes of cell phone technology, which is anything but foolproof. Although the incidence of affairs may not have changed, the revelation of them has; many affairs are discovered when one spouse examines the cell phone activity of the other.

There are myriad ways boundary issues constrain implementing solution sequences. For example, a couple presented a lack of sexual intimacy as a problem and informed the therapist that their children came in and out of their bedroom until late into the evening. They never closed their bedroom door and "locking it would make the kids feel rejected." In another example, a physician husband, disengaged within his marriage, encouraged his patients to call his cell phone at all hours of the day and night, continually interrupting his time with his wife. For these couples, solution sequences must address the couple boundary.

Boundaries always exist in a context; therefore, therapists must be cautious not to judge the health of a client system's boundaries without accounting for that context. For instance, maintaining the safety of teenagers in a disadvantaged urban community requires fairly rigid boundaries between family and community. A porous boundary exists between the nuclear and extended families, as evidenced by Sarah's contact time with her mother. Postdivorce families have complex boundaries that include the rules of two households. The boundary around the client system regulates its contact with the environment. A homeless family living in a shelter is protected by a flimsy boundary, whereas a family with wealth living in a gated community may be too walled off.

Leadership

Leadership is required for any living system to function well and to avoid problems. In a client system, the leaders' functions include the following: mediate conflicts among members; assure that the needs of each client are met; make each client feel valued; allocate resources, responsibilities, and influence fairly; provide firm and fair limits and control; encourage the growth of each member while considering the needs of the group; represent the needs of the client system in interactions with other systems; and plan for the client system's future (Breunlin et al., 1997). Clearly, leadership involves much more than telling other members of the client system what they can and cannot do. In fact, serious leadership constraints emerge if the leaders do not take seriously all the functions of their job.

Families and Leadership. Early on, family therapy emphasized the power and control aspect of leadership expressed through the construct of hierarchy: Who is in charge? Minuchin (1974), Haley (1987), and Madanes (1981) all provided organizational models for family therapy that located the problem in the family organization and were designed to correct hierarchical problems. Hierarchical problems exist when parents fail to be in charge of their family. This failure can result from an abdication of leadership (the alcoholic parent), conflict between parents about how to be in charge (the strict vs. the nurturing parent), sabotage of one parent's ability to be in charge (a postdivorce battle for control), or lack of clarity about who is in charge (an older sibling or grandparent given control without authority). For the early models, troubled youth presenting with a variety of problems were thought to improve when the family hierarchy was improved. Correcting the hierarchy remains an important part of solution sequences designed to address problems of acting out children, adolescents, and adults.

Early theories of family therapy also confounded hierarchy with patriarchy by accepting the traditional view of families that placed men in the role of leaders of their families (Goldner, 1985). These family therapy models obscured the resulting gender inequity associated with patriarchy, making it harder to see how the status of women in families created problems that were part of every problem sequence. Issues about gender and leadership are also addressed in the gender metaframework, discussed later.

The emphasis on hierarchy obscured other vital aspects of leadership such as balance and harmony. A client system has balance when the resources, responsibilities, and influence are allocated appropriately according to the needs and talents of the members of the client system. When the members of the client system believe the leaders are attending to balance, the client system is in harmony. Harmonious client systems require less hierarchical attention because members feel secure.

Twenty-first-century families tend to prefer more democratic leadership styles. Parents today are more likely to believe that balance includes input from children and adolescents regarding the allocation of resources, responsibilities, and influence. This includes giving children choices. This type of leadership flattens the hierarchy (Taffel, 2012). Democratic leadership, however, only works well when parents put in the time and energy to make it work. Parents must engage patiently in the conversations needed to reach consensus. Whatever the issue and its resolution, as leaders, parents must still enforce consequences. For example, although modern families are likely to negotiate curfews, consequences must still exist for curfew violations.

Twenty-first-century views of leadership are also influenced by *attachment theory* (Whiffen, 2003). Attachment theory purports that children thrive when they experience their families as a safe haven that provides a secure base from which they can explore their development and their environment. Further, children feel secure when they experience their parents being attuned to their feelings. Attachment ruptures can damage this security and contribute to problem sequences involving "acting out" (delinquency, substance abuse) or "acting in" (depression and anxiety). Repair of these ruptures is frequently an important part of the solution sequence.

Today, the pendulum may be swinging back again as experts are beginning to recognize that too much democratic leadership and too much attunement and nurturing may look right during the child-rearing years, but can produce young adults who experience frustration with the demands of emerging adulthood, particularly the response to authority and the frustration of not being the best or even failing at something. The question is, has modern parental leadership prepared children for adult life (Gottlieb, 2011)? The goal of parenting is to produce happy, well-adjusted adults, but the data have suggested that for many young adults, happiness can be elusive, and many are experiencing anxiety and depression (Drum, Brownson, Burton Denmark, & Smith, 2009). Experts on parenting are searching for a better balance between nurturance and limit setting and between dependency and autonomy. For example, the concept of "free range parenting" (Skenazy, 2009) advocates that parents encourage children, in a developmentally appropriate way, to explore and encounter their environment, thereby sometimes succeeding and sometimes failing. The net effect is a more resilient young adult who can better weather the challenges of life.

Leadership in Couples. Most partners in a relationship experience themselves first as an individual in their relationship. Their sense of "we-ness" is secondary (Skerrett, 2016). Leadership struggles, therefore, are cast as struggles for power and resources between individuals. Because the relationship cannot advocate for itself, in the absence of couple leadership, the relationship frequently suffers. For example, most people contend they should engage in sex only when each desires to do so. The result can be extended periods of time when sex is absent from the relationship. Today, some sex therapists advocate for partners to consider what is good for the relationship; therefore, sometimes one partner agrees to sex when personally that would not be their choice. The result, however, is that both the relationship and the partners benefit (Perel, 2006).

Couples can also ascribe leadership functions to the person with the greater expertise. For example, if one partner is a financial planner, that partner might exercise greater leadership in decisions regarding the couple's assets. In the end, two well-matched partners will have an equal number of areas in which each exercises some degree of leadership.

Gender can also affect leadership for couples. The women's movement has called attention to the shift from patriarchy to egalitarianism in couple leadership (Goldner, 1988). Today, most couples aspire to egalitarian power sharing; however, daily life frequently falls short (for further elaboration of this idea, see the gender metaframework). These power dynamics play out in both same-sex and heterosexual relationships.

Couple leadership also changes over time. For instance, while raising children, partners may opt for one partner to be the stay-at-home parent while the other maximizes earning power. When couples become "empty nesters," however, stay-at-home partners may reenergize their careers and expect more coleadership at home. Retiring partners must be integrated into the areas requiring domestic leadership. When couples have to renegotiate the rules governing their relationship, they must share leadership or risk becoming polarized over whatever the change necessitates.

Development

Jan, a woman in her mid-50s, sought therapy for depression. The depression, which appeared to be dysthymic in nature, had come on a year earlier. Jan had started taking an antidepressant 6 months earlier and reported that some of the depressive symptoms had marginally improved, but there had been no improvement in her lack of energy.

The IST therapist encouraged her husband, Bruce, to also attend therapy. The couple could not identify a precipitant. The therapist learned that Jan had been to her internist and received a clean bill of health. They described their marriage as stable but bland. Having been empty nesters for 4 years, they both admitted they had hoped to breathe new life into a marriage that had been career- and child-focused. When asked what kept them from succeeding, Jan at first blamed Bruce for still being tied up with his work. Bruce countered that he had considered cutting back his practice but lamented that every time he suggested something for the couple to do, Jan would decline, saying she had too much to do. Puzzled, the therapist asked Jan what took up her time. Jan looked down, clenched her fist and spat out the words:

> Jan: I waited 25 years for this to be my time to enjoy life, and now it is never going to happen.

> Therapist: Tell us, Jan, what's going to keep it from happening?

Jan then laid out a web of constraints that she felt kept her trapped and depressed in the current state of her life. The therapist opened the development hypothesizing metaframework to understand this web. For decades Jan had worked part time helping her father with his rare book business. The father had professed many times that he was ready to sell the business or give it to Jan, but when Jan's mother died, the father clung to the business as his last vestige of dignity. Jan had no interest in rare books and dreamed of opening her own business, but lamented that her father would die were he to close or sell the business. She claimed she would not take that risk and, therefore, believed she had to stay in the business until he died.

Next, she reported that her daughter, Sandy, had returned home to live with them a year earlier following a breakup of a long-term relationship and the loss of her job. The daughter moped around the house, and Jan felt compelled to spend time with her and to attend to the daughter's personal business. Jan would drive her to appointments and solve problems for Sandy, all of which proved time consuming. Sandy showed no signs of getting a job or making a plan to move out. Jan again felt trapped because she feared Sandy could once again become depressed, as she had as a teenager.

Using the development metaframework, the therapist quickly synthesized Jan's predicament as an extreme example of the sandwich generation: boomer adults who are caught between the needs of their elderly parents and of their own children (Hamill & Goldberg, 1997). Caught in this way, adults like Jan are developmentally stuck because they feel they must either sacrifice their age-appropriate needs or bear the guilt of not meeting the needs of their parents and/or children. Understandably, depression and attendant marital distress are frequent occurrences in these situations.

Bruce empathized with Jan's predicament but did not volunteer to alter his life for the sake of hers. Although Jan felt resentful about this, when asked, she stated that he could not change his work hours anyway because the couple had been poor shepherds of their money and were a long way from being able to retire.

As this clinical vignette illustrates, the development metaframework is much more than knowing something about the stages of individual, couple, and family development. Knowledge of these stages is frequently necessary but not sufficient to see how developmental constraints can block the effectiveness of solution sequences. For example, a couple entered therapy with conflict about their life goals. The therapist immediately noted the husband must be at least a decade older than the wife. They had been married for 20 years, having both been previously divorced. The husband, a successful business owner, wanted to retire and travel. The wife had just completed a degree in accounting and wanted to enter the workforce. As individuals, both were developmentally on time; however, the fit between them was off because of their age difference. This lack of fit was putting their marriage at risk.

Development and the Biopsychosocial System

The development metaframework posits that for client systems to be healthy, each level of the biopsychosocial system must possess the requisite developmentally appropriate competencies. This includes the biological, individual, relational, family, and community levels. When these competencies exist at each level, the levels develop synergistically, and all levels thrive. When a developmental constraint emerges at one level, it can affect development at all other levels. This can trigger an escalating spiral of developmental constraints that produce a negative developmental synergy that further complicates problem sequences. For example, if a couple has a child with Down syndrome early in their marriage, before they have worked out their relational rules, they will struggle to adapt to challenges they face, thus putting the marriage and the family at risk. As another example, young adult men living in communities with few employment opportunities will struggle to address the developmental task of finding and holding a job.

Developmental competencies are acquired in two time frames. Large leaps forward, called *macrotransitions*, occur over months and sometimes years and involve the entire client system. Smaller leaps, called *microtransitions* (Breunlin, 1988), involve the acquisition of individual competencies. Microtransitions begin at a point in time, but mastery of them takes place over a period of months and sometimes longer.

Macrotransitions and Family Development

Transitions associated with the predictable stages of the family life cycle are examples of macrotransitions. Research has shown that problems frequently occur at these times as the family searches for solution sequences to facilitate the transition to the next stage of family development (Neugarten, 1968; Terkelson, 1980). These macrotransitions involve changes in the composition or living arrangement of a family; hence, births, deaths, marriages, divorces, retirement, and leaving home are typically times of developmental challenge for everyone in the family. Macrotransitions are also marked by events that take time to unfold and resolve. Examples are an episode of illness or the coming out of a family member.

Families face myriad life cycle demands: the out-of-work downsized parent, the young-adult son failing at college, the aging parent with Alzheimer's. Families can attempt to "carve out" these developmental challenges in an effort to protect the family, but inevitably they always have some impact. Developmental demands can compete for a family's scarce resources (time and money).

When a developmental instability of any sort is combined with a psychiatric disorder (anxiety, depression, mood swings), the concoction can be lethal. For instance, intense anxiety may prevent emerging adults from meeting potential partners, or unmanaged mood swings may prevent them from holding a job.

Microtransitions and Individual Development

Microtransitions are a ubiquitous part of family life because each family member is always expected to develop new competencies. As these competencies are mastered, both the individual and the rest of the client system become more competent and complex. A microtransition occurs through a process of oscillation (Breunlin, 1988, 1989). When the new competency first emerges, it exists simultaneously with the lesser competency. For example, when children are first learning to do their homework, they generally get assistance from a parent (lesser competency). Usually, by the fourth grade, teachers encourage children to do their homework on their own (a greater competency), but most parents will still occasionally offer help. Hence, a period of oscillation ensues. By the fifth grade, the oscillation should have dampened as competent students do their homework on their own and only seek the help of a parent when they are stuck. The benefits of this new competence are enormous for all levels of the client system. Children gain a sense of mastery over their schoolwork. Parents have extra time to do other things—sometimes even nurturing their marriage—and the family feels more harmonious.

In some circumstances, the oscillation fails to dampen; consequently, the new competency never fully takes hold and a stable oscillation results. As time passes and it becomes less clear how homework is completed, both parent and child begin to battle over it. At this point, the child has generally performed below potential and in extreme cases formed a loathing for school. All of this delays the child's development. This was the case with Jan's daughter, Sandy. She had never learned to master small adversity; hence, she felt crippling anxiety when her relationship failed and she lost her job and ended up living at home, dependent on her mother.

Stages of Relational Development

Wynne (1984) and Breunlin, Schwartz, and Mac Kune-Karrer (1992, 1997) hypothesized stages of relational development and argued that couples will be challenged to master later stages if they fail to achieve mastery of earlier stages. For example, both models hypothesize that couples must learn to communicate before they can engage in joint problem solving. Later in life, when it becomes necessary to redefine the rules of their relationship, they are likely to fail in this exercise if problem solving has not been mastered. Depending on what tasks the solution sequence calls for, failure to succeed could be associated with a constraint of relational development.

Identifying developmental constraints can help therapists see where the couple and/or partners are "stuck" as well as the developmental work that has to occur. Couples frequently present in the midst of their developmental "mess." Labeling and contextualizing the mess developmentally creates empathic understanding and illuminates solutions.

By development at the community and societal levels, we mean the norms and expectations of development established at these levels. At one point in our history, small, somewhat homogenous communities existed in which the participants all knew each other and shared many of the same values, including what was developmentally appropriate. An adolescent or young adult in such communities could not stray far before members of the community would question that person's behavior. Of course, some would view this context as oppressive.

In large urban and heterogeneous communities, consensus about developmental norms does not exist. At what age should a young girl be allowed to wear makeup? When does dating begin? At what age do adolescents become sexually active? Confusion about these and many other issues engenders uncertainty among parents and dissension between parents and their children and adolescents. Lacking clear developmental norms, therapists can struggle to help families find solution sequences that include clear developmental markers.

Culture

Corey, a 55-year-old White man employed as a surgeon, first came to therapy when he began to experience debilitating anxiety before performing surgery. He decided to stop operating and eventually retired. Although he enjoyed his retirement, he felt a crippling sense of failure that he could not shake off. When asked about his family of origin, Corey emphasized that he came from a working class background that made him feel like an outsider among his physician peers. This feeling arose when he first left his working-class neighborhood to attend a prestigious college. It followed him through medical school and into his career. He had met and married a woman from a wealthy family, and they settled in an affluent suburb. There, Corey felt out of place, even when he went into Starbucks.

Corey's therapy progressed well, but he still reported experiences in which he felt he could never get on the inside of the dominant group. These experiences intensified again when his oldest son, Jason, received an MBA but had not been hired. Corey reported that Jason seemed immobilized and unable to engage in networking. Corey overfunctioned for Jason by spending hours searching the web for opportunities for him that Jason would fail to contact. The father–son relationship became strained. When the therapist explored it further, the following exchange occurred.

> *Therapist:* Corey, it sounds like you are still struggling to step back and let Jason handle his own job search.
>
> *Corey:* I just can't step back. I see him paralyzed and not taking action. He's so talented. He'd be great for any company.
>
> *Therapist:* What do you think prevents him from taking action?
>
> *Corey:* I could never get "in," and years of being on the outside damaged me. It has to stop with me. My kids are going to get in.

The therapist and Corey returned to the theme of class and how Corey's upward mobility had placed him among people with high socioeconomic status, but he still did not feel he belonged. The therapist suggested the whole family attend one or more sessions as needed to address this concern.

Contexts of Membership

Without a culture metaframework, the therapist could easily overlook or deem irrelevant the way social class distressed both Corey and his son. The culture metaframework is built on the premise that individuals, relationships, families, and groups of humans draw their identity, in part, from simultaneous membership in a multitude of human groups and exclusion from others. Identifiers of these groups are socioeconomic status, ethnicity, race, religion, class, geographic region, economic status, education, gender identity, sexual preference, and age. These groups specify normative beliefs and behaviors and frequently prescribe how to act and react in a given situation. The culture metaframework serves both as a clearinghouse of information about these "contexts of membership" and as a template for understanding how client experience associated with membership in a group can generate distress that creates constraints to solving problems.

The concept of *intersectionality*, drawn from feminist and critical race theories, is closely associated with the concept of contexts of membership (Cole, 2009; Watts-Jones, 2010). Intersectionality analyzes both the meaning and consequences of multiple contexts of identity, including the disadvantages that accrue from both membership and the intersection of memberships in contexts. Using intersectionality, therapists must be willing to reconceptualize the meaning and significance of membership within multiple contexts both for the individual and the client system. For example, what is the experience of a gay man of color who lives in a disadvantaged community and lacks a high school diploma? How might his life be different if one of those contexts were different?

Constraints of Context of Membership

Cultural constraints create distress in several ways. First, membership in a group can create risk factors for the members of that group. For example, two female teenagers seek therapy for the problem of obesity. They are identical in every way except that one comes from a middle-class family and the other from a low-income family. Opening the culture metaframework, the therapist recognizes that the low-income client faces a major constraint to weight loss created by the fact that her parents can only afford to feed her inexpensive foods that are high in sugar and fats. Any weight loss program would have to address this constraint. Second, being a member of one group can lead to oppression from another group. For example, most persons of color have been profiled in some way. Being pulled over in a White neighborhood, turned down for a loan, or passed over for a job corrodes one's sense of self and outlook on life. The oppression need not be blatant. The repeated experience of microaggressions can have the same effect (Sue et al., 2007). Members of disadvantaged groups face challenges to success every day that are not experienced by more privileged people. For example, good jobs are often located in suburban communities where housing costs are beyond the reach of low-income workers. Paying for public transportation and commuting for several hours each way to and from work is exhausting and comes at the expense of self-care and family time.

Third, membership in a group can lead to internalized oppression. Repeatedly faced with the relentless constraints associated with membership in a group, that member can begin to feel that the oppression is deserved. A 7-year-old Asian child attending a predominantly White school presents for therapy with high levels of anxiety. He reports that daily he is subjected to some form of bullying. His parents' English is poor, and they do not know how to approach the principal, and so the bullying continues. The therapist, in this case, would recognize the cultural constraint and assist the family in getting the bullying to stop. An African American teenager comes from a family in which the parents have high expectations for success in school. The teenager also wants to be successful but struggles at school because peers see school success as "acting White."

Fourth, the fit between a member and members of two groups can produce distress. The fit can involve members of the same level of the psychosocial system or different levels. An example of members on the same level is a married couple. Couples possess a "goodness of fit" depending on how many contexts they share in common. Research has established that the more similar the background of a couple, the more likely their relationship will be stable (Decuyper, De Bolle, & De Fruyt, 2012). Conversely, couples with dissimilar backgrounds are more likely to struggle to achieve a stable relationship.

Corey, the retired doctor, possessed the intelligence, education, and economic resources to belong to high socioeconomic status (SES) groups, but he lacked the easy familiarity that came with growing up in those circumstances. Although his son had grown up immersed in a high SES community, a transgenerational sequence seemed to connect him to the experiences of his father and made him feel inferior to his peers.

Constraints of Acculturation

In a culturally diverse society, the stage and rate of acculturation produce normative stresses associated with immigration. For example, in families from a Mexican heritage in the United States, teenagers tend to acculturate faster than parents and mothers faster than fathers. A wife's expectations about relationship equality can easily surpass that of her husband, leading to battles between them about the issue of individual autonomy. She may believe it is normal to have a male coworker as a friend, whereas he may feel quite threatened. Similarly, when a first-generation Mexican American teenager attempts to live a mainstream-American adolescence that privileges autonomy, serious tensions created by different norms in the family can constrain the adolescent's development.

Social Justice

The culture metaframework grounds IST within the paradigm of social justice by acknowledging that disadvantaged client systems experience a multitude of constraints triggered by a lack of access to power and authority that is not experienced by privileged clients. It recognizes and discusses the constraints that these injustices place on clients. The therapist's attendant empathy strengthens the therapeutic alliance. To address the constraints within the culture metaframework, therapists extend their hypothesizing and planning outside the consulting room. This work can include advocating for clients and helping them identify and access resources. Although therapy cannot lift some cultural constraints, the therapist's compassion and commitment strengthen clients' resolve to manage their lives as best they can.

The culture metaframework also serves as a template to understand the therapeutic relationship when therapist and clients have membership in different groups. These differences must be acknowledged and addressed whether it is a White therapist working with clients of color, a straight therapist working with a same-sex couple, or a young therapist working with seniors. These differences can only be bridged if the therapist privileges the "local" knowledge of the clients. The life experience of clients from different backgrounds must be understood and celebrated as relevant to the understanding of the problem and the problem sequence. Moreover, solution sequences must be adapted to the cultural norms of the clients.

The Knowledge Base Needed for Understanding Contexts of Membership

It is beyond the scope of this chapter to thoroughly explicate the knowledge needed to understand all the contexts of membership therapists will encounter. What is vital is that IST therapists assume the responsibility to learn about these contexts of membership. Listening with cultural humility creates openness to the local knowledge of clients who educate therapists and gradually expand their fund of knowledge. Working with a diverse population and having friends from diverse backgrounds speeds this process. Curiosity about diversity speeds the acquisition of knowledge through reading, the media, and conversation.

Mind

The organization, development, and culture metaframeworks described thus far provide templates that enable IST therapists to hypothesize about macro data reflecting how client systems function. These metaframeworks assure that hypothesizing is systemic and considers the entire biopsychosocial system, particularly the levels of relationship, family, and community.

On another level, client systems are composed of humans, each of whom has mental processes that affect how the client system works. Every therapy session, therefore, consists of verbal and nonverbal utterances that reflect clients' internal experiences. These microdata reveal clients' emotional and meaning worlds that become involved in the problem sequence in two ways. First, each client has an inner dialogue that is a sequence. For example, a wife may think, "What he said just now is so not true, and it is making me very angry. I'm not going to put up with this. Why can't the therapist see through his calm, reasonable demeanor?" All the other clients in the session experience their own internal sequences. Second, these internal sequences contribute to the problem sequence in the room. The therapist's challenge is to attend to the observable sequence while hypothesizing about each client's internal sequences. To manage this part of the therapeutic process, IST uses a mind metaframework.

Consider the following vignette. A family entered therapy to deal with the acting out behavior of Evan, age 14. Trying to understand their leadership style, the therapist asked the parents, Joe and Sharon, to discuss how they deal with Evan when he misbehaves.

Joe: Well, the first thing we try to do is understand the circumstances surrounding any given infraction.

Sharon: That's the problem right there, Joe. All you do is try to understand. You never stand up to Evan. I think you are afraid of him.

Therapist: Joe, what do you think of what Sharon just said?

Joe: It's not that I am afraid of Evan. I am afraid of what Evan might do. My brother drove the family car into the side of a bridge when my father cracked down on him. Hell yes, I'm afraid.

From this exchange, the therapist hypothesized that the parents were split regarding how to parent Evan and that Joe's perspective on disciplining him is constrained by his fear that Evan, like his uncle, will react to consequences by harming himself. At this moment, the therapist had to choose whether to continue hypothesizing and planning using the organization metaframework or to expand the work by opening the mind metaframework by focusing on Joe's fear. The two directions are interrelated, but the planning and conversation for each are different. Whether the therapist knows it or not, at this moment in the therapy, a choice must be made. In IST, it is better to make that choice proactively. A choice to focus on Joe's fear would result in defocusing on leadership between the parents. The therapist bridged this dilemma:

Joe, it sounds like your fear is very much on your mind when you think about Evan. I do not want to lose our focus on how you and Sharon work together to do what is best for Evan, but for the moment, can you tell me more about what happened to your brother and your fear of what might happen to Evan?

If the therapist decided to focus on Joe's fear, he or she must hypothesize about it by drawing on some theory of mind. This theory would tell the therapist how to hypothesize about the fear and how to reduce it so it does not keep Joe from setting limits for Evan. The myriad models of individual therapy propose many theories to understand Joe's fear. Because the mind metaframework contains all the theories, the IST therapist could potentially choose from any of them. For example, a psychodynamic perspective might purport that Joe uses the defense of denial to keep him from accurately assessing the seriousness of Evan's behavior and focus on the roots of this denial. Alternatively, a cognitive behavior therapy approach might hypothesize that Joe's catastrophic thinking keeps him from holding Evan accountable and would use cognitive restructuring to change this thinking and thus diffuse the fear (Beck, 2011).

The mind metaframework guides hypothesizing about internal experience by cataloging the theories of mind to help therapists decide which theory to use in which clinical situation. IST's principle of minimal complexity calls for therapists to use basic theories of mind first and only to use more complex theories when basic theories prove insufficient. This principle also enables therapists to stay systemic by maintaining focus on all relevant metaframeworks while still addressing the internal processes of clients. In this way, internal process does not dominate therapy until it is necessary.

IST proposes three levels of complexity, progressing from the least to the most complex depending on the strength and organization of the constraints. We label these levels M1, M2, and M3. The therapist begins hypothesizing and intervening at the M1 level of complexity and moves to M2 or M3 hypotheses and interventions only when the less complex level is not working.

The M1 Level of Mind

The M1 level of mind recognizes that emotion and meaning are part of human experience and can, therefore, be part of a problem sequence or constrain the implementation of the solution sequence. At the M1 level of complexity, emotion and meaning are taken at face value: Clients have and express them, and they can sometimes be constraining. When clients express an emotion and/or a cognition, at this level, the therapist might say, "That seems to really upset you." So long as the client responds appropriately, "Yes, I felt devastated when he said that to me," there is no need to evoke, discuss, and use a model of mind that explains the feeling's origin.

In the earlier example, Joe's fear was an emotion that connected his view of parenting to the death of his brother. If the therapist discussed that connection with Joe and he recognized that his fear was not appropriate to the present, he could let go of his fear, so it no longer constrained his parenting. In another example, a wife may say she feels lonely in the marriage. If the solution sequence successfully improves the marital connection and she reports no longer feeling lonely, the M1 level will have been sufficient. M1 analyses of mind lead to the use of strategies that access adaptive emotions and regulate or reappraise constraining emotions to implement solution sequences.

Likewise, at the M1 level of complexity, clients' meaning can be part of the problem sequence and/or constrain implementation of the solution sequences. M1 interventions can be drawn from therapies that privilege meaning, such as cognitive behavior therapy that works in part by replacing constraining automatic thoughts with thoughts that facilitate the solution sequence. Reframing is another intervention that can change client attributions.

Mindfulness practices have also emerged as a way to calm the mind so that intrusive thoughts and/or feelings do not persist as part of the problem sequence. When the mind is calm, it is easier for individuals to know what they are thinking and feeling and, in a relationship, to hear the perspective of another person. Some therapies now introduce mindfulness practices at the outset of therapy and begin every session with a mindfulness exercise. In IST, when the client system cannot use action in a solution sequence and emotion and/or meaning constraints persist despite attempts to remove or modify them, mindfulness practices can be indicated.

At the M1 level, personal narratives can also be addressed. At this level, these narratives are thought to be malleable. A client can have a problem-saturated narrative and have a successful re-storying experience by choosing a different narrative. For example, clients who have experienced sexual abuse can shift their narrative from being a victim to being a survivor. At the M1 level, IST focuses on McAdams's (2006) narrative level of personality— "I am my story." Clients have more or less conscious narratives about all of the levels in the web (Solomon, 2001). These narratives address "Who am I?" "Who are we as a couple?" and "Who are we as a family?" IST asks to what extent their self, couple, or family narratives facilitate or constrain problem resolution.

The M2 Level of Mind

When a straightforward examination and discussion of meaning and emotion fails to alter the problem sequence or lift constraints, the therapist shifts to the second level of complexity, M2. At this level, the therapist introduces a model of mind that helps the clients understand, cope with, and change their emotions and meanings. These are structurally simple models of mind that explain mental process. Examples are object relations (Kernberg, 1976) and internal family systems (IFS; R. Schwartz, 2013). The M2 level enables clients to understand better themselves and others. The wife's loneliness, for example, may persist despite the husband's greater attentiveness. Using IFS, the therapist can identify a part of her that believes she is not entitled to marital closeness so that part minimizes the extent of the change or even rebuffs her husband's efforts.

When clients are cut off from their emotions or cannot understand them or locate their source, M2 draws on such formulations as *object relations* (J. Greenberg & Mitchell, 1983; Savege-Scharff & Scharff, 2002; Summers, 1994). Object relations link current emotion and meaning to early family-of-origin experience. Emotions and meanings constellate as internalizations of early family relationships. Self-objects are beings (e.g., people, animals) and things (e.g., house or home, business, cars) that become part of the person's sense of who they are. In the old language of psychoanalysis, they are cathected or charged with self-energy. In attachment language, they are objects of attachment. A wife's loneliness may persist despite her husband's loving attention because her mother was insufficiently attentive to her.

IFS uses a model of mind composed of a self and groups of parts (R. Schwartz, 2013). Problematic thoughts and feelings are felt by and expressed by the parts. The parts can become extreme because the self's leadership has been compromised. The goal of therapy is to restore the self-leadership so the parts can be calmed. Because people often refer to parts of themselves in common parlance, many clients readily identify with this model. R. Schwartz (2013) hypothesized that clients have groups of parts he called *managers* and *firefighters* that protect a person from painful thoughts and feelings held by another group of parts call the *exiles*. Firefighters and managers must be convinced by the self to allow the exiles to come forth and express their pain.

Another M2 model of mind is the five-factor model of personality theory or the Big Five: Openness, Conscientiousness, Extraversion, Agreeableness, and Neuroticism (McAdams, 2006). Each exists on a continuum from low to high. High Conscientiousness people are organized, dependable, and self-disciplined, whereas people low on that continuum can be described as unreliable and sloppy. Personality characteristics are derived primarily from genetics and secondarily from environment. One's personality can be "tweaked" but not fundamentally altered. Problem sequences are often fueled by a poor "fit" between the personality traits of two clients. For example, a high Conscientiousness spouse might struggle with the perceived unreliability of a low Conscientiousness partner. In this instance, some degree of acceptance is essential if the couple is to be stable. Nonacceptance and disrespect generate pernicious sequences, but complete acceptance is not necessarily ideal. A partner's nonhostile criticism (Zinbarg, Lee, & Yoon, 2007) can result in successful personality "tweaking." For instance, a husband may criticize his wife's extreme extroversion, and she may tone it down.

When the symptoms of psychiatric disorders such as major depression and bipolar disorder can be stabilized and managed with medication, the disorders can be framed with M2 language. Clients can accept the oppressive nature of the disorder and appreciate a model of mind that includes a belief that the disorder has a genetic component. The therapist must always remain alert that failure to implement a solution sequence could involve the constraint of the disorder.

In addition to psychiatric disorders, present trauma, which happens in adulthood, can also be framed with M2 language. Parents can lose a child, a spouse can experience infidelity, a serious accident may occur. These traumas have remediable sequelae. The key question is, What prevents the client system from dealing optimally with the trauma? Some of the M1 answers are lack of information, beliefs about the trauma, or powerful emotions such as fear, guilt, or shame. An M2 analysis can be used to help clients explain and clarify the often conflicting or intolerable internal responses they experience. For example, Arthur and Samantha were coping with the death of their adult son. Part of the problem sequence was that they were disconnected because they each occupied their own silo of grief. The therapist used an IFS formulation to address this disconnection.

> *Therapist:* For each of you, the pain of loss is so great that you are trapped in your own silo. I understand why that is happening, but it is sad because it prevents you from supporting each other. I wonder if there is a courageous part of each of you that wants to at least peek out of the silo to see if you can see your spouse?
>
> *Arthur:* I have that part, but I am so afraid that if I do peek, I will see that her grief is so great that she won't be able to see me.
>
> *Therapist:* So another part of you is afraid.
>
> *Arthur:* Yes.
>
> *Therapist:* [To Samantha] What do you think would happen, Samantha, if Arthur's courageous part did help him peek?
>
> *Samantha:* Part of me is terrified that I would let him down as I have so many times before.
>
> *Therapist:* Arthur, are you up for trying right now?

The M3 Level of Mind

When therapy does not progress, and clients remain mired in their constraints of meaning and emotion despite M2-related interventions, the therapist next questions whether one or more of the clients are too fragile to modify their internal process. The theoretical core of this level of mind is *self psychology*, which defines the self as the most basic psychological unit— the cell of human identity (Kohut, 1977, 1984; Pinsof, 1995). This self is conceptualized as the container of the internal representations or psychological objects or parts. This self is fundamentally psychosocial—it needs its self-objects over the entire life course. *Self-objects*, through a set of transferences, perform self-development and maintenance functions. The transferences involve *mirroring* (positively reflecting the self), *idealizing* (looking up to and using core self-objects as role models), and *twinning* (feeling connected to others as "like me"). The self grows in relationship to its self-objects by manageable disruptions or ruptures of the transferences, which are followed by empathic repairs. When these transferences are significantly or traumatically disrupted in childhood and adolescence, the self does not develop adequately and becomes extraordinarily vulnerable.

Narcissistic vulnerability constrains a person's psychological flexibility, resilience, and emotional availability. This vulnerability limits their ability to appropriately engage in certain kinds of psychosocial tasks and solution sequences. For instance, a narcissistically vulnerable man struggled to tolerate his wife's or his daughter's needs to differentiate developmentally. His wife decided to pursue a master's degree in drama, and the daughter just completed her first year at college where she fell in love with a girl. He experienced these differentiating steps as betrayals that threaten his narcissistic equilibrium. He demeaned his wife's initiative and threatened to cut off the daughter financially. The wife dragged him into couples therapy, after multiple unsuccessful attempts, by threatening to divorce him.

When clients have such vulnerable or less-developed selves that rigidly require the people to whom they are attached to fulfill specific and immutable roles, the M3 level of mind addresses such "self" constraints. This M3 work focuses on strengthening the fragile client's self so that eventually the solution sequence can be implemented. Similarly, a couple has a "couple self" that defines them as a conjoint system. Like the narcissistic homeostasis of individuals, a couple's narcissistic homeostasis can constrain them from making progress in therapy.

The modus operandi of M3 work is to increase therapeutic support. This is achieved in several ways. First, the pace of therapy is slowed and the frequency of sessions increased. Second, the alliance is viewed as the pathway through which change must first occur. The focus of such therapies becomes the successful management of the vicissitudes of the alliance over time. Strengthening the alliance may require giving the vulnerable client additional sessions or referring the client to an individual therapist. Third, the therapist offers contact between sessions through phone calls or texts. Although an M3 formulation of mind will necessitate careful attention to the nuances of the therapeutic alliance and the effects of the client's narcissistic vulnerability, it does not preclude the implementation of new patterns of action or the use of interventions targeting M1 or M2 formulations of constraints.

An M3 level of mind is needed when personality substantially constrains problem solving. Extreme and rigid behaviors are key indicators of such personality constraints that diagnostically are referred to as personality disorders. These behaviors render M1 and M2 interventions ineffective. When a husband's lack of empathy and guilt about his critical and personally attacking behavior does not respond to his wife's entreaties or his therapist's interventions, the husband's self-constraints must be addressed. Historical trauma experienced in early childhood also requires an M3 level of intervention. When clients report historical trauma early in therapy, the therapist either shifts immediately to an M3 level of mind or plans to make historical trauma one of the problems to be addressed at a later time.

When the symptoms of a serious psychiatric disorder are persistent or ebb and flow over time, the disorder poses major constraints. The approach to the client would include M3 formulations because of the damage that such disorders do to the self. Over time, the ebb and flow of each exacerbation of the disorder can sap the resiliency of the client with the disorder and other clients who are part of the system. Multiple hospitalizations and suicide attempts can ultimately infuse the system with despair, such as feeling that "we are never going to get beyond this problem." Here the therapy must both strive to stabilize the symptoms and build hope that meaningful lives can be lived despite it.

It is easy to conclude that the more severe the psychiatric disorder, the more a complex level of mind is called for; however, contemporary therapies such as cognitive behavior therapy and dialectical behavior therapy use M1 level interventions to address the symptoms of the disorder such as depression, anxiety, and emotion dysregulation. At the M3 level, however, the therapist must join the client on a long journey in search of a combination of acceptance and harmony that facilitate strengthening the self and making the best of difficult and potentially incurable disorders.

Gender

For most of history, gender was considered a biological fact that divided humans into the nonoverlapping categories of male and female. Membership in one or the other of these categories was assumed to determine a great deal about the skills, preferences, potential, and traits of a person. Beginning in the early 20th century and accelerating since then, many assumptions about the meaning of gender have come under scrutiny (Goldner, 1985; Malpas, 2011). The lesbian, gay, bisexual, transgender, and queer or questioning (LGBTQ) community and more recent social science have challenged assumptions about what constitutes "real" maleness and femaleness, whether gender is binary, and even whether it is an essential category of human identity (Blume & Blume, 2003).

The feminist movement has challenged the connection between gender and male privilege, resulting in a cultural transformation that has significantly altered both the public and domestic landscape of male–female relationships. Beginning in the 1970s, feminism has influenced the conduct of couple and family therapy.

These challenges to gender as a singular, inalterable, biological fact have resulted in gender being accepted as a construct that is culturally as well as biologically determined. Because gender has profound and complex influences on human relationships, because it is embedded in all cultures (albeit not always with the same meanings and role prescriptions), and because advances in science continue to raise questions about the biology of gender, IST regards gender as a metaframework in itself.

The significance of gender in psychotherapy emerges most frequently in one of two ways. In the first case, either an individual client or someone who is participating in therapy with a partner or other family members experiences distress about his or her gender identity, gender assignment, gender expression, or sexual orientation or that of another family member. The second common way that gender becomes relevant in therapy is when one or both members of an intimate partnership feel constrained by their own or their partner's gender role expectations, resulting in conflict or distress in the relationship. Either of these presentations will signal the IST therapist to open the gender metaframework to explore and lift the gender-based constraints that prevent the problem from being resolved.

Gender As a Nonbinary Category

The following clinical vignette illustrates the way IST lifts the constraints created by nuanced gender differences. Franny and Noel met late in college, where they were both active in the LGBTQ community. Both were assigned the female gender at birth. Franny had come out as a lesbian in junior high and been politically active on behalf of LGBTQ rights ever since. Noel (born Noelle) had first identified as a lesbian, but by college was identifying as transgender. When the couple met, Noelle's gender expression was still female, but she was open with Franny about her plan to undergo hormonal treatment and surgery to transition her identity to male. Despite the uncertainty of how this change would affect their relationship, the two fell in love and decided to live together after college. Over the next 2 years, Noelle transitioned to becoming Noel. As the transition proceeded, Noel felt increasingly better about himself, more comfortable in his identity, and less depressed. Throughout the process Franny had been unwaveringly supportive, assuring Noel that she loved him as a person, not because of his gender. The couple initiated therapy after Franny engaged in a brief affair with a female coworker. When Noel discovered the affair, he was hurt, but he also became concerned that it signified some unacknowledged discomfort in Franny about Noel's transformation.

The therapist was impressed by the openness and care the partners showed each other and by their reluctance to make each other the problem. Franny declared that she loved Noel, and the only things that had changed in their relationship pertained to the secondary sex characteristics he had acquired—a lower voice, facial hair, and more obvious musculature. She said she could not explain the affair except as a brief infatuation, something she had "fallen into" while on a business trip. Given their unique history, the therapist decided to use the couple's ideas and feelings about gender to explore how Noel's transition to becoming a transgender man had affected their relationship. To ask the couple about the ways that Noel's transition had affected the relationship, the therapist adopted a "not-knowing" stance. Such a stance presupposes there are multiple meanings attached to their problem sequence and that the therapist is sensitive to not imposing meaning. "Not knowing" differs from "knowing nothing." The therapist may well possess knowledge about gender identity transition, but this is shared only when the couple clarifies their beliefs.

Franny and Noel had long been committed to the idea that gender is not a binary concept and that gender identity can be fluid. They loved and respected each other as people, and Noel found Franny as attractive a sexual partner now as he had when they met. Over the course of a few sessions, it became clear that Franny had undergone some change in her feelings of attraction to Noel. She was conflicted about these feelings because she was fully supportive of Noel's new gender identity, loved him as a person, and wanted it to make no difference in their relationship. But it did make a difference to her. By opening the gender metaframework the therapist asked questions that led Franny to acknowledge that her affair was not just a lapse of judgment, but that she missed Noelle, that she still thought of herself as a lesbian, a woman who loved women, and that identity was hard to reconcile with the person Noel had become. She did not want to leave Noel, but she wanted the freedom to clarify her sexual orientation. She was able to admit to herself and Noel that her affair had been an attempt to make that discernment, but she regretted that she had not felt able to talk to Noel about her discomfort rather than acting on it. Once they felt free from the constraint for gender not to matter, Franny and Noel were able to discuss it in a new and deeper way that allowed for all of their feelings to be acknowledged. They left therapy having renewed their commitment to be monogamous, not yet certain about exactly how their relationship would proceed but more confident that they could face it openly and in ways that respected each of their identities.

Gender in Heterosexual Relationships

The salience of gender for heterosexual couples lies principally in its connection to power (Goodrich, 1991; Goodrich, Rampage, Ellman, & Halstead, 1988). Same-sex couples also have power dynamics, but these are less often driven by gender roles. Power is the ability to have an effect, the right to have an opinion and to make it count. Historically and across cultures, power has been unequally distributed in marriage, with men having much more of it (Coontz, 2005). In Western societies since the beginning of the 20th century, this imbalance has been decreasing. As women have accrued legal and social power (e.g., the right to vote, access to birth control, greater educational and work opportunities), they have also sought and acquired domestic power. The dominant discourse about marriage in the United States shifted from a "head of household and helpmate" structure to a "partnership of equals." At least, that is the aspirational ideal. Exceptions to this egalitarian aspiration include (mostly older) couples who have long-established, traditional gender roles, as well as couples whose religious faith prescribes such role division.

The reality of gender equality is seldom so simple. Most couples struggle with gender constraints (both conscious and unconscious) that can lock them into a problem sequence and render solution sequences highly elusive. They struggle, sometimes endlessly, over who is getting more from the relationship and who is carrying more of the burden. Research on marital satisfaction overwhelmingly supports the benefit of an egalitarian marriage (Rampage, 2002a, 2002b), but the constraints that work against such an arrangement remain formidable, even when the partners themselves believe in it. As just one example, most couples without children share the distribution of responsibilities and privileges quite equally and often without stress. They each generate income and feel authorized to make decisions about how to spend it, they share (or outsource) domestic responsibilities, and they have equal degrees of freedom about how to use leisure time. This satisfying arrangement is inevitably challenged in the transition to parenthood when the amount of responsibility increases exponentially and the degrees of freedom are reduced correspondingly.

In most contemporary heterosexual families, it is still the woman who assumes more of the responsibility for child care and household responsibilities (whether she continues to work outside the home or not), whereas the male partner's attachment to his job or career remains steady or increases. This pattern continues to place a constraint on how closely couples with children can come to realizing the ideal of a truly egalitarian, peer marriage (P. Schwartz, 1995). The implications of these changes are profound, usually including a decrease in marital satisfaction and frequently accompanied by an increase in conflict. Couples come to therapy seeking relief from their distress, often without any awareness of how their shift from an egalitarian partnership to more stereotypic gender roles constrains the relationship.

Joi and Lamar met at work a few years after college. He worked in sales and she in marketing for the same athletic clothing company. Following a courtship of 2 years, they married, and both continued to work for the same company, where they were each successful. The marriage was gratifying to both of them. They both worked long hours, but they were able to eat dinner together most evenings (usually take-out), keep housekeeping time to a minimum by hiring a cleaning service, and reserve a lot of time on weekends to be together. When they decided to start a family one of their major considerations was Joi's desire to continue at her job, a decision that Lamar fully supported, both because he knew how important her career was to her and because her income provided a level of security they both valued.

The pregnancy was uncomplicated, but the baby had both eating and sleeping difficulties and was hard to soothe. Joi returned to work when the baby was 2 months old, but she felt exhausted and irritable most of the time. She felt that most of the responsibility for taking care of the baby fell to her because Lamar had less patience with the baby than she did (which she resented) and because his working hours were longer and less flexible. She also felt guilty leaving the baby at day care. Lamar felt Joi had completely lost interest in him both as a person and as a sexual partner, and her threats to quit her job terrified him. They fought frequently and finally decided to come to therapy as a couple.

Following the IST approach, the therapist assumed that Joi and Lamar were capable of having a satisfying relationship because they had done so for several years. During the initial interview, the conversation focused on the number of things that had changed in the marriage following the birth of their child. Several themes emerged. There was far less "couple time" than before the baby was born, a situation that seemed more immediately distressing to Lamar than to Joi. The house was messier than ever, a change about which Joi felt particularly upset. The partners were more often disappointed in or irritated by each other. Joi was experiencing less job satisfaction, and Lamar worried more about their financial future. Like many couples, the transition to parenting had led to shifts in the relationship that were consistent with traditional gender roles. Moreover, each partner felt conflicted about this shift, and yet compelled to enact it.

By encouraging the couple to overtly acknowledge both the changes they were struggling with and their mixed feelings about these changes, the therapist was able to engage them in a conversation in which they were able to consider alternatives and resist the pull to polarize and reflexively adopt more traditional gender roles. Instead of engaging in a problem sequence of blame and counterblame, they were able to discuss the problem as something they shared and to collaborate about solutions that allowed them to feel they were choosing the changes parenthood required instead of feeling the changes were being imposed on each of them by the other.

Biology

Jordan, a 55-year-old African American man, sought individual therapy to address his inability to leave his marriage to Rhonda, which he felt had died years ago. For several years he had been having an affair with Shantell. He considered Shantell to be his soul mate. His wife knew of the affair but had not given him an ultimatum, nor did Shantell press him to leave his marriage. Both women were, however, perpetually upset with him, so Jordan found himself in a dysfunctional triangle. He maintained that he had to sort through his dilemma himself. The therapist kept focusing on what kept Jordan from taking steps to resolve his dysfunctional triangle. The therapist identified many constraints, but the work did nothing to resolve the triangle. Finally, Jordan agreed to go into couples therapy with the goal to either improve his marriage or leave. He reported no progress in the therapy and stated that going just magnified his stress.

One day he came to his session and reported he had contracted a serious and painful case of shingles. For several weeks, Jordan canceled his appointments, claiming he was in too much pain. When he returned 6 weeks later, he still had shingles (shingles should remit in about a month). The therapist knew that although it does not cause shingles, stress can weaken the immune system, making a person more susceptible to the shingles virus. After sharing this information with Jordan, the therapist had the following exchange with him.

> Therapist: Jordan, have you thought that your body might be sending you a message with shingles?
>
> Jordan: What sort of message?
>
> Therapist: Let's think about it: The stress you have been under for years may have weakened your immune system and left you vulnerable to shingles.
>
> Jordan: I agree, but I still can't see what you are getting at.
>
> Therapist: I wonder if your body is telling you that you can't tolerate the stress any longer and that you must reduce your stress or face even more dire health problems.
>
> Jordan: Like what problems?
>
> Therapist: Frankly, I fear you are becoming a candidate for a heart attack or a stroke.

This conversation got Jordan's attention like no other, and after a few more sessions, he told his wife he was moving out. In this example, the therapist did more than empathize with Jordan's medical condition. He opened the biology metaframework and used his knowledge about shingles to focus Jordan on the need to take action to resolve the triangle and reduce his stress.

Biological constraints can be woven into problem sequences in sometimes obvious and sometimes subtle ways not fully understood by clients. Biology can profoundly affect quality of life that in turn functions recursively with clients' moods. Sleep deprivation, pain, and physical and mental limitations from illnesses are examples of biological constraints. They interact with daily life and sap clients' resiliency. Sometimes the relevance of the biological constraint is obvious. The therapist may choose to focus on it or make a note to return to it later. For example, John, a building contractor, sought a consultation regarding how he would handle succession in his business. As they walked to the office, the therapist noticed that John's gait was quite uneven and as part of the settling-in conversation made note of it:

> Therapist: John, you seem to be moving a little slow today. Did you hurt yourself?
>
> John: I wish. I have a bulging disc that should be operated on, but I can't afford to be laid up for 6 weeks recovering from surgery.
>
> Therapist: I am really sorry to hear that. How much pain do you have?
>
> John: Quite a bit, but I can't let my competitors see that I am down, nor do I want my son, who is my successor, to believe he has to take over before he's ready.
>
> Therapist: I see. So we seem to have stumbled on to one of the factors related to your goal of being here: to talk about succession.

Incorporating biology into psychotherapy is a challenge for most psychotherapists who usually have received little formal training in this domain of human experience. Learning about biological factors is a lifelong endeavor for therapists. Therapists should ask clients about their health and when they last saw a doctor. If they report health-related concerns, therapists should explore them and assess the impact of the concern on clients' lives as well as their plans to deal with the concern. Nonmedical therapists must often recommend that clients seek medical opinions about their health concerns. However they are identified, biological constraints must often be addressed if solution sequences are to be effective. The following is a brief overview of the factors making up the biology metaframework.

Wellness

In the modern world, health is primarily understood through the concept of wellness. All physical conditions—cardiovascular, weight, and so forth—have been extensively studied through the lens of risk and protective factors (World Health Organization, 2002). To stay healthy, clients must maximize their protective factors and minimize their risk factors. For example, people should maintain a healthy diet, get regular exercise, have good sleep hygiene, lower their level of stress, and so forth. Unfortunately, there is often a correlation between coming to therapy and failing to get this balance right; therefore, therapy is always on solid ground when it encourages clients to take wellness seriously. When clients present problems that have physical components, therapists should know the risk and protective factors for that condition. Often the protective factors have been absent, and the solution sequence involves adding them.

For example, Angie presented for individual therapy with depression. The therapist soon learned that she was obese and sleep deprived and had not exercised in years. The synergism of these three factors rendered her perpetually exhausted and unable to function well at work. As part of the plan to address her depression, Angie agreed to work toward a healthier weight, establish better sleep hygiene, and begin an exercise program. She started slowly and for several months reported little headway. But over time she lost weight, began sleeping better, and found good outlets for exercise. Combined with cognitive behavior therapy and an antidepressant, these wellness practices gradually lifted the depression. Toward the end of therapy, she remarked how much more active and engaged in life she had become.

Mindfulness

A growing body of research has established the efficacy of mindfulness practices in the treatment of a range of physical problems (Kabat-Zinn, 2003). The common denominator of these studies is that mindfulness helps to create a calm mental state that is of therapeutic benefit, but more so that a calm mental state facilitates the way the mind addresses a physical illness. Client systems whose web of constraints includes a physical illness can benefit from the introduction of mindfulness to help manage that illness.

Medication

For better or worse, the pharmaceutical industry has showered society with myriad drugs that improve the quality of life. People with life-threatening cardiac conditions can take medicine that allows them to lead life without the persistent fear of a cardiac event. At the same time, clients on medication must contend with side effects that can adversely affect the quality of life and/or be dangerous. Therapists can help clients understand their medicines and evaluate the trade-offs of taking them. Of course, the final decisions regarding medicine always rest with the prescribing physician and client.

Of all classes of medication, psychotropic medications are the most likely to become part of the solution sequence for problems necessitating psychotherapy. Sometimes the therapist "inherits" the medicine because one or more clients are taking it at the outset of therapy. In other instances, medication becomes part of the solution sequence worked out during the course of therapy. IST therapists, therefore, must possess a basic knowledge about psychotropic medications, including the classes of drugs (e.g., antidepressants, mood stabilizers, stimulants), how they are designed to work (including how long they should be taken), their effectiveness, and their side effects. The therapist cannot assume the client knows this information. Physicians often do not share information about medicines, more than half of all psychotropic medicine is prescribed by physicians other than psychiatrists (Mark, Levit, & Buck, 2009; Mojtabai & Olfson, 2010), and the client may not have listened to and/or comprehended what was said. A psychotropic medication can be an important solution sequence. Occasionally, though, the therapist may hypothesize that it is constraining a client. For example, clients engaged in artistic pursuits sometimes complain that their creativity is blunted by the medication, so they face a trade-off between managing their mood and maximizing their talent.

Sleep Hygiene

According to the National Institute of Neurological Disorders and Stroke (2014), 40 million Americans suffer from chronic sleep disorders. Another 20 million have intermittent sleep problems. Persons experiencing sleep insufficiency are more likely to suffer from chronic diseases such as hypertension, diabetes, depression, and obesity, as well as from cancer, increased mortality, and reduced quality of life and productivity. Depending on the particulars of the case, sleep problems can be a presenting problem, part of the problem sequence, or one of the constraints to problem solving. The solution sequence often addresses a sleep problem using better sleep hygiene, medication (although current practice calls for time limits on such medication), or an evaluation for sleep apnea.

Sexual Health

Good sexual health is a predictor of personal and relational well-being. In addition, there are many other benefits to having satisfying and regular sex: a stronger immune system, lower blood pressure, lower risk of heart attack, lessening pain, improved sleep, and less stress (Brody, 2010; Jannini, Fisher, Bitzer, & McMahon, 2009). Couples often have difficulty discussing their sex lives, so therapists must possess the requisite knowledge and skills to guide these conversations. This requires knowledge about sex and the comfort to engage clients in such conversations. Having common ground in the form of reading material helps to create language and bridge the awkwardness—Bernie Zilbergeld's (1999) book on male sexuality and Emily Nagoski's (2015) book on female sexuality cover the waterfront of topics. Couples therapists do not have to be certified sex therapists to help couples with sexual difficulties so long as they can recognize problem sequences within sexual activity, as well as how a sexual pattern can function as a constraint or as part of a problem sequence. When a sexual dysfunction is outside of their expertise, therapists should refer clients to a certified sex therapist.

Illness

We often hear the expression "at least we have our health." Everyone understands how illness can turn worlds upside down. Unfortunately, virtually every client system we encounter will have dealt with a significant episode of illness currently or in the past. Consider just cancer. Forty-one percent of Americans will get cancer during their lifetime (American Cancer Society, 2009; Horner et al., 2009). Factor in the number of marriages, families, and extended family members affected by those cancers and virtually no one escapes. For example, when a couple reports that a parent has recently died, after offering condolences, the therapist should ask about the experience because the individuals and relationships might still be recovering from caregiving stress, the experience of seeing a parent die, and/or the grief associated with the loss. Further, if the disease had a genetic link, the client system lives in fear that another family member might fall ill.

Illnesses come in many forms and with varying degrees of severity (Rolland, 1994a). The impact of illness on a client and the client system will vary accordingly. Regardless of the illness, it can be part of the problem sequence or constrain implementing the solution sequence. A bout of flu or a cold can keep harried parents from that agreed-on date night designed to improve their connection. More serious illness can present significant challenges to the organization of the client system and profoundly compromise a family's resources. As such, poor adaptation to illness may be the presenting problem that brings clients to therapy.

Rolland (1994a, 1994b) classified illnesses as acute, chronic, relapsing, and degenerative. The physical and psychological impact of the illness on the client and other clients varies depending on the form of the illness. Rolland (1994b) referred to chronic illness as the uninvited family guest. He estimated that by 2020, 134 million Americans will be dealing with a chronic condition, 39 million of whom will have limitations in major activities. Chronic illness is relentless and over time progressively taxes clients' resilience.

Acute illnesses create a crisis for the client system. For example, a diagnosis of meningitis forces clients to put their lives on hold to address the medical crisis. The high-stress environment includes ambiguity about the initial diagnosis, uncertainty about the prognosis, tolerating anxiety when the course of the illness may be uncertain, and preparing for any long-term impact the illness may have on the quality of life.

Relapsing illnesses generate ebb-and-flow sequences that create constraints for the client system. After multiple cycles of relapse and recovery, clients begin to lose their resiliency. Increasingly, they have difficulty embracing the symptom-free part of the cycle because they know the illness is going to return and when it does, there is the sickening feeling of "here we go again."

Degenerative illnesses get worse over time. The client system is living with a "ticking time bomb" that progressively takes its toll and will ultimately end in death. The various types of dementia are examples of degenerative illnesses. Clients with these illnesses must prepare themselves to gradually lose their ability to participate in their own lives and to accept the need for caregiving. Their loved ones must come to accept loss long before death.

Increased life expectancy has added another stage to the life cycle: extended caregiving. It takes an enormous toll on the caregiver. It is estimated that women spend over 18 years providing caregiving to a parent (U.S. Senate Special Committee on Aging, 2002). This caregiving takes its toll on the well-being of the caregiver and also affects the caregiver's family of procreation. When the caregiver is an adult in therapy for a different problem, the therapist should consider whether caregiving is a constraint and, if so, how it is distributed among the primary caregiver's siblings (who are part of the indirect system). Renegotiating caregiving responsibility can be part of the solution sequence that helps solve the client's presenting problem. This renegotiation is challenging because it requires the caregiver to relinquish control over a role that may be syntonic with a part of the caregiver; the caregiver must develop a new approach to siblings that activates their involvement.

Mental Illness

Although debates among psychotherapists remain regarding the extent to which mental illnesses have biological underpinnings, IST embraces current science that strongly supports that major mental illnesses do have a biological component. Clients with illnesses such as bipolar disorder, major depressive disorders, and schizophrenia struggle to live adaptive lives. The illness can result in such incapacitation as to necessitate hospitalization. Sometimes the cyclical nature of the illness can result in multiple hospitalizations. The impact of these illnesses on the clients who have them and the clients whose lives are affected by them cannot be underestimated. IST therapists, therefore, must be versed in both the knowledge about mental illnesses and their various treatments.

Because the vast majority of psychotherapy is practiced on an outpatient basis, therapists must know how to maintain a therapeutic relationship with a client system when a client has to be hospitalized. Understanding both the legal and insurance issues associated with psychiatric hospitalization is necessary for the therapist to help the clients. Because risk to life is always a factor in hospitalization, discharge can be complicated. Similarly, extending hospital stays requires negotiations with insurance managers. All of these issues are better navigated when the IST therapist for the client system establishes a relationship with the psychiatrist and/or the treatment team at the hospital.

Addictions

Estimates are that one in 12 Americans over the age of 12 has a substance use disorder (Substance Abuse and Mental Health Services Administration, 2014). In the United States, drug and alcohol addictions are considered to be diseases. This has created a societal view that alcoholics and drug addicts are sick and must be treated as such; hence, an enormous industry has been created that uses a medical model to treat addictions. These treatments involve various levels of care: inpatient programs, day hospital programs, specialized addiction psychotherapy, and Alcoholics Anonymous. When an addiction is defined as the primary presenting problem, the treatment of choice is generally one of the aforementioned. Interestingly, other than initial detoxification and the possible prescription of medication to prevent the usage of a substance (e.g., Suboxone prescribed to replace heroin), the treatments are decidedly nonmedical, specialized talk therapy. IST therapists sometimes work in these contexts and bring a systemic, integrative approach to their work.

Concerns about addiction are often presented as part of the problem sequence or a constraint to the solution sequence. The use of substances and clients' concern about them often ebb and flow as a part of a problem. In these instances, IST therapists consider the biology (in addition to the psychology) of addiction. To do this with success requires that IST therapists possess a skill set that includes the following: ability to talk candidly about substance use, ability to perform preliminary screening to determine the severity of the substance use, ability to reconcile differences of opinion among the clients regarding the severity of the substance use, ability to use motivational interviewing (Miller & Rollnick, 2012) to bring the "using client" to a state of readiness to address the substance use, ability to walk the path of recovery with the using client, and ability to handle the reactions of the nonusing clients, particularly any who have codependency issues. IST requires that therapists possess knowledge about the nature of addiction and recovery, including risk factors for addiction; the trajectory of an addiction, including the stages of the addictive process; the biological impact of addiction; the struggle to seek treatment; and living a sober life.

Brain Functioning

Until recently, scientists had to treat the brain like a "black box"—they could note inputs and outputs, but they possessed no instruments to measure how the brain works. Only when neurologists began to study the effects of traumatic brain injury did they begin to learn about how particular parts of the brain regulate aspects of human consciousness. The dramatic departure from normal mental functioning caused by traumatic brain injury signaled that brain damage can serve as a powerful constraint.

For example, Tom's parents brought him to therapy because of his explosive temper. When the therapist inquired and learned that Tom had sustained multiple concussions playing football, she encouraged his parents to seek a neuropsychological evaluation for Tom that confirmed injury to his prefrontal cortex. Later in life, changes in cognitive functioning can be predictive of aging and/or the onset of some organic brain syndrome. Working with clients through these challenging times is more effective and rewarding when therapists possess knowledge about brain functioning.

Recent advances in the neurosciences using functional magnetic resonance imaging technology to image parts of the brain while they are being stimulated have created a deeper understanding of brain functioning. Applied to psychotherapy, these advances enable therapists to understand better how the brain creates cognition and influences emotion, stores and retrieves memories, interprets our senses, and regulates our organ systems. Further, understanding the habitual nature of brain functioning coupled with brain neuroplasticity reveal both constraints and pathways to change.

These insights have led to therapies rooted in neurobiology. Even relational therapies are now incorporating neurobiology (Fishbane, 2007, 2013). The methods proposed in this therapy are helpful in dealing with many aspects of relational dysfunction, including emotion dysregulation and couple reactivity. Sharing knowledge of brain functioning with couples is a form of reframing that removes much of the blame attached to problem sequences. It is much easier to accept that a partner's angry outburst occurs because his prefrontal cortex that guides rational thought cannot get the upper hand on the faster amygdala that is responding to some perceived danger that activates the fight-or-flight response. This fascination with the brain is here to stay. Nonetheless, IST therapists, grounded in systemic thinking, are quick to recognize that attributing human functioning to the biology of the brain can lead to reductionist thinking that blinds us to the contributions of the other levels of the biopsychosocial system.

Aging

In the lifespan of a couple, many biological issues will arise that can pose constraints to relational stability. Along the way, they encounter nodal physical events, such as pregnancies and major illnesses, as well as changes in appearance and shifts in hormone levels, such as menopause. The physical and mental health of each partner, how their health-related issues interact, and how all of this affects the relationship are all within the purview of the biology metaframework.

Some couples are transparent about their physical well-being and are supportive when an illness arises. Others know virtually nothing about the other's health. Even worse, one partner might hold secrets about his or her health, thereby also hiding the sometimes enormous psychological stress accompanying illness. All of the biological issues described previously can constrain couples from addressing the problems for which they seek help.

Death is the final biological event. Knowledge about the biological aspects of death enables therapists to prepare clients for what they, or a loved one they are caring for, must experience. Eventually, all therapists will experience death through the loss of someone close to them, but those who have not experienced a personal loss can be removed from the immediacy of death. They should gather at least a rudimentary understanding of the dying process. Witnessing death is but one part of the journey.

Hormones

Modern science is advancing the importance of hormones in the maintenance of physical and psychological well-being. Healthy levels of hormones contribute to healthy living. Inadequate hormone levels (too much or too little) contribute to distress. For example, cortisol is released in our system in response to stress. The right amount of cortisol facilitates stress management. Excessive release of cortisol can affect the brain and result in weight gain. Another hormone, oxytocin, competes with cortisol by lowering stress and creating a sense of well-being. Estrogen and testosterone fuel sexual desire in the first adult stages of the life cycle, but as they wane with aging, physical changes occur, including lowered sex drive. A wife struggling with premenstrual hormonal shifts may find it harder to regulate her irritability and soothe herself during certain times. An antidepressant with a cyclical dose regimen may ameliorate her irritability. Conversely, a husband addressing his depression with antidepressant medication (particularly with selective serotonin reuptake inhibitors) may experience reduced libido that impairs the couple's sexual relationship.

Genetics

In the great debate about whether nature (genetic endowment) or nurture (environmental factors) contributes more to define who we are as humans, the current wisdom seems to be not only that both contribute substantially but also that nature and nurture are involved in close feedback loops in which they influence each other constantly. In fields such as epigenetics, there is no dividing line between inherited and acquired traits. Hence, even though the field of psychotherapy has been strongly slanted toward affecting environmental factors as a way to produce change, modern psychotherapy must pay closer attention to genetics and the constraints and opportunities it presents. This is particularly true because the mapping of the human genome was completed in 2003, making it possible to study the relationship between DNA and many illnesses, both physical and mental (Oksenberg & Hauser, 2010).

Therapists can now engage in a set of questions regarding genetic illness. Who is at risk of particular illnesses? Who is affected psychologically? What are the interpersonal ramifications of the illness (McDaniel, 2005)? For example, the wife in a couple in therapy learned that her mother has breast cancer. She was terrified she would contract the disease as well. The therapist discussed with the couple the merits of genetic testing and arranged for them to have a consultation. The testing confirmed a high risk, and the woman elected to have a double mastectomy. The therapist supported the couple through the ordeal of the surgery.

We have presented biology largely independent of the other metaframeworks, but we must always be mindful that biology is located in the web of human experience and, therefore, influences and is influenced by the other metaframeworks. Hence, for example, culture mediates biology. A child living in a disadvantaged neighborhood is at higher risk of obesity than a child growing up in an affluent community. Twenty-first-century science is escaping mind–body dualism as their interconnected nature is being revealed through more sophisticated technology and research. IST embraces these advances and recognizes the need to incorporate biology into hypothesizing as it relates to the problem sequence, the success or failure of implementing the solution sequence, and the way constraints are preventing success.

Spirituality

George and Shirley, an African American couple in their mid-60s, first came to therapy when the school expressed concerns about their grandson, Jerome, who was exhibiting aggressive behavior in his fourth-grade classroom. George and Shirley were legal guardians of Jerome and their 8-year-old granddaughter, Alice. Jerome was their son's child, and Alice was their daughter's child. Their son, Michael, was currently in prison, where he was serving time for selling drugs. Jerome's mother had never been involved in his life. Their daughter, Sandy, had been cited by family services for drug use and had lost custody of Alice. Sandy lived in the area and sometimes visited Alice.

George and Shirley had been meeting with an IST therapist for over a year. The therapist sometimes met with George, Shirley, and the children; sometimes with just George and Shirley; and sometimes with one or both of the children. The therapist had worked with the school to get Jerome tested and diagnosed with attention-deficit/hyperactivity disorder. Jerome's outbursts diminished when he started taking medication and after a period of talking in sessions about missing his father. Alice had been diagnosed with sickle cell anemia. Exacerbations of the illness resulted in periods of time when she was in pain and missed school.

George and Shirley had been through a lot, and they showed signs of strain dealing with two grandchildren in an underresourced household at their age. But they were always upbeat in session, smiling and laughing frequently. Whenever the therapist expressed amazement at their capacity to handle adversity, they always replied the same: "God never gives you more than you can handle." To this, the therapist would reply, "You are blessed to have such strong faith."

One day George and Shirley arrived for their session carrying a heavy burden. Shirley burst into tears and reported that Michael, who had been recently paroled, was murdered in a drive-by shooting. Jerome had not yet been given the news. The therapist was speechless and barely able to say, "I am so sorry for your loss." In a moment of awkward silence, Shirley looked at the therapist and said, "It will be all right; the good Lord never gives us more than we can handle." As the therapist sat helpless, feeling an internal rage at the social injustice that had brought the family to this terrible moment, it became clear that George and Shirley were taking the lead and that the therapist's job at that moment was to honor and respect the deep faith that enabled the couple to cope with their tragedy. For the next two sessions, the couple used their time in therapy to talk about how their faith was helping them stay strong and how their church community had surrounded them with support and love.

Reactions to adversity in which spirituality organizes clients' response to human suffering happen all the time. In fact, in 2015, 52% of U.S. Americans reported that religion is "very important" to their lives, whereas 26% rated it "fairly important" (Gallup, 2016). Likewise, surveys have indicated that 52% of people believe religion can answer "all or most of today's problems" (Gallup, 2016). The United States is, to a great degree, a nation of faith. The statistics lead us to a position that spirituality, when desired by clients, should be allowed to find a place in the therapy. Although the incidence of religiosity and spirituality varies among countries and some countries have significantly lower levels than the United States, when spiritual beliefs and practices are important to clients, they can positively affect therapy.

Spirituality involves "a relationship with God, or whatever is held to be the Ultimate that fosters a sense of meaning, purpose and mission in life" (Hodge, 2001, p. 204). It involves "transcendent beliefs and practices, within or outside formal religion" (Walsh, 2009, p. 3). IST maintains that therapists should be open to discussions of spirituality, able to identify spiritual strengths and constraints, considerate of client spirituality in planning interventions, and mindful of a therapist role, boundaries, and ethics in spiritual work.

Designating spirituality as a metaframework acknowledges the special significance that spirituality has in the lives of many people and its impact on the problems they bring to therapy. Although not a mainstream position among the many psychotherapies, there are authors who also champion this position (Walsh, 2009). Sometimes working in the spiritual realm involves helping clients draw on their relationship with a higher power to persevere in their problem solving. Alternatively, clients can benefit from transcending the struggle and "letting go." Spirituality can also constrain problem solving, such as when a client excessively defers to a higher power or when a person's spirituality has been damaged or diminished.

Mainstream psychotherapy, however, has traditionally eschewed spiritual matters. Several arguments have supported this position. First is the premise that psychotherapy is grounded in science that is limited to the observable. Consequently, spiritual matters that are outside the realm of the observable should not be in its purview. Second is the position that spiritual beliefs are a creation of humans designed to shield humanity from the reality of the finality of death. Spiritual beliefs are constructions and, therefore, should not be encouraged in the practice of therapy. Moreover, psychotherapy has sometimes designated reports of intense spiritual experiences as evidence of a psychiatric disorder. Third, psychotherapy and spirituality are separate realities that cannot be reconciled in one practice; therefore, spirituality should remain outside the purview of psychotherapy.

Generations of psychotherapists have been trained to ignore spirituality or to politely deflect client references to their spirituality. A cyclical process, therefore, has built up in which clients, to some extent, know their spiritual beliefs are not welcome in therapy, and therapists do not ask about them. The outcome is that spirituality is seldom addressed substantively in mainstream psychotherapy. Exceptions do exist: pastoral counseling, therapy offered by Christian and other religion-based therapists, and the work of therapists who integrate Eastern religions into their practice. In fact, clients who have strong spiritual beliefs often seek out therapists who are sympathetic to spirituality.

Because IST harnesses clients' strengths to solve problems, all clients' experiences, including spiritual experiences, are welcomed as resources in the service of therapy. IST therapists must, therefore, be conversant with the many manifestations of spirituality and be able to incorporate them respectfully into therapy. IST therapists need not share clients' spiritual views to do this.

It can be asked whether spirituality warrants its own metaframework. Just as we have made gender a metaframework because we believe its importance cannot be addressed adequately by making it part of the culture metaframework, we also recognize that spirituality cannot be addressed adequately as part of religion, which is one of the of the contexts of membership in the culture metaframework. The reasoning behind this is twofold. First, spirituality cannot be adequately subsumed under religion because the spiritual experiences of many people are not connected to any formal religion and, second, spirituality involves transcendent experiences that seem to occur in all religions and cannot be fully explained by descriptions of the practices of particular religions.

The spirituality metaframework includes a definition and understanding of transcendent experience, how transcendent experiences are reported, typical ways that clients discuss spirituality in relation to the goals of therapy, and, finally, the therapist role and ethical issues in spiritual discussions.

Transcendent Experience

The basis of spirituality is *transcendent experience*, defined as any experience that stands outside the world of observable and logically understandable experience. Spirituality transcends the universe of material existence in which humans live out their lives. Transcendent experiences include such things as the felt presence of a supreme being (usually referred to as God), the perceived interventions of this being into the lives of humans, and a sense of connection to something larger than the self. For George and Shirley, transcendent experience was expressed as a deep faith in a loving God who has a plan for each individual: "God will never give you more than you can handle." The senseless murder of their son, though extraordinarily painful, was experienced as tolerable and ultimately forgiven. That humans have transcendent experiences cannot be established scientifically despite many efforts to do so. Rather, acceptance of transcendent experience is taken as a matter of faith.

Undoubtedly, this perspective feels foreign for some therapists. The idea that "God will never give you more than you can handle" can seem unhelpful or even repugnant—why should God single out some people and not others for illness and tragedy? Why ignore the impact of oppressive societal structures? When clients indicate that their faith guides them in a different direction, it is not the job of the therapist to try to change their views.

Encountering Spirituality in Therapy

Therapists can find themselves having to access the spirituality metaframework in the course of treating any client system. While exploring clients' social context at the beginning of therapy, it is important to ask, in a nonjudgmental way, whether the clients have religious or spiritual involvement. If they describe a religious affiliation or spiritual practice, it is reasonable to ask whether they think it might influence their approach to solving the presenting problem. If so, further inquiry will shed light on how spirituality may affect the problem-solving process. If not, the therapist then moves on to other areas of discussion. This typically brief exchange is meant to open a space for clients' experience, establishing that spiritual matters can be discussed in therapy, but need not necessarily be part of the conversation.

Although spiritual resources might be accessed to deepen meaning, strengthen resolve, or find acceptance in relation to many different problems, there are several situations in which the spirituality metaframework can be particularly helpful. These include moments of loss, situations that call for forgiveness, overwhelmingly challenging life circumstances, and addictions. George and Shirley chose to embrace and live their faith rather than be crushed by their life circumstances. They believed devoutly that God cared about them and hence they possessed self-worth (Aponte, 2009). When Michael was murdered, they grieved together and with their faith community. The person who murdered Michael was ultimately caught and convicted. George and Shirley attended the trial and felt justice was served; however, they reported that their greatest peace came when they both forgave the young man who had robbed them of their son.

The power of addiction is such that many addicts spend a lifetime believing they can defeat their addiction only to be proven wrong time and again. Success within a program such as Alcoholics Anonymous (AA) depends in large measure on addicts' recognition that they are powerless against the addiction; consequently, the path out of addiction is to turn their lives over to a higher power and trust that the relationship formed with this higher power will create the strength needed to defeat the addiction. IST therapists partner with AA in many ways. They may commence treatment with a client who has been sober for decades and still uses AA as a resource. IST therapists would embrace AA as a strength in the client's life. An addiction might be the presenting problem or one of the constraints to implementing the solution sequence. In this case, AA is viewed as part of a solution sequence, and the IST therapist supports the client's approach to treating the addiction. This is not to say that IST endorses twelve-step programs as the only possible solution for addictive problems. Rather, IST strongly supports the spiritual practices of these programs (AA, Narcotics Anonymous) for the many people who find them beneficial.

Spirituality can be thought of as a personal experience and/or a shared experience, as when a family or couple shares similar spirituality. In these cases, accessing spiritual resources has benefit for all members. Clients can also be constrained by their spirituality. For example, when problem solving involves excessive deferral to a higher power, clients can be blinded to solution sequences that involve their own agency. Some clients may "hide out" in their spirituality, avoiding anger, pain, and sadness by using it as a defense. When spirituality is a constraint, the therapist can supportively and non-judgmentally describe the dilemma the client faces about the problem-solving process. The challenge is to sensitively and respectfully evaluate spirituality's role as a constraint or resource and work to diminish the former and strengthen the latter.

Spirituality can be a challenge when clients have discrepant views about it. In this case, there is a problem of fit between the spiritual views of a couple or among family members. An example would be spouses who are both spiritual but from different traditions. A working coexistence of their respective beliefs and practices may have prevailed until a particular life cycle stage or a crisis is reached, such as a serious illness of one of their children. At other times, only one partner embraces spirituality. The other partner may have strong negative views about spirituality. During times of stability, the spiritual partner may devote time and energy to practices such as praying, going to church, or affiliating with other believers without affecting the relationship; however, when the believer needs to embrace spirituality in a time of need and the other partner is not available or even hostile, a crisis of disconnection can occur. Moreover, these circumstances present an alliance dilemma for the therapist who must navigate different levels of spirituality without creating a split alliance.

Therapist Role and Ethical Issues

Whenever spirituality is being discussed, the focus of the conversation should be on the client's experience. Therapists should be careful not to impose their beliefs or put any spiritual expectations on the clients. This is a challenge for therapists with strong religious or spiritual backgrounds in that the way they cope is influenced by their particular beliefs, and by extension they may attempt to help the client cope in a like manner. Something as simple and caring as saying "God bless you" or "God loves you" can be an abuse of power in that it expects clients to subscribe to something with which they may not be comfortable in order to have a good alliance with the therapist. Incorporating recommendations about the therapist's role in spiritual matters, the IST therapist does not indoctrinate or impose beliefs on clients (Curlin et al., 2007; O'Dell, 2003) or make assumptions about what their spirituality means to them (Faiver, Ingersoll, O'Brien, & McNally, 2001; Griffith, 1995, 1999). Rather, as the therapist hears spiritual language or is informed of a client's religious denomination, this presents the opportunity to find out what this means to the client and how any beliefs or practices relate to the problems they are experiencing or the solutions they seek. The IST therapist does not disclose personal spiritual beliefs without careful attention to the therapeutic alliance and the possible benefits or harm that may result from disclosure. Doherty (2009) proposed helpful guidelines for levels of intensity of spiritual intervention, including when self-disclosure is warranted and how it can be approached.

6

WHAT TO DO, WHEN, AND WHY: PLANNING AND THE PLANNING METAFRAMEWORKS

A depressed husband calls for an appointment with the therapist. Should the therapist see him alone or with his wife? A couple has been in weekly therapy for 2 months. The focus has been on changing the painful criticize–defend–escalate conflict sequence that drove them to therapy. The therapist has been teaching them active listening and healthy conflict skills. Recently she has addressed their negative attributions and victim narratives. Nothing seems to have any lasting effect on their conflict sequence. A defiant and drug-involved adolescent is failing in his second year of high school. The therapist has helped the parents provide a loving but firm structure to support his work at school and encourage him to find new friends who might share his prosocial interests. The therapy is not working. Last, a 28-year-old single woman has been in individual therapy for 9 months working on social anxiety, fears of intimacy, and lack of communication with her family of origin. She remains stuck.

http://dx.doi.org/10.1037/0000055-006
Integrative Systemic Therapy: Metaframeworks for Problem Solving With Individuals, Couples, and Families,
by W. M. Pinsof, D. C. Breunlin, W. P. Russell, J. L. Lebow, C. Rampage, and A. L. Chambers

These brief therapy scenarios present the therapist (and the clients) with critical decisions about how to proceed. The first example asks who should be involved in the therapy from the beginning—the individual client or the client and his wife? The other examples deal with cases that have not been making progress and lead to the question of whether the therapists should stick with what they have been doing or try something different. If they opt for something different, what should that be? In the overall decision-making process of the blueprint, the planning component provides guidelines and strategies for answering these questions. These guidelines and strategies, the focus of this chapter, address what to do, when, and with whom, delineating the logic of clinical decision making in integrative systemic therapy (IST).

PLANNING AND THERAPY

Therapy is and should be planful. This is apparent in the problem-solving tasks of the essence diagram and the decision-making function of the blueprint, which are used over the entire course of therapy. Intervention is a mindful activity that perpetually involves some degree of planning. That planning derives from the therapist's hypotheses about solution sequences and the primary constraints that prevent the client system from implementing them.

Planning entails the construction of macro and micro clinical experiments to test the therapist's and clients' hypotheses about the constraints that prevent change. On the macro level, those experiments address the hypothesized "primary" constraints that prevent clients from implementing the solution sequence. With the 28-year-old "stalled" woman, action or behavioral strategies could be used to address the hypothesized organizational and developmental constraints preventing her from moving on. On the micro level, experiments address hypothesized secondary constraints on the path to resolving the primary constraints. For example, the therapist hypothesizes that the client passive aggressively sabotages her growth. Can she allow herself to experience (and eventually express) her hypothesized anger toward her parents for overprotecting her while they supported her brother's adventures and independence?

As with all the components of the blueprint, planning must be collaborative. Much of it goes on within the therapist's mind, but ultimately the planning process has to become part of the explicit conversation with the clients. This collaborative planning empowers clients, making them better problem solvers.

THE INTEGRATIVE SYSTEMIC THERAPY PLANNING MATRIX

The planning guidelines and metaframeworks, as well as their linkage to the hypothesizing metaframeworks, are embodied in the matrix presented in Figure 6.1, which we discuss over the course of this chapter. The planning metaframeworks house and organize the many and varied strategies and interventions available to an IST therapist. The matrix also classifies the contexts of therapy (family, couple, and individual). The organization of the matrix is predicated on a number of planning guidelines that suggest what to do when over the course of therapy. The matrix embodies these guidelines and addresses the question of what to do when what you are doing is not working.

WHY LOOK BEYOND SPECIFIC MODELS OF THERAPY?

Most specific therapy models, such as cognitive behavior therapy for anxiety, depression, or marital distress or emotion-focused therapy for individuals or couples, present themselves as "sufficient" therapies—sufficient to

Metaframeworks (MFs)		Contexts of therapy		
Hypothesizing MFs	Planning MFs	Family/ community	Couple/ coparent	Individual
Sequences, organization, development	Action			
Culture, gender, spirituality, sequences of mind	Meaning/emotion			
Biology	Biobehavioral			
Intergenerational patterns: sequences, organization, mind	Family of origin			
Organization of mind	Internal representation			
Development of self	Self			

Figure 6.1. Integrative systemic therapy planning matrix. From "Integrative Problem-Centered Metaframeworks Therapy II: Planning, Conversing, and Reading Feedback," by W. M. Pinsof, D. C. Breunlin, W. P. Russell, and J. L. Lebow, 2011, *Family Process*, *50*, p. 318. Copyright 2011 by John Wiley & Sons. Adapted with permission.

resolve the problems they were designed to address. The research literature on psychotherapy over the last 30 years, including specific studies and meta-analyses, has consistently shown that virtually every specific therapy model facilitates significant improvement, if not full remediation, of symptoms (a more stringent goal) in approximately two thirds of clients seeking help. Follow-up studies show varying degrees of maintenance of change in these "improved clients" posttherapy, ranging from 50% to 90%. Typically, this initial success rate of two thirds, even with some subsequent deterioration, is better than what emerges in studies of therapies that are tested away from their initial sites of development in more standard practice settings (Nathan & Gorman, 2007). Thus, at least one third of clients are not helped by specific models, and many more deteriorate posttherapy.

The critical problem is what to do when these models do not work. The solution of many of the model developers and adherents is to increase treatment adherence—ensure that therapists do a better job of providing the treatment (Perepletchikova, Hilt, Chereji, & Kazdin, 2009). That may improve outcomes, but it is not enough. Psychotherapy needs a metamodel that moves beyond the limitations and foci of specific models.

That movement can occur at least in two ways. The first is to sequence specific models. After working with a cognitive behavior model, unresponsive depressed clients might be offered antidepressant medication and/or emotion-focused therapy for depression (L. S. Greenberg, 2011; Pos, Greenberg, & Warwar, 2009). When emotion-focused therapy does not work, clients may be offered a trauma-focused psychodynamic therapy that deepens and historicizes the emotional work. In other words, unresponsive clients receive a sequence of specific model treatments until they begin to improve.

With IST, we propose a more fundamental and comprehensive shift that integrates common factor and generic approaches to transcend the use of specific models. A mature psychotherapeutic field has to move beyond specific models and the sequencing of specific models to a perspective that incorporates strategies and techniques from specific models into a coherent and integrated metamodel. The IST planning matrix and metaframeworks represent this next step.

In articulating this new perspective or metamodel, we integrate principles, strategies, and techniques from specific models, but do not constrain or confine ourselves to the theoretical and clinical assumptions of those specific models. The preceding chapters in this book laid out the theoretical framework for thinking within this new perspective or metamodel, and this chapter lays out its specific, generically defined intervention strategies.

The matrix in Figure 6.1 integrates three core dimensions: (a) the hypothesizing metaframeworks, (b) the planning metaframeworks, and (c) the contexts of therapy. The first column on the left presents the hypothesizing metaframeworks, the second column depicts the planning metaframeworks, and the last three columns on the right delineate the therapy contexts. This chapter focuses on the planning metaframeworks and therapy contexts. The planning guidelines, which integrate them, are presented as a group after the metaframeworks and contexts.

FINDING THE BEST-FIT STRATEGY FOR EACH CONSTRAINT

A planning metaframework organizes and delineates a set of therapeutic strategies and interventions that share a common theory of problem formation and problem resolution. Specifically, they share a common focus (e.g., behavior, emotion, cognition, family of origin) regarding what they attempt to change. IST has evolved over the years from thinking about the planning metaframeworks as umbrella structures for pure form models to conceptualizing them as structures for transcending models (Breunlin, Pinsof, Russell, & Lebow, 2011; Pinsof, Breunlin, Russell, & Lebow, 2011). The proliferation of pure form models characterized a phase of the development of psychotherapy as a clinical science that was necessary to legitimate the field, but now constrains the emergence of a more mature clinical science. The articulation and development of more inclusive, generic, and common factors and strategies herald the emergence of this new developmental phase (Sprenkle, Davis, & Lebow, 2009).

Each planning metaframework provides a categorical structure for organizing therapeutic strategies and interventions that aim to change particular types of constraints. The strategies and techniques within a metaframework, to some extent, are less important than the particular types of constraints that are addressed by the metaframework. This constraint focus reflects IST's endorsement of the systemic principle of *equifinality*, which asserts that different strategies and interventions ("inputs" or "causes") can, and more often than not, lead to similar outcomes ("outputs" or "effects"). For instance, encouraging a wife to talk directly to her husband in therapy may have the same impact (she talks directly to her husband and feels less frightened of him) as helping her understand that her fear of her husband has more to do with her relationship with her abusive father when she was growing up than with her husband today (who has never been abusive). Thus, the direct stimulation of interaction (a behavioral or action technique) may have the same effect as a transference interpretation (a psychodynamic or internal representation technique). Equifinality justifies disconnecting strategies and techniques from the theoretical context in which they were articulated—their "home theory." For instance, "exposure" is a strategy with a long history in cognitive and behavioral therapies. However, many, if not most, therapies encourage clients to expose themselves to frightening situations, feelings, and thoughts. Confining a generic and common factor strategy like exposure to one type or category of therapy limits its value and impact.

This line of thinking, reflected in the two left columns of the matrix in Figure 6.1, means that strategies and interventions from a single planning metaframework can address constraints from multiple hypothesizing metaframeworks. This is not to say that the strategies and interventions emphasized in certain planning metaframeworks do not fit better with the constraints addressed by certain hypothesizing metaframeworks. Using the earlier example, directly stimulating interaction, a strategy that falls most appropriately within the action planning metaframework, most appropriately targets or addresses organizational and developmental constraints. However, there is a significant and unavoidable degree of flexibility and plasticity between planning and hypothesizing metaframeworks, just as there is between different types of interventions and similar outcomes.

THE PLANNING METAFRAMEWORKS

The presentation of the planning metaframeworks focuses on the constraints they address and the way in which they address them. The emphasis within each metaframework is on the primary intervention strategies that address its particular constraints. Our presentation of the planning metaframeworks rests on the distinction between strategies and interventions (Goldfried, 1982). A strategy is a broader category that includes different interventions. For instance, exposure is a primary strategy of the meaning/emotion metaframework that involves encouraging clients to expose themselves to historically frightening but necessary or unavoidable situations or tasks. Building an exposure task hierarchy, encouraging in-session exposure ("do it now"), or asking clients to imagine what they fear happening (imaginal exposure) are all variants of exposure. Next, ways in which strategies are implemented are mentioned, but a detailed presentation of the myriad interventions available to therapists within a strategy exceeds the scope of this chapter. The intervention level is the point at which each therapist brings his or her unique style, values, and personality (genuine self) into the strategic implementation process. Different therapists draw on different interventions to implement a strategy, typically selecting those that fit their personalities and preferred styles of interacting.

It is important to clarify three things about the strategies within the planning metaframeworks. First, we have not discovered or created the strategies or interventions within each metaframework. Most, if not all, of them have been identified and/or created within specific therapy models. The way in which we organize them and attempt to define them in a generic, nonmodel specific language represents our unique contribution. Second, the strategies listed for each planning metaframework are not meant to be a complete list of all possible strategies or interventions within these metaframeworks. Rather, they represent a reasonably comprehensive list of strategies that can be integrated into each planning metaframework. IST is an open theoretical system that incorporates new ideas and strategies for intervention as they are developed. Third, though each planning metaframework includes an ordered list of strategies, the strategies do not have to be used in any particular order. The strategy chosen from a planning metaframework at a given point is based on a specific hypothesis about the constraints and the feedback in the therapeutic conversation, including key clients' viewpoints.

Although the first two planning metaframeworks are action and meaning/ emotion, it is important to note that action, meaning, and emotion pervade every conversation in therapy. Further, although we describe the first three planning metaframeworks as being present focused to indicate their temporal emphasis, therapists and clients may reflect on the past in the implementation of the present-focused strategies. In this way, the conversation is not rigidly constrained, but the therapist's strategic emphasis is clear.

Action Planning Metaframework

As mentioned earlier, behind planning rests hypothesizing. Each planning metaframework has certain key hypotheses about what prevents the client system from solving its problem. The major working and prioritized hypotheses in the action metaframework are that the clients have been unable to resolve their presenting problems and change their problem sequences because the sequences are dominated primarily by behavioral constraints such as inertia, bad habits, and not knowing what to do. The corollary problem solution hypothesis is that these action constraints should be addressed by helping clients change the way they are acting—by helping them interrupt the problem sequence and replace it with a mutually agreed-on solution sequence. The action metaframework can be thought of as a distillation of "just-do-it" strategies and techniques. On the way to "just doing it," the therapeutic conversation will deal substantively in the realm of meaning to establish a reason for the action strategy and will address emotion to build the therapeutic alliance and motivate action and interaction. In this way, from the beginning of therapy, the action and meaning/emotion planning metaframeworks work closely together.

The action planning metaframework is the "go-to" metaframework when clients are constrained by organization and/or development because organization and development are so often revealed and changed through interaction. Often, with respect to organization, there are constraints of leadership and/or boundaries. How do parents exercise leadership in their family? How do they share leadership? What happens when leadership is disrupted by divorce or loss? Simply asking one parent to not undercut the leadership of the other in the presence of the children can have a powerful impact on leadership. Are boundaries appropriately established for the circumstances? For example, when a parent repeatedly interferes with the conflict between siblings, the therapist can request that the parent refrain from interfering so the siblings can solve their own conflict. Without parental interference, the siblings may be able to sort out the conflict themselves.

Likewise, development unfolds in the context of interaction. Parents are constantly trying to determine what is age appropriate for children and are prone to create interactions that produce oscillations. This challenge is exacerbated by the relentless march of development through which all members of a family grow and change. For example, a parent might continue to offer excessive help with homework long after the time children should be doing it on their own. Finding strategies to phase out the parent's involvement can help to dampen the oscillation around schoolwork. When a family member's development is constrained by a disability, the entire family has to organize and interact through that disability. Achieving maximum potential from the disabled family member is one goal, but another is to create organization and interaction that also attends to the development of other family members. For example, marriages are at risk when a couple cannot handle the disability of a child, and they can end in divorce, further affecting all members. Parents sometimes have to be guided to give more attention to the so-called well sibling lest his or her resentment and sense of neglect contribute to more problems.

The following strategies fall primarily within the action metaframework.

1. *Identifying, labeling, and interrupting the problem sequence—who is doing what when.* This strategy initially involves helping clients sequentialize their problem (Breunlin & Schwartz, 1986). What precedes its emergence? What does it look like when it emerges? What happens after it emerges? This process explicitly or implicitly labels the sequence or problem—what needs to change. This labeling may or may not label the problem sequence as "bad," "destructive," or "not a good thing." This strategy involves the therapist interrupting and stopping the sequence if clients cannot do so on their own. Eventually, it involves the therapist teaching the clients to stop or interrupt the sequence themselves.

2. *Identifying a solution sequence and encouraging clients to implement it* (Pinsof, 1995; Russell, Pinsof, Breunlin, & Lebow, 2016). Frequently, clients do not know what to do—or they do know but have been unable to do it. Unlike the nondirective stance of many therapists, IST therapists direct or encourage clients to do what has to be done to solve the problem. IST therapists are not afraid to take an "expert" stance and use their knowledge of human problem solving and human development to "tell clients what to do." This instructive stance is not authoritarian or dictatorial, but it is authoritative. A wife who effectively runs her own business with 200 employees but puts up with lies and excuses from her "underadequate" husband can be asked, "What stops you from holding the line with your husband the way you do with your employees?" Parents who negotiate with their 3-year-old daughter about every decision may have to be told, "She needs you to take leadership and be clear about what has to be done. She is too young to be the opposing attorney." The directed solution has to be discussed with and ultimately "bought" and adopted by the clients. It should not be imposed. Similarly, if it does not work, the therapist and the clients should embrace the failure and use it as an opportunity to better understand the web of constraints and what might be a better solution.

3. *Creating enactments* (Minuchin, 1974). This refers to the process of getting clients to talk to each other. Enactments have several purposes, about which IST therapists are generally transparent and which form, with greater or lesser specificity, the justification or "frame" for the interaction. First, they allow the therapist to observe the ways family members interact, which display strengths, problem sequence(s), and constraints. In a session, if the therapist gets the father to ask his adolescent son about the kind of things he worries about, she or he has a dual opportunity: to see how the father and son communicate (an interaction assessment opportunity) and to hear what the son has to say about his anxieties (an information-gathering opportunity). Enactments create intensity and spontaneity, particularly with couples and families. It is easy when talking with a therapist individually to present oneself in a more normal and measured way, whereas in couple or family contexts, enactments trigger powerful and ingrained patterns of interaction that tend to reveal "what really goes on at home."

Therapists may be so blunt in deploying this strategy that they say, "Show me now. Tell him that you disagree with what he's saying, and let's see how he reacts."

A second purpose of creating an enactment is to strengthen the adaptive capacity of the system by asking members to do some of the work together. This is consistent with the IST goal of empowering clients to engage directly in the solution sequence or the behaviors it comprises. Interventions range from "OK, do it now" through "What do you think would happen if you asked him right now?" to sitting passively until the husband passes the box of tissues to his weeping wife. A third purpose of having clients talk with each other in session is to develop new adaptive patterns and solution sequences. The therapist suggests a reason for a particular communication and encourages the parties to engage in it in a particular way. He or she might ask a husband who had been unfaithful to see the depth of his wife's pain about the affair and listen carefully and empathically to her description of what it is like to live with it. The wife would then be encouraged to share her experience. Often clients need assistance enacting new patterns, which brings us to the next strategy.

4. *Teaching or coaching new patterns for clients to enact in session (and later at home).* This strategy involves everything from specifying behaviors that clients can or should engage in to modeling and practicing those behaviors in session (Bandura, 1969). It might involve the therapist demonstrating active listening with a wife while her husband listens and then asking him to try or it might involve practicing how parents will apply reinforcement contingencies with their children. Compared with enactments, this strategy tends to be more directive and specific. It may involve "shadowing" clients by sitting next to them and speaking for them until they can take over the conversation. The goal of this strategy is to directly and actively facilitate clients' engagement in specific interactions that will lead to or be part of the solution sequence.

5. *Developing between-session behavioral experiments* ("homework"; Haley, 1976; Kazantzis & L'Abate, 2007; Reid & Epstein, 1972). This strategy involves the therapist and clients agreeing to try certain new and more adaptive behaviors linked to or that are part of the solution sequence outside the office. For instance, "date night" with a couple, taking time for one parent to be alone with a child doing something fun, or asking clients to try

active or open-hearted listening at home after learning to do it in session are all interventions derived from this strategy. The implicit message of an experiment is "I expect you to change and try new things despite your ambivalence." It is important that the therapist follow up on the experiment in the next session by asking for feedback about how it went. If the clients did not do it or failed, it is important to not be critical, judgmental, or disappointed but to use the failure as a learning opportunity to explore what prevented them from doing it—that is, to identify constraints. Suggesting experiments early in therapy gives clients hope that the therapist thinks they can change and defines the therapy as doing something different and not just talking about it. Whether an experiment is suggested by the therapist, developed by the clients, or coconstructed, client buy-in is essential to a successful experimental process.

6. *Teaching clients about behavioral principles and action strategies for ameliorating problems* (Lucksted, McFarlane, Downing, & Dixon, 2012). This psychoeducation strategy may involve teaching parents about the power of ignoring bad behavior (extinction) or the value of acknowledging and praising prosocial behavior (positive reinforcement). Another example is teaching clients about the negative impact of hostile criticism ("expressed emotion") and the positive impact of nonhostile criticism (Zinbarg, Lee, & Yoon, 2007).

    Psychoeducation about behavioral principles and action strategies typically involves providing plain language minilectures that provide "hot" information that supports the implementation of a solution sequence. For instance, the nonhostile criticism information would be timely and appropriate when working with a couple with a mentally ill son who becomes clearly dysregulated in the face of any kind of hostility. The goal is to use the research findings to help parents understand the impact of their irritation and then find a nonirritated way to communicate their concerns to their son.

7. *Facilitating behavioral exposure* (Barlow, Raffa, & Cohen, 2002). This strategy involves encouraging clients to expose themselves to frightening or difficult situations. Exposure within the action metaframework emphasizes doing or action (vs. imaginal) exposure. Can a husband stop defending or explaining himself when his wife criticizes him and see how he feels and how she reacts? Can a socially phobic adolescent push herself to sit with one or two other people at lunch and see

how she feels and what happens? Typically, behavioral exposure is not implosive—going to the most frightening activity first. Behaviorists create fear or anxiety hierarchies to structure the exposure process in gradually increasing increments. IST exposure is a collaborative activity in which the client and therapist decide together how the exposure process should be structured and paced. This collaborative interaction ideally forms a template that clients can eventually use on their own to deal with frightening tasks and situations.

8. *Facilitating behavioral activation* (Hopko, Robertson, & Lejuez, 2006; Jacobson, Martell, & Dimidjian, 2001). This strategy encourages clients to engage in activity that is either reinforcing from a behavioral perspective or that bypasses constraining coping mechanisms (e.g., avoidance, rumination, alcohol or drug use) that reinforce the problem. In either case, the emphasis is on the performance of specific activities that manage, reduce, or eliminate a problem. For example, a depressed man may be encouraged to get up and exercise instead of staying in bed and ruminating. He may also be encouraged to engage in a productive, generative, or interesting activity instead of watching TV all day.

9. *Developing adaptive routines.* This strategy involves helping clients develop and institute positive routines that are solution sequences or that will facilitate solution sequences. For instance, for a couple immersed in work and child rearing, a regular "date night" each week would give them some time alone together as husband and wife—the aspect of their lives and roles that has been lost to being "mom" and "dad." Similarly, the institution of a family dinner at home without computers, cell phones, or television at least a few nights a week can facilitate cohesion, communication, and sharing across generations. Last, the institution of a nightly routine of preparing for the work or school day may help clients be better prepared for the next day and sleep better at night. Ideally, the therapist creates and plans the routine with the key system members to maximize their ownership and commitment to the new behavior. Routines can bring comfort, facilitate connection, clarify expectations, and facilitate the accomplishment of life tasks.

10. *Facilitating rituals* (Fiese, 2006; Imber-Black, Roberts, & Whiting, 1988). Although family routines and rituals overlap, we separate them because of their differential impact. A

couple's routine of having dinner together each week may become a ritual to the extent it begins to help define who they are as a couple or deepens their emotional connection. Rituals can be distinguished from routines by their more obvious link to factors such as identity and belonging and their capacity to produce a more lasting emotional experience (Fiese et al., 2002). Rituals can provide healing, deepen relationships, and address rites of passage. For example, an extended family may hold a yearly reunion that sustains connectedness and reaffirms their identity as a family. Or a family may have a tradition of a ceremonial tree planting in honor of a deceased member. Therapists often support families in enlivening existing rituals or creating new ones that strengthen their relationships and bring meaning to challenging or celebratory events and circumstances.

This list of action strategies is not meant to be exhaustive or limiting but rather to provide a sense of the type of strategies that fall in this planning metaframework. The critical component of all of the strategies is that they are designed to address constraints or establish a solution sequence as simply and directly as possible. They presume that clients are capable of adaptive action at that moment. As mentioned previously, the strategies and techniques of the action planning metaframework are ideally suited to addressing problems and constraints from the organization and development hypothesizing metaframeworks.

Specific models that contain more detailed information about action strategies and interventions include social learning, behavioral, and cognitive–behavioral approaches (Bandura, 1989, 1991; Barlow, Craske, Cerny, & Klosko, 1989; Baucom, Epstein, & Norman, 1990; Craske, 1999; Jacobson & Margolin, 1979; Patterson, Reid, & Dishion, 1992); structural family therapy (Minuchin, 1974; Minuchin & Fishman, 1981); strategic family and couples therapy (Haley & Erickson, 1973; Watzlawick, Weakland, & Fisch, 1974); solution-focused therapy (Berg, 1994; Miller, Hubble, & Duncan, 1996); and the use of family rituals and routines (Fiese, Foley, & Spagnola, 2006).

Meaning/Emotion Planning Metaframework

This planning metaframework rests on the hypothesis that the client system has been unable to implement the solution sequence because of constraining feelings and/or thoughts. The intervention hypothesis asserts that implementation of the solution sequence requires replacing the constraining thoughts and/or feelings with alternative adaptive thoughts and/or feelings.

Whereas the action metaframework focuses on behavior, the meaning/emotion metaframework is experiential, focusing on thoughts and feelings experienced by clients.

Meaning/emotion strategies and techniques also address client narratives—the stories that clients develop about themselves and their important others (Tarragona, 2008). Narratives are elaborate and organized cognitive and affective structures that can either constrain or facilitate the solution sequence. For instance, if a husband believes that if he reaches out to others for emotional support they will reject and shame him (a narrative that was true in his family of origin, but is not true in his marriage), it will be hard for him to talk with his wife about his fears and anxieties about his problems at work.

IST's action facilitation theory of emotion (Pinsof, 1983, 1995) asserts that emotions play key roles in constraining or facilitating implementation of the solution sequence. Emotion (except sadness and grief) is not addressed as an end in itself but rather as a constraint or facilitator of the solution sequence. Emotion adds intensity, genuineness, and power to psychological experience and interpersonal behavior. Emotions that constrain the adaptive sequence are reduced or replaced by emotions that facilitate its implementation. Emotions are not inherently constraining or facilitating, but are evaluated and treated as such because of how they emerge within particular client systems in regard to specific problems. In one client system, anger may constrain the solution sequence, and in another, it may facilitate it.

In terms of action strategies and techniques, the hypothesis is that although constraining feelings, thoughts, and narratives may be present, they do not have to be addressed directly or in depth because they do not play a central role in constraining implementation of the solution sequence. Rather, the focus on emotion and meaning at that point in therapy aims to build the therapeutic alliance and support adaptive action. When action strategies and techniques fail to facilitate the solution sequence, it raises the possibility that meaning/emotion constraints are more powerful than initially hypothesized and have to be addressed directly and substantively in their own right, with strategies that explicitly aim to change them. The following planning strategies explicitly address feelings, thoughts, and narratives that constrain and facilitate solution sequences.

1. *Identifying and labeling thoughts, feelings, and narratives that constrain implementation of the solution sequence* (Beck, 2011; L. S. Greenberg, 2011). This strategy aims to help clients see and understand how particular thoughts, feelings, and narratives constrain the implementation of the solution sequence. It involves identifying the thoughts, feelings, or narratives and labeling them as maladaptive or constraining. For instance, a mother

who feels helpless and bursts into tears when her 4-year-old daughter becomes defiant would be helped to understand that these feelings constrain her ability to deal effectively with her daughter. Alternatively, a father who can only feel anger at his son's growing disengagement and withdrawal would be helped to see how his anger just drives his son further away. Last, in regard to maladaptive narratives, for a 33-year-old woman who continually enters into unsatisfying and self-depreciating roles with the men she dates, the goal would be to help her understand how she permits herself to be victimized. How does she find and engage in relationships with men who take advantage of her, and what emotions and narratives does she experience that constrain her from extricating herself from those interactions and/or relationships?

2. *Interrupting or challenging constraining thoughts, feelings, and narratives that contribute to a problem sequence* (Pinsof, 1995). This strategy entails actively intervening with constraining emotions or meanings to stop the problem sequence from playing out. For instance, a couple starts to engage in an escalating criticize–defend sequence in which both of them get increasingly angry and alienated, ultimately culminating in destructive name-calling and withdrawal. The therapist may step in and stop it as they are starting to get angry and help them explore their "deeper" feelings at that moment. Similarly, a wife who sees her husband as uninterested and disengaged may attribute a lack of authenticity to his new efforts to engage with her ("He is just doing it because you told him to"). The therapist may help her see how that attribution discourages his new behavior and undermines his efforts to change. This may involve Socratic questioning aimed at challenging such dysfunctional beliefs. For instance, the therapist may ask her what she thinks the effect of disqualifying his efforts may have on his desire to continue trying to connect with her.

This strategy also helps clients stop engaging in hostile criticism or "expressed emotion" in general, but especially with other system members struggling with anxiety, depression, and bipolar and psychotic disorders. Asking a mother how she thinks telling her 16-year-old son he is acting like a baby when he withdraws to his room will affect their relationship may help her see the negative consequences of her shaming behavior.

This strategy would help the 33-year-old woman "victim" mentioned earlier notice her anger at being exploited and her fear of being alone or abandoned if she stands up or sets limits on her partner's behavior. In fact, the therapist may have to help her see how she "freezes" and "numbs" herself, before helping her explore the anger and fear underneath the numbness.

3. *Identifying, accessing, and/or heightening contextually appropriate and adaptive thoughts* (Wile, 2002). This strategy aims to help clients notice, experience, and express thoughts that facilitate the implementation of the solution sequence. For instance, a shy, lonely, and avoidant young man may be helped to notice and experience the fleeting thought that a woman who smiled and conversed with him at work might be interested in getting to know him. Or a husband may be encouraged to consider that his wife's complaining may be her way of reaching out to him. This strategy includes such interventions as Socratic questioning, circular questioning (Tomm, 1987b), motivational interviewing (Miller & Rollnick, 2012), externalizing the problem (White & Epston, 2004), and reframing (Watzlawick et al., 1974).

4. *Identifying and facilitating the development and use of adaptive narratives* (White & Epston, 1990). This strategy helps clients find within themselves or create new adaptive narratives to facilitate solution sequences. In working with a depressed, retirement-age man whose business was at a crossroads, the therapist learned that the man had formerly had a passion for teaching engineering concepts and related manufacturing applications to his employees. Over several sessions, the therapist led a careful discussion that gave the man the opportunity to elevate the narrative that his calling was to teach others. Then they worked on ways in his business and with his adult son (in the business) he could begin again to offer his knowledge and wisdom. Helping the parents of a young man with schizophrenia understand that his general withdrawal and avoidance of large family gatherings is his way of regulating his propensity to feeling overstimulated and then decompensating may help them permit or even facilitate his withdrawal without rancor or guilt induction.

5. *Identifying, accessing, and/or heightening contextually adaptive emotions.* This strategy accesses and augments emotions that are likely to facilitate solution implementation. For example, it might be important for a wife to access her anger (as opposed to her shame or fear) when her husband sarcastically depreciates her in front of their children. Alternatively, a husband who "armors" and moves to anger whenever he feels frightened or sad may be helped to experience and express his fear and/or

sadness. Identifying and heightening "buried" or frightening emotions may take time, patience, and persistence on the part of the therapist before clients can allow themselves to acknowledge and experience contextually appropriate emotions that have been denied or repressed for much of their life.

6. *Offering psychoeducation on emotion* (Gottman, 2001). This strategy teaches clients about healthy emotion management and expression in regard to implementing solution sequences. For instance, in trying to transform escalating hostile confrontations between family members and a mentally disordered family member, the therapist may explain the way in which hostile criticism fuels escalation and how nonhostile criticism would give the disordered member feedback that might be heard and integrated. Similarly, the therapist may explain the salutary benefit of "attacking" the behavior, not the person doing the behavior. Last, the therapist may help clients understand the destructive nature of emotional triangulating sequences—telling a family member how you feel about another family member—and the importance of detriangulating—telling the person directly.

7. *Regulating constraining emotions* (Gross & Thompson, 2007). This strategy is important both in managing certain painful emotions and in modifying the interactional sequences in which they are embedded. Strong feelings of fear, anger, shame, or guilt that are not contextually adaptive and interfere with solution sequences have to be regulated. There are many specific interventions within this strategy, but they typically involve change in how a situation is seen or understood or modification of the emotional response to it. For example, a young woman who damages her relationships with recurrent strong anger might be helped to look differently at the situations that stimulate her rage. The therapist may also teach her to attend to the sensations that precede outbursts and practice a time-out or self-calming procedure when they occur. Further, the therapist may teach her to assert herself in a manner that is effective, but significantly less intense.

8. *Facilitating healthy and direct emotional expression* (L. S. Greenberg, 2011). This strategy is the action corollary of emotional psychoeducation. It entails actively helping system members express adaptive, primary emotions directly and appropriately to each other and/or the therapist. IST's emphasis on getting clients to do as much of the work as possible, as well as on creating enactments, encourages therapists to help clients express emotions directly to each other in their sessions. For instance, a husband

telling the therapist about the terrible shame he feels for having betrayed his wife would be encouraged to directly express that shame to her in the session. Similarly, an adolescent telling the therapist about his anger at his father for betraying his mother would be directed to "tell your father about your anger" right in the session.

Complex Meaning/Emotion Strategies

Some strategies address a more complex formulation of constraints and require multiple meaning/emotion strategies as well as strategies from other metaframeworks for their implementation. Examples of these larger arc plans, which typically unfold over multiple sessions, are discussed in this section because of the prominence of the meaning and emotion strategies in their implementation.

9. *Identifying, exploring, and integrating recent traumatic experiences, the sequelae of which constrain solution sequences* (Johnson, 2002). Frequently, clients' engagement in solution sequences is constrained by the posttraumatic sequelae of traumatic experiences that have occurred in their relationships with each other or in other aspects of their life. This strategy aims to identify and neutralize these sequelae. Typically, this entails identifying the traumatic experience, labeling it as such, helping the client describe the trauma and helping other key clients respond with empathy, patience, and warmth. Trauma may range from the revelation of an affair all the way to the pain and terror of being physically assaulted by a drunk or enraged family member and fearing for one's life. Last, this strategy may involve helping a client talk about an extrafamilial trauma, such as being sexually assaulted by a stranger, with trusted others who can offer their love and support.

10. *Facilitating acceptance and forgiveness* (Christensen, Doss, & Jacobson, 2014). This strategy aims to help clients accept their own and each other's limitations and mistakes and forgive themselves and each other. Interpersonally, forgiveness is typically facilitated by the genuine expression of shame and remorse on the part of the offender and acceptance of this emotional "owning up" on the part of the injured party (L. S. Greenberg & Iwakabe, 2011). Although this process occasionally may play out in one episode, it typically plays out over time in multiple mini-episodes that confirm the validity of the process. It cannot and should not be legislated or

imposed. It should emerge over time out of a genuine interpersonal process that has its own logic, rhythm, and pacing. This strategy is particularly important in the resolution of emotional injuries that prevent implementation of the solution sequence. In addition, it is relevant when desired change cannot happen (e.g., a husband cannot empathize with his wife's distress after repeated efforts on the part of the therapist and the wife) in regard to a solution sequence. At this point, accepting the reality of what is and making the best of it becomes the new solution sequence.

This strategy can also be usefully applied to understand and/or redefine interpersonal differences in couples and/or families as deriving from endogenous personality characteristics as opposed to stubbornness or intentionality. For instance, a wife's extrovert tendencies may annoy her introverted husband, putting him in challenging interpersonal situations that make him anxious or uncomfortable. If he can understand that her social outreach is part of her "nature" rather than her desire to make him more social, and if she can understand that his social discomfort is not a psychological defect but part of his "nature," it may be easier for each of them to accept and live amicably with each other.

11. *Facilitating grief and adaptation to loss* (Walsh & McGoldrick, 2004). This strategy involves helping clients deal with loss and grief. This strategy becomes relevant under two circumstances. The first is when coming to terms with loss is the presenting problem. This is typically the case when a client system has experienced the traumatic loss of a family member or an individual member has lost a key activity or role (e.g., job) or capacity (cognitive, emotional, or physical function). For instance, a married couple may come into therapy dealing with the loss of their adolescent daughter after a long and complex battle with her cancer. The second circumstance occurs when grieving or the resolution of loss is not the presenting problem, but constrains the client system's capacity to implement the solution sequence. For instance, a family may present with extraordinary levels of conflict between a mother and her adolescent son after the death of the father in a car accident. In the first session it becomes clear that the conflict functions to help the entire family avoid dealing with their sadness and anger about their loss. Conjoint grief work (grieving together) is particularly important for client systems after

loss to fight the all-too-frequent propensity of client systems to fragment into separate grief silos. Grief work typically entails exploring both the sadness and anger involved in coming to terms with loss. Modern Western societies typically minimize, depreciate, and pathologize grieving, adding a powerful cultural constraint to normal and necessary grieving, which may have to be neutralized by the therapist with psychoeducation and exposure facilitation.

12. *Identifying and transforming emotion recognition and management in addiction.* Dealing with addiction typically encompasses a number of planning metaframeworks. However, virtually all forms of addiction work (substance addictions, eating disorders, sex and gambling addictions) are predicated on the hypothesis that the addiction has developed in part to help the client (as well as the client system) avoid dealing with painful and distressing feelings, especially anxiety. The typical problem sequence involves the emergence of the painful feeling, which is rapidly followed by engagement in the addictive behavior. Subsequently, the client system gets embroiled in a variety of codependent behaviors that facilitate the avoidance. The solution sequence begins with the emergence of the painful or distressing feeling and is followed by appropriate intrapsychic and interpersonal processing of the feeling, which may also entail using the feeling as an initiator of appropriate action. A wife binges and purges in part to avoid her feelings of fear, anger, and abandonment at her husband's withdrawal and possible engagement in an extramarital affair. The couple's therapy focuses on helping her identify these feelings and using them to confront her husband and address his physical and emotional withdrawal. A drug addicted emerging adult has to learn how to experience and manage the fear, shame, and guilt that prevent him from getting the help he needs to become sober and face the developmental challenges he has avoided for years (e.g., finishing school, getting a job, creating meaningful interpersonal relationships).

13. *Identifying constellations of emotions and cognitions as distinct "parts" of a person that may facilitate or constrain solution implementation.* This strategy involves the therapist in helping clients differentiate within themselves and each other distinct cognitive and/or emotional parts of themselves. For instance, helping an angry adolescent son see his anger as one part of himself along with other parts (e.g., a compassionate part, a

frightened part) may allow him to not feel so overwhelmed by his anger and facilitate within him a greater capacity to manage his anger. It may also help his parents see him as more than his angry self. Differentiating parts within individuals helps them to not "totalize" themselves so much ("I am an angry person" or "I am a sad person") and have a greater sense of personal options and alternatives.

Meaning/Emotion and Other Metaframeworks

Meaning/emotion commonly accesses the mind, gender, culture, and spirituality hypothesizing metaframeworks. Mind, gender, and culture, although sources of many strengths, are also obvious sources of constraint in human problem solving as they define what is appropriate and tolerable for people to think and feel. In contrast, spirituality, although a source of constraint at times, is more often relevant as a strength or a component of the solution sequence. Particularly in regard to acceptance, forgiveness, grief, and addiction work, spirituality provides the possibility of some kind of personally transcendent experience that can facilitate problem resolution and the quest for serenity.

The internal process theory that guides the selection of strategies and foci in the meaning/emotion planning metaframework falls primarily within the M1 and secondarily within the M2 categories of the mind hypothesizing metaframework. Within M1, emotions and cognitions are taken at face value and dealt with directly and simply. They are not historicized beyond current relationships and are explored, heightened, or reduced depending on the way they function in regard to the problem and solution sequences. At this level of work, a wife's fear of expressing her anger toward her husband would be dealt with regarding her fears of how he might respond. She would be encouraged to ask him directly how he might respond if she expressed her anger at him. If his response is encouraging, she would then be encouraged to express her anger directly to him in the couple session. If he responds negatively, the therapist would focus on the thoughts and feelings that might be preventing the husband from responding more constructively to his wife's anger. If historical constraints or determinants are addressed at this level of work, they are touched on but do not become the primary foci of the work.

Certain ahistorical aspects of the models of mind discussed in M2 in Chapter 5 also fall within the meaning/emotion planning metaframework. For instance, using aspects of the five-factor personality theory of mind would fall in this category, insofar as it is used to facilitate understanding and acceptance of interpersonal differences. Similarly, the identification of parts within individuals that are not historicized (linked to their pasts) with the use of internal family systems or gestalt therapy models of mind can be relatively simple, straightforward, and helpful in facilitating solution implementation.

Specific models that contain more detailed information about meaning/emotion strategies and techniques include cognitive behavior therapy (Beck, 2011; Meichenbaum, 1977), integrative behavioral couples therapy (Baucom, Epstein, LaTaillade, & Kirby, 2002; Christensen, Jacobson, & Babcock, 1995), emotion-focused therapy for individuals and couples (L. S. Greenberg, 2011; Johnson, 2015), narrative therapy (Freedman & Combs, 1996; White & Epston, 1990), and acceptance and commitment therapy (Hayes, Strosahl, & Wilson, 1999). Fishbane's (2013) work on vulnerability cycles elaborates strategies and techniques for transforming couples' problem sequences.

Biobehavioral Planning Metaframework

The biobehavioral planning metaframework rests on the hypothesis that clients have been unable to resolve their presenting problems because they engage in problem sequences that are dominated by biological constraints. Implementation of their solution sequences requires lifting or modifying these biological constraints. This metaframework involves behavioral and biological strategies aimed at these constraints.

This metaframework is typically drawn on after initial intervention with action and meaning/emotion strategies has not proven successful. Sometimes in the face of overwhelming evidence (e.g., a profoundly depressed and suicidal client who cannot engage in talk therapy or an overwhelmingly anxious client whose capacity to listen or respond appropriately is not available), it might be prudent and appropriate to draw on this planning metaframework earlier in the intervention process along with the action and/or meaning/emotion strategies.

The following strategies fall primarily within the biobehavioral metaframework.

1. *Biobehavioral psychoeducation* (Patterson & Vakili, 2014). This strategy entails teaching client system members about the role of physiological constraints in regard to their problem-solving processes. This not only entails teaching system members about physical disorders and illnesses, but it can also involve helping clients understand the role of biological processes in their problem sequences. For instance, if a couple can understand how their fight-or-flight arousal systems dominate their conflict problem sequences, they may feel less blamed and at fault for their conflict problems and more able to address them without guilt, shame, or blaming. Calming and time-out interventions can be used effectively to reduce arousal and facilitate implementation of solution sequences.

2. *Exercise and fitness* (Blumenthal et al., 2007). This strategy uses exercise and fitness programs to address biological constraints to solution sequence implementation. Cardiovascular exercise (e.g., walking, hiking, running, biking) has been shown to improve mood disorders, anxiety, and attention-deficit/hyperactivity disorder (ADHD). Many clients feel they would rather engage in an exercise and fitness program than take psychotropic medication, and if they can it may well obviate the need for medication and increase overall health and well-being.

3. *Mindfulness*. Mindfulness includes, for example, meditation, yoga, and tai chi (Baer, 2003). This strategy attempts to increase *mindfulness*—a state of personal serenity, awareness, and non-obsessive self-observation. In this strategy, clients can be taught meditation, yoga, or tai chi techniques in session if their therapist knows how. If not, they can be referred to knowledgeable professionals for training. Mindfulness can be useful when the implementation of the solution sequence requires clients to have greater self-awareness (e.g., of holding their breath, heart rate increase, muscular tension), serenity, emotional equilibrium, and self-regulation.

4. *Physical assessment*. This strategy typically involves a referral from the mental health professional (therapist) to a physician or medical institution that can conduct a comprehensive medical "check-up" or evaluation. It is used to determine the extent to which the solution sequence may be constrained by a medical or physical constraint, the resolution of which would require some kind of medical intervention. This strategy should almost always be used when there are any so-called psychosomatic symptoms—physical complaints or symptoms that allegedly derive from or are symptomatic of some kind of psychological process (e.g., anxiety). Physical assessment in this situation is used to confirm or rule out that the problem or symptom does or does not have major physical determinants. A client who complains of gastrointestinal pain for which his primary care physician has been unable to determine any cause should probably be referred for a complete gastrointestinal workup before therapy addresses psychosocial constraints. Similarly, a client complaining of chronic headaches should be referred for a complete headache or migraine assessment as well as a complete neurological assessment to rule out brain tumors or other neurological disorders.

5. *Neuropsychological evaluation and counseling* (Clarkin, Hurt, & Mattis, 1994). This strategy involves the neuropsychological

evaluation of members of the client system who might have some type of chronic and/or degenerative neuropsychological disorder that constrains their ability to participate appropriately in the solution sequence. At least two situations clearly warrant the therapist referring a client for such an evaluation. The first involves a hypothesis that a client might have a cognitive and/or social learning disability. Historically, children and adolescents have been most commonly referred for this type of assessment, although in recent years more adults have been identified as potentially experiencing these disorders. The cognitive disabilities typically manifest themselves primarily but not exclusively in academic domains, whereas the social learning disabilities usually appear in social relations. A variant of social learning disabilities concerns clients who might be undiagnosed and experiencing an autism spectrum disorder. Frequently, people with social learning and autism spectrum disorders are seen as being socially insensitive, stubborn, obsessive, unempathic, or extraordinarily persistent in pursuing certain activities. These characteristics can severely constrain solution sequences.

The second common referral situation concerns older adult clients who might be experiencing the onset of some form of dementia. The unjustifiably jealous 76-year-old wife who becomes obsessed with the notion that her 78-year-old husband is having affairs with her best friends and begins cutting off from them may be experiencing early Alzheimer's. If the evaluation identifies a neuropsychological disorder, the next step entails addressing the disorder, which may involve medication, tutoring, coaching, and the use of technology to supplant deficits. In addition, couples or family therapy is an ideal context to help system members learn the best ways to manage and help the member with the disorder.

6. *Psychopharmacological intervention* (Holtzheimer, Snowden, & Roy-Byrne, 2010). In the United States this is currently the most common intervention for mental disorders and problems. Psychotropic medications have been developed and widely used to treat anxiety, mood disorders, and emotion-regulation problems. Unfortunately, most of these medications have side effects that complicate their use. However, with certain individuals, they can have close to miraculous effects. Because most therapists are not psychiatrists or physicians, the use of psychotropic medications requires referral to a physician with expertise in the use of these medications. Good communication and a good interprofessional alliance facilitate the use of these medications in the context

of IST. In terms of sequencing, these medications would typically be considered after action and/or meaning/emotion strategies have failed to moderate or lift the depressive, anxiety, or emotion-regulation problems sufficiently to permit implementation of the solution sequence. However, as mentioned earlier, if a client's anxiety, depression, or emotion-regulation problems are so extreme that the client cannot appropriately engage or participate in the action and/or meaning/emotion intervention, psychopharmacological intervention may be turned to earlier in the treatment process. In such situations, the medication may make it easier for the client to take advantage of the talk therapy.

7. *Nutritional and allergy evaluation and intervention.* This strategy addresses nutritional and dietary constraints preventing implementation of the solution sequence. Clients may have trouble engaging in solution sequences because they are allergic to certain foods (e.g., peanuts, wheat, dairy, sugars) and the allergic consequences constrain them from acting, feeling, and thinking adaptively. Similarly, certain foods may make it harder for them to function appropriately, although their reaction may fall short of an allergic one. Last, certain nutritional requirements may restrict their ability to engage in normal activities. For instance, having to avoid certain foods may require children to be alone during lunchtime at school, leaving them feeling isolated and lonely. Clients and other system members with allergic and/or nutritional constraints need proper evaluation, education, and training to deal effectively with these constraints.

8. *Addiction evaluation, detoxification, and treatment* (Haaga, McCrady, & Lebow, 2006). This strategy addresses the biological aspects of addiction in client systems in which addiction is a presenting problem and/or a constraint to the implementation of a solution sequence addressing another problem. Typically, clients with substance addictions have to go through some kind of controlled and supervised detoxification process that involves hospitalization or residential treatment. Subsequently, they will often have to continue in some kind of intensive treatment to develop new habits and be physically restricted from their addiction until the new habits and routines take hold. Frequently, they may also need some kind of psychotropic medication as they address the depression or anxiety that drove the addiction. Last, they need "sober time" for their brains and nervous systems to readjust to sobriety, which may also require more residential treatment and/or engagement in a twelve-step program or living in a recovery residence setting.

There are a host of other existing and emerging biobehavioral strategies and techniques (e.g., eye movement desensitization and reprocessing, neurofeedback, transcranial magnetic stimulation, massage, acupuncture), and enumerating them is beyond the scope of this chapter. From the delineation of the aforementioned strategies, it should be clear that "many roads lead to Rome," meaning that biological constraints can be addressed in many different ways with both behavioral and biological interventions. Once again, the use of these strategies by IST therapists usually requires a consultation and collaboration with other health professionals with particular expertise in the specific strategy. The development of coprofessional alliances with these professionals typically facilitates their engagement with clients. Last, biology, mind, and development are the most commonly addressed hypothesizing metaframeworks by the biobehavioral planning metaframework.

A number of specific assessment and intervention models provide more detailed descriptions of strategies and interventions to understand and transform biological constraints, including Fishbane's (2013) work on the role of neurobiology in couples' functioning and couples therapy; mindfulness and meditation (Kabat-Zinn, 2003; Langer, 1992); the use of psychotropic medications (Stahl, 2013); exercise and mental health (Weinberg & Gould, 2014); addiction treatment (McCrady & Epstein, 2013; Morgan & Litzke, 2008, 2013); and collaborative therapeutic neuropsychological assessment (Gorske & Smith, 2009).

Family-of-Origin Planning Metaframework

The major organizing hypothesis for the family-of-origin planning metaframework is that adult clients have been unable to transform their presenting problems because constraints from multigenerational problem sequences concerning their family of origin interfere with the solution sequence. Although these family-of-origin problem sequences have a historical and longitudinal component, they are currently active and function to constrain problem resolution in the here and now. Implementation of the solution sequence requires modifying or lifting these constraints. In some cases, the action and meaning/emotion metaframeworks are sufficient for intervening with these constraints. In other cases, the therapist has to draw also on family-of-origin planning strategies to address the more complex or embedded constraints related to estrangement or the lack of differentiation.

Typically, family-of-origin planning strategies are used under two types of circumstances. The first pertains to clients presenting the family-of-origin problems as their presenting problems. For instance, a mid-40s couple presented for therapy. He worked for his father and was a member of the third generation in their family business. He was depressed and felt marginalized and disrespected by his "dominating and narcissistic" father, but had never confronted his father with his feelings and concerns. His wife was furious at both her father-in-law for what he was doing to her husband and at her husband for being so passive and weak.

The second circumstance pertains to the emergence of family-of-origin problems as constraints to the implementation of a solution sequence to a problem that does not directly involve the adult client's family of origin. For example, a couple in their late 30s presented for therapy. They had two children. The wife had not spoken to anyone from her family of origin for the last 3 years. The couple's presenting problems concerned chronic conflict about money and what the husband described as his wife's constant negativity and criticism. They wanted to work on improving their communication and resolving their conflicts about money. In working with the couple, it became clear that the wife's negativity and insecurity about money related in part to being cut off from her family of origin. She felt hurt by her family's willingness to cut her loose and felt utterly dependent on her husband for financial and emotional support. The therapist cautiously raised the possibility of inviting her parents to come into therapy with the couple to see whether the rupture could be repaired, knowing the suggestion would probably not be received well. This suggestion initiated a conversation between the couple and the therapist that played out over a number of sessions, culminating in the wife inviting her parents to join her and her husband (and the therapist) in a three-session episode of direct family-of-origin work.

The following strategies fall primarily within the family-of-origin metaframework.

1. *Genogram work* (McGoldrick, Gerson, & Petry, 2008). When family-of-origin issues emerge as significant foci in therapy (or at the beginning of therapy with large and complex families), it can be useful to do a *genogram* (multigenerational family diagram). Clients can be asked (after brief instruction) to prepare a genogram at home and bring it in, or the genogram can be done together in therapy. The exploration and discussion of the genogram with a client in a conjoint (couple or family) context provides new and valuable information for the other clients as it simultaneously provides opportunities to dive into certain historical events, alliances, and cutoffs that represent psychosocial nodes in a client's familial history. It also provides a visual aid in assessing transgenerational sequences that may affect, for better or worse, the client system's capacity to implement solution sequences.

2. *Identifying problem sequences from an adult client's family of origin that currently constrain solution sequence implementation* (Kerr &

Bowen, 1988). This strategy involves helping clients see and understand how historical patterns from their family of origin are currently constraining problem sequence identification and/or solution sequence implementation. For instance, a wife–mother in couples therapy with major, objectively unwarranted trust problems may not clearly see how the fact that her mother, grandmother, and great-grandmother were divorced as their families entered the child-launching stage predispose her to fear that will happen to her. Also, she may not understand (opening the gender hypothesizing metaframework) how men have been defined within her family of origin as unreliable and untrustworthy. Alternatively, an overburdened husband–father, the oldest of three brothers, may not see how his widowed mother's need for him to take care of her constrains his capacity to invest in his relationship with his wife and how it also leads both him and his wife to resent his siblings for their lack of involvement with the mother.

3. *Helping clients differentiate themselves from their families of origin* (Bowen, 1978). This broad strategy involves helping adult clients become more differentiated in regard to their family of origin to better transform family-of-origin problem sequences. The key to differentiation is the ability to increasingly be and appropriately express one's "true self" within relationships with an adult's family-of-origin members. For instance, can an enmeshed and overresponsible daughter express her need to take care of herself, her husband, and her children to her dependent mother who has "existed" within a disengaged and unfulfilling marriage for 30 years? Or can a 50-year-old wife–mother tell her father that if he does not turn over the reins of the family business to her within the next couple of years, she will leave and pursue other business opportunities?

4. *Developing, implementing, and evaluating between-session family-of-origin experiments* (Bowen, 1978). This strategy, a specific variant of differentiation of self, entails at least three stages. The first is working with adult clients to develop a plan for them to implement solution sequences with family-of-origin members outside therapy. The second is encouraging, instructing, and supporting them to implement the planned solution sequence. The last stage is evaluating the process (how events played out) and outcome (what worked and what did not) of the implementation. Other clients ideally should be involved in each of these steps. The "untrusting" wife–mother mentioned earlier, in couples therapy, planned with her husband and the therapist to have a

conversation with her mother and grandmother when she went home over the Thanksgiving holidays about their awareness of this pattern and their attitudes toward the men in their lives. They explicitly agreed that the husband should not be present during this conversation. In the session after the Thanksgiving trip, they debriefed. The wife and husband described the difficulty the wife had in getting time alone with her mother and grandmother and how she and her husband strategized on the spot to make it happen. The wife described the honest and painful discussion between the three women that eventually occurred and her sense afterward of having shed a cloak of loneliness and hopelessness. The wife and the therapist helped the overburdened adult son mentioned earlier script the conversations he needed to have with his siblings. He subsequently described how the phone calls went and the subsequent decisions that resulted in a more even and fair distribution of responsibility among the siblings for their mother.

5. *In-session work with family-of-origin members* (Framo, 1992; Pinsof, 1995). This strategy involves facilitating an adult client's work with his or her family of origin in therapy. As with homework, this strategy has at least three stages. The first involves helping the adult client invite his or her family-of-origin members, usually parents, to join his or her individual or couples therapy for an episode of family-of-origin work, which typically involves three sessions with the family-of-origin members, interspersed with regular therapy sessions with the client (and his or her partner if they are in couples therapy). The family-of-origin members are invited by the client to join the therapy as "guests" to improve the client's relationship with the family-of-origin members. The stage also involves planning the family-of-origin sessions, particularly the first one. This planning focuses on the "work" the adult client has to do with his or her family of origin, which consists of extricating himself or herself from the problem sequence and implementing the solution sequence with the family-of-origin member.

   The second stage involves conducting the sessions with the client, his or her partner (who functions primarily as a "witness" to his or her partner's work with his or her family of origin), and the family-of-origin members. The therapist's role in these sessions is to coach and support the client to do the work directly with their family-of-origin members, rather than the therapist doing the work for them. With adequate preparation, the client becomes the leader of the sessions with his or her family of origin. In-between sessions with the client(s) are used to review what happened in the preceding family-of-origin session and plan what will be worked on in the upcoming family-of-origin session.

The last stage involves integrating the family-of-origin work into the primary direct client system—the individual, couple, or family. Typically, this entails integrating the positive changes with the family of origin or, if the family-of-origin members were not able to engage or change appropriately, accepting who they are and making the best of it. The latter may necessitate grief work. The integration aspect of this stage also involves "bringing it home"—taking advantage of loosened or lifted constraints (as a result of the family-of-origin work) to facilitate implementation of the primary solution sequence with the clients. As well as working with the parents of the clients, family-of-origin sessions can be productive with clients' siblings.

The most commonly accessed hypothesizing metaframeworks by the family-of-origin planning metaframework are organization, mind, development, gender, and culture. Family-of-origin sessions are also particularly useful as a prelude to the work within the next planning metaframework, internal representation. Compared with the other planning metaframeworks, there are relatively few, if any, specific therapy models that primarily target family-of-origin constraints. However, numerous authors have written about this type of work as part of their overall therapy program. For instance, Paul and Paul (1986) used a combination of video and family pictures to facilitate imaginal confrontations in the here and now with deceased or unavailable family-of-origin members. Framo (1976, 1992) developed a complete methodology for the engagement of family-of-origin members in therapy. Pinsof (1995) elaborated and expanded Framo's methodology as part of his integrative problem-centered model. Many therapists have written about the use of genograms, but McGoldrick and colleagues' (2008) work is particularly useful and systematic. Of course, Bowen's (1974, 2004) work on differentiation of self within one's family of origin represents one, if not the most, seminal work in regard to family-of-origin therapy. Last, contextual therapy (Boszormenyi-Nagy & Krasner, 1986; Boszormenyi-Nagy & Spark, 1973) addresses how to understand and work with transgenerational loyalties and obligations in family systems.

Internal Representation Planning Metaframework

The guiding hypothesis for this planning metaframework is that clients have not been able to implement their solution sequences because of constraints from internalized (mental) representations of themselves and others (primarily from their family of origin). Typically, these internalized representations derive from repeated experiences in their childhood and adolescence. The general planning hypothesis is that implementation of the solution sequence requires modifying these internalized representations. These representations are best addressed as internalized problem sequences.

The family-of-origin strategies identified previously facilitate identification of internal representations of self and other by differentiating them from the external representations of current self and others (family members). The 70-year-old father of today who just participated in three family therapy sessions with his son and his wife is not the intimidating and powerful father of 35 years ago. Nor is the strong and competent 40-year-old client of today the vulnerable and dependent 5-year-old of times past. After family-of-origin work, it is easier to see that the adult client of today is primarily struggling with the internal as opposed to the external family-of-origin objects. This is not to deny the real complications of dealing with the parents or siblings of today, but these people do not typically have the power and authority attributed to their internal representations.

Internal representation typically works with and "historicizes" the parts of clients that were initially identified in parts of internal family systems work pertaining to the meaning/emotion planning metaframework. It now takes those parts of self and looks at them through a historical lens that links them to early experiences in childhood and assesses their appropriateness or lack thereof in regard to current individual and interpersonal functioning.

The following strategies fall primarily within the internal representation metaframework.

1. *Helping clients identify internal representations of themselves and others.* This strategy involves helping clients become aware of their internalized representations of themselves and/or others (J. P. Siegel, 2015). The key hypothesis (mind metaframework, M2) is that past experiences have left an imprint or representation of those experiences that constrains solution sequences. For example, encouraging a man to invite his mother and father into therapy will "flush out" the internalized representations of himself and his parents. His fear that his father may become enraged at him for challenging him directly depicts the powerful internalized father and the helpless little boy in his mind. The distortion of the self and others is the tip of the iceberg of the internal representations.

    Independent of family-of-origin work, parts of the client may emerge in family, couples, or individual therapy, which suggests the presence of an internal representation. Their emergence is typically associated with some kind of extreme or contextually inappropriate response. A father reported becoming unchar-acteristically punitive in reaction to his son's misbehavior. The therapist asked him when he had seen this part of himself before. He responded, "It is my father. That's the way he used to treat me."

2. *Identifying key events (sequences) associated with the emergence or development of the internalized representations.* The strategy delineates a traumatic or important event in the client's adoles-cence or childhood and/or a series of events that "produced" or crystallized key internal representations. In the earlier example, the father described an incident in which he had lied about something when he was 8 or 9 and his father screamed at him that he would never amount to anything and his life would be one big lie. He felt shamed and hopeless. A woman talked about how she would come home from school and find her mother drunk and unconscious on the living room couch with her little sister playing on the floor. She would get her mother to bed and make dinner for her sister and do her homework after getting her sister to bed. That sequence repeated multiple times, and she developed her "little mother" self who could take care of everyone else and do what needed to be done regardless of what she was feeling or thinking. In fact, her little mother had no feelings or thoughts (they were dissociated and denied); she just rose to the occasion no matter how challenging it was.

3. *Identifying and working with parts of the self* (Perls, 1969; R. Schwartz, 2013) linked to historical relationships and/or events that constrain solution implementation. The little mother part of the woman mentioned before later stopped her from asking her husband or her adolescent children to take care of her when she was tired or upset. Parts interact. One part may "protect" another (the angry part protects the sad part or vice versa), or certain parts may be more available to consciousness than others. This strategy may entail identifying parts of self that constrain solution sequences and modifying or balancing them with alternative parts that facilitate the solution sequence. For instance, asking a man overwhelmed with feelings of inadequacy and incompetence whether there was or ever had been any part of him that felt adequate or competent may elicit some aware-ness of a more adaptive and resilient part of him. If his mother was the over-adequate little mother mentioned earlier, asking him whether there was any part of her in him may facilitate a positive and mobilizing identification with her competence.

Parts work can also involve guided imagery or empty-chair interactions between the parts as means of bringing greater balance and harmony (Breunlin, Schwartz, & Mac Kune-Karrer, 1992) to the self. Internal family systems (R. Schwartz, 2013) elevates and strengthens the self to guide and nurture other parts.

4. *Transference interpretation* (Luborsky & Barrett, 2006). This strategy links and contrasts internalized representations of self and others with current relationships. Typically, this strategy focuses on maladaptive transferences that constrain adaptive problem solving. For instance, a husband experienced his wife as his excessively critical and demanding mother when she asked him to pick his clothes up off the floor. He became inappropriately enraged and defiant, and she withdrew with feelings of fear and contempt. After discussing several of these painful problem sequences, the therapist suggested he might be transferring his feelings of worthlessness and anger in relation to his mother toward his wife. He acknowledged the inappropriateness of his behavior with his wife and began to understand that he is projecting his internalized critical mother onto his wife and experiencing himself as her "bad" and helpless child. His wife felt relieved to see his awakening and his validation of his overreaction to her.

5. *Helping clients understand how internalized representations constrain implementation of the solution sequence within the current client system* (Luborsky & Barrett, 2006; Scharff & Scharff, 2005). In the case of the aforementioned husband, this strategy helped him see how his extreme reactivity to his wife's appropriate criticism alienated, angered, and frustrated her. Recently, rather than go through this problem sequence over and over, she just withdrew from him. He began to worry that she may leave him. He clearly saw that she was not his mother and that his propensity to see her that way constrained him from being a better partner and husband. Similarly, a woman who was physically abused by an older brother may see that she can stand up to her husband when he is angry and that he will not abuse her the way her brother did. She sees that her fear of what her anger may unleash in her husband (her brother's abusiveness) has led her to defer and avoid conflict at almost all costs, which has devitalized their marriage and left her feeling powerless and resentful.

6. *Helping clients take responsibility for their internalized representations* (Gurman, 2008). This strategy helps clients "own" the parts of themselves they transfer or project onto others. The father takes responsibility for his punitive part and commits to

managing it more adaptively when it emerges. The wife–mother takes responsibility for her "little mother" part and reduces her compulsive and exhausting caretaking of others at her own expense. She works on being constructively and appropriately selfish. Taking responsibility typically involves understanding that "this is a part of me that I must understand and manage more adaptively."

7. *Helping clients understand and cope with the internal representations of other family members* (Scharff & de Varela, 2005). This strategy helps the wife understand why her husband is responding to her so inappropriately and helps her point out to him when it may be happening without shaming him for it. This strategy embeds within the client system knowledge about their internal representations and how they maladaptively constrain solution sequence implementation. Internal representation work with a client in front of other clients maximizes the strategy's learning potential.

8. *Helping clients see how certain internal representations can be beneficial* (Scheinkman & DeKoven Fishbane, 2004). An example of this strategy is helping the wife–mother see how her "little mother" helped her survive as a young adolescent and even today comes in handy at tough times. The problem is when it becomes so dominant in her life that she becomes depleted, angry, and resentful. Similarly, a man who grew up with an abusive father and a loving mother who tried to protect him may see his wife as a loving and protective force in his life.

Mind (particularly M2), gender, culture, and development are the most commonly addressed hypothesizing metaframeworks with the strategies of the internal representation planning metaframework. These strategies aim to elucidate and transform internal representations within clients that constrain their ability to implement solution sequences. When the clients are able to reliably implement the solution sequence, internal representation work can be discontinued. Within IST, transformation of internal representations is not a goal in itself, but primarily a vehicle for lifting constraints that prevent problem resolution.

Internal representation strategies and interventions have historically been articulated in psychoanalysis and psychodynamic therapies over the last 100 years. IST draws on more modern versions of these approaches that have been articulated within object relations theory and therapy (Guntrip, 1969; Guntrip & Rudnytsky, 2013; Scharff, 1995; Summers, 1994, 2013) as well as brief psychodynamic therapies that tend to use more here-and-now active strategies (Levenson, 2010; Messer & Warren, 1995). The internal family systems model (Breunlin et al., 1992; R. Schwartz, 2013) has brought a family system's perspective to the understanding of internal representation theory and therapy, viewing the different parts of the psyche (including the self) as a malleable family system.

Self-Planning Metaframework

The chief hypothesis of the self-planning metaframework is that clients have been unable to implement their solution sequence because of constraints that derive from their narcissistic vulnerability and rigidity. Implementing the solution sequence requires increasing their narcissistic resiliency and flexibility. The theoretical core of this planning metaframework, presented in Chapter 5 in regard to the M3 level of mind, views the self as the "cell" of human identity. The self contains the internal representations or psychological objects or parts. The weaker the self, the more rigid and unchangeable the relationships between the objects or parts.

The self needs self-objects (e.g., attachments, important others) over the life course. Self-objects perform self-development and maintenance functions through what Kohut (1971, 1977) called *narcissistic transferences*: mirroring, idealizing, and twinning. In contrast to the classic sense of transference in psychoanalysis as negative and distortive, Kohut's narcissistic transferences are positive, necessary, and sustaining. The self grows in relationship with self-objects through manageable transference disruptions or ruptures, which are followed by empathic repairs. Self-work uses clients' natural and manageable transference disruptions with the therapist or significant others as opportunities for empathic repair and self-growth. Typically, self-strategies are deployed in an individual intervention context. It is difficult to create a sufficiently strong alliance (set of positive narcissistic transferences) with a client in a conjoint context to do sustained narcissistic repair work. Occasionally, the intensely personal work required by this planning metaframework can be done conjointly, but only when the other client(s) is (are) extraordinarily empathic and attuned.

The following strategies fall primarily within the self-planning metaframework.

1. *Helping clients understand how their narcissistic vulnerability constrains implementation of the adaptive solution* (Pinsof, 1995). With a divorced mother, this strategy aims to help her become aware of how her narcissistic vulnerability impedes her capacity to support her daughter's developmentally healthy and appropriate separation. The therapist empathizes with her pain from feeling abandoned and betrayed by her daughter. Using the techniques

of motivational interviewing (Miller & Rollnick, 2012), the therapist might help her see how her efforts to constrain and punish her daughter only drive her further away, leaving her more abandoned and resentful. Typically, this strategy involves two major steps. The first is empathic outreach (mirroring) to the narcissistically constrained client. As this outreach strengthens the alliance, the second step helps the client see her role in the problem sequence and its potentially devastating consequences. In essence, the therapist becomes the empathic self-object that strengthens the client's crumbling sense of self so she can participate in the solution sequence.

2. *Using the vicissitudes of the therapist–client relationship to strengthen vulnerable clients' selves* (Kohut, 1968). This strategy also involves two stages. The first is the construction of a relationship in which the therapist becomes a self-object for the vulnerable client. This means that the therapist and the client have had enough experience with each other so that the therapist becomes a self-object or psychologically significant for the client. The achievement of this goal typically requires time together as well as the occurrence of emotionally significant events or interactions in which the therapist is experienced as a safe, trusted, and competent "other." Achieving the goal of becoming a self-object cannot be dictated ("trust me") or the product of intentional action but occurs as the byproduct of meaningful interactions that progressively test and reveal the trustworthiness and competence of the therapist.

The second stage is the unintentional rupture and the intentional repair by the therapist of the self-object relationship between the client and therapist (Pinsof, 1995). Inevitably, over the course of therapy, the therapist will fail to be properly empathic (mirror failure); will "fall off his or her pedestal" by being late, forgetting something, or saying something "stupid" (de-idealization); or will differentiate himself or herself from the client so that the client feels "different" (twin rupture). These are breaks or ruptures in the narcissistic transference. Their repair involves at least five steps: (a) coidentifying the rupture, (b) taking responsibility for or owning the error ("I really missed the boat with that comment"), (c) empathizing with the client's experience of the rupture, (d) apologizing, and (e) planning with the client to avoid a repeat of the rupture.

The core of IST self-work is the repeated working through of rupture-repair episodes, which progressively strengthen the client's self and diminish his or her narcissistic vulnerability. The ideal is that the clients can function in this way for each other, but by the time the therapist has moved down the matrix to the self-planning metaframework, the client system has demonstrated that the necessary self-development work cannot occur between the clients. It must play out between the therapist and the client in an individual context.

3. *Teaching rupture-repair skills to the client through the therapist–client relationship that can then be used between the client and others.* The hope in the rupture-repair experience between the therapist and the individual client is that as the client's self strengthens, he or she will be more capable of using others as "facilitating" self-objects and vice versa. Rupture-repair experiences between the therapist and client are teaching moments that pave the way for the client to carry their growing emotional and relationship intelligence to others. For instance, a previously narcissistically brittle, domineering, and authoritarian father can learn to deal with his inevitable and understandable failures with his adolescent son as rupture-repair opportunities to help his son become more narcissistically resilient.

4. *Deepening the bond component of the alliance with the client through effective use of self.* With this strategy the therapist makes the relationship with the client more personal, idiosyncratic or unique, and "real" (as a human relationship). This involves being present and caring without losing personal boundaries. For instance, as a client describes a horrendously painful experience in his or her life (e.g., rape, death of a child, a younger brother dying tragically in the arms of his sister) the therapist might cry empathically. Or a therapist might call a client to find out the outcome of a major life event (e.g., surgery of a severely ill child, a doctoral dissertation oral exam, a dreaded confrontation). Under rare circumstances, the therapist might allow the client to be of solace and support. For instance, a therapist who just tragically lost a chronically ill child might allow the client to comfort him or her. This experience can validate the client in that he or she is being treated as a trusted resource by the therapist. This self-work requires emotional maturity and responsibility on the part of the therapist to not turn the client into a self-object.

5. *Developing and tolerating dependency and emotional intensity with the client.* This strategy is to some extent behaviorally silent— it does not have clear behavioral dimensions. It is primarily

experiential. It involves the capacity of the therapist to tolerate being the target or object of the intense feelings and needs of the client without fusing with or cutting off from the client. The therapist must be able to be the target of the client's sadness, desire, pain, need, hope, anger, or fear without "freaking out" and behaving in ways that might shame, reject, or injure the client. For instance, a female client may express intense sexual desire for a male therapist. The therapist must tolerate this experience without gratifying or shaming the client. Similarly, a client's expression of intense need for the therapist ("How can you go away and leave me for 2 weeks?") should trigger empathic versus defensive or aggressive behavior toward the client.

6. *Awakening the self to embrace disowned or dissociated parts*. When solution implementation is constrained by the failure of certain parts or aspects of a person's mind to be integrated or connected to other parts or aspects, the therapist should facilitate the integration. In the language of internal family systems, this entails helping the constrained client's self take leadership and restore connection and harmony between its parts. This may entail helping the client see that something she has projected on others (e.g., anger, fear, vulnerability, despair, greediness) is actually a part of her that should be included in her internal family. Frequently, the therapist may act as the bridge that connects the disconnected parts, empathically accepting what must be faced. This empathic bridging models for the client how to break down the psychic silos that prevent integrated functioning and adaptive action. This strategy is particularly important with clients with personality disorders and historical trauma sequelae that prevent solution implementation.

7. *Integrating spirituality to facilitate acceptance and transcendence*. This strategy builds on the use of mindfulness as a strategy for facilitating acceptance and serenity. However, the use of mindfulness in regard to the here-and-now planning metaframeworks views it more as a technique for self-calming and meditation. The self-planning metaframework involves a deeper and more profound use of spirituality to address psychic pain, loss, and self-constriction. Hard to articulate and specify, this strategy involves facilitating clients' acceptance of themselves, their lives, their injuries, and their own and each other's limitations. It frequently involves a felt awareness of a higher power or force that transcends the individual and an acceptance of death, with-

out losing joy, pleasure, and connection. This strategy involves a nonverbal wisdom and grace on the part of the therapist of which clients can avail themselves almost osmotically. This level of spiritual awareness expands the self (not the ego) and facilitates the solution sequence as well as awareness and graceful management of constraints.

THE INTERVENTION CONTEXTS

IST focuses primarily on natural systems with a history and future that respectively precede and follow the therapeutic episode. This focus embodies the legacy of family therapy. The assumption in individual and group therapy is that clients will transfer what they have learned in therapy to their natural systems—their family, marriage, and/or other important relationships. Unfortunately, this is rarely the case. When children and adolescents are treated individually, no matter how much progress they make, if their family does not support or welcome their changes, they seldom persist. Similarly, a married client in group or individual therapy who has a troubled marriage and who is unsupportive of the changes he or she makes with the therapist and/or group is likely to regress or get divorced posttherapy.

Recognizing the challenges associated with what early behaviorists called *transfer of learning*, family therapists decided to work with the "system"—the interpersonal context in which the client was embedded. If the system changed or if the individual changed in the context of a system that welcomed the change, the likelihood of maintaining the changes posttherapy increased. This profound shift was at the core of family therapy and is at the core of IST. This is not to say that individual therapy or group therapy are not useful. They have a place in IST, but we prefer, when feasible and appropriate, to change the problem sequences by working directly with the couple or family system.

Direct Intervention Contexts

An intervention context defines which members of the client system are directly involved in the session—the direct system context. As reflected in Figure 6.1, the context and planning metaframework matrix, there are three primary intervention contexts in IST: (a) family, (b) couple, and (c) individual. IST aims to transcend the concept of what are frequently referred to as *therapeutic modalities* with the concept of intervention contexts. We view context as a more flexible and less theoretically laden concept than modality. IST therapists frequently use multiple contexts during the treatment of a single case or client system.

The integrative component of IST is at the core of the modality–context distinction. IST is not a family, couples, or an individual therapy approach. It uses all three contexts as appropriately and flexibly as possible to transform the problem sequences of the client system. As such, IST integrates family, couples, and individual therapy into a unified, multimodal approach that uses the most appropriate context to facilitate change.

Family Context

The family context includes two or more family members (excluding couple sessions, which define the couple context). It is often multigenerational—involving members from different generations—but may consist of adult siblings or important friends within the same generation. In such cases, the role expectations tend to be symmetrical or similar. Often, though, some degree of role complementarity (different but reciprocal role expectations) characterizes the family context, in that one or more family members function in some parental role and the others in a more dependent role. This complementarity is evident in dealing with parents and their young children as well as with midlife and older adult children caring for aging parents.

Although two or more family members define a family context, it does not follow that any one subsystem of the family is the ideal group to convene. For example, much current child and adolescent therapy involves the child or adolescent and a caregiver. More often than not, that caregiver is the mother. The experience of early family therapists was that involving the mother and allowing the father to remain extraneous to the therapy was a clinical mistake (Minuchin, 1974). Beyond marginalizing fathers as a resource and overburdening mothers, it overlooked the extent to which the child or adolescent's problem may perform a homeostatic or regulatory function for the couple—regardless of whether the parents were married or cohabitating. By defining the family context as two or more members, we do not condone the failure to engage both parents, as well as other family members, directly in the treatment of a child.

Couple Context

The couple context involves two people who consider themselves to have a committed relationship—a relationship with a past and potentially a future. This inclusive definition covers married couples, dating couples, unmarried cohabiting couples, and unmarried cohabiting coparents. Couple partners may be straight, gay, lesbian, or transgender.

Individual Context

The individual context involves one individual from the client system directly in therapy. In IST, this context is appropriate when the rest of the client system is not available (e.g., student at university, client living in a different location), when the other members refuse therapy, when the person initiating therapy insists on being seen individually, and when constraints to the solution sequence cannot be adequately addressed in any other context (e.g., an adolescent struggling with coming out, a wife in an affair who cannot decide what she wants to do with her marriage, mind-M3 constraints). The critical distinction between individual context work in IST and more conventional individual therapy is the "map." As articulated in Chapter 2, the IST therapist sees the individual client as part of a client system. Chapter 11 further elaborates individual context work in IST.

PLANNING GUIDELINES

IST embodies a set of guidelines that sequence intervention contexts and planning metaframeworks over the course of therapy—guiding the therapist as to what to do when. The large arrow (and to a lesser extent by the small arrow) in Figure 6.1 expresses these guidelines.

Failure-Driven Guideline

The first principle that sequences interventions in IST is the failure-driven guideline, which states: Therapeutic shifts occur when the current interventions fail to modify the web of constraints sufficiently to permit implementation of the solution sequence. This guideline directly addresses the question, What should I (we) do when what we are doing is not working? The sequence of presentation of the planning metaframeworks is the sequence in which they should be deployed in practice. This order of deployment is subject to exceptions based on special circumstances or compelling hypotheses. The shift from one metaframework to the next occurs in the face of the higher or preceding metaframeworks' strategies' failure to remove or ameliorate the constraints to the solution sequence. The following guidelines elaborate the rationale for the progressive use of therapy contexts and planning metaframeworks.

Interpersonal Guideline

The large arrow in the planning matrix (Figure 6.1) operationalizes a number of critical features of IST. Beyond the failure-driven guideline, the second core principle that drives the IST progression, particularly the progression of planning contexts, is the interpersonal guideline. It asserts that when possible and appropriate it is always preferable to do an intervention, regardless of its nature, within an interpersonal (family or couple) as opposed to an individual context. Multiple advantages derive from this guideline. First, it maximizes the direct impact and transformative power of the intervention. For instance, if an emotionally constricted husband in individual therapy connects with and expresses his grief (with tears) about the death of his father, the breakthrough affects him and possibly the therapist. However, if the same breakthrough occurs in a couple context, his wife has the direct experience of seeing and feeling her husband transformed. The rules of their relationship (she feels, and he thinks) change, at least momentarily. If he comes home from his individual session and tells her what happened, it has less impact than if she witnessed it directly. That opportunity is lost if she is not present.

Second, the interpersonal guideline increases the learning and assessment opportunities for the therapist (and clients) by providing direct observation of clients in action. When the emotionally constricted husband has his emotional breakthrough in the presence of his wife, the therapist has the opportunity to observe directly her reaction. Does she get tears in her eyes and touch him, or does she look out the window and fidget uncomfortably? The tears or outreach response suggests that she has the desire and capacity to welcome the change in her husband and that her reaction will not constrain further change. In contrast, the look away or fidget response would lead the therapist to hypothesize that the wife is uncomfortable with the change and that exploration of what constrains her from responding more adaptively would be in order.

Another advantage is that it facilitates the expansion of the "observing ego" and psychological mindedness of the client system. A 14-year-old girl with an eating disorder tells her therapist that when she feels anxious, she is afraid to reach out to her parents for fear of burdening them. It is easier to binge and purge to forget her feelings because "no one knows about it." If that interaction occurs in the presence of her parents, their understanding of their role in her disorder increases and has direct action potential. They can address and hopefully replace her "overburdened attribution" with a demonstration of their interest in hearing what she feels. The members of the client system now understand a central driver of their problem sequence and can work together to implement a new solution sequence.

Similarly, a husband realizes that his intense feelings of shame and worthlessness when his wife does not want to make love derive from his mother's sexual provocativeness to him after his parents divorced. If he even looked at her when she would walk around in her underwear, she would shame him and accuse him of being sick and perverse. If his wife is present when this insight and the feelings linked to it emerge, she is far more likely to respond to him empathically when he expresses disappointment and distress when she says "not tonight." The critical concept is that when insights, new meanings, and deeper understanding emerge if client system members are present, the new understanding and meaning rests on a broader cognitive foundation. This builds the collective observing ego of the client system and the observing ego of the client.

Clinical Implications of the Interpersonal Guideline

The interpersonal guideline has a number of direct clinical implications. For instance, if a married or partnered adult presents for therapy, regardless of his or her presenting problem (with certain exceptions delineated as follows), he or she should ideally be seen with his or her partner for the first session (couple context). A child or adolescent presenting for therapy, regardless of the presenting problem, should ideally be seen with his or her parents and possibly siblings. A therapist in couples therapy who has to explore a wife's early trauma history should initially attempt to do so in the presence of her husband. In IST it is always better to do work in an interpersonal context if possible and appropriate.

A second clinical implication of the interpersonal guideline involves the concept of "key" clients. A *key client* is a member of the client system who plays a major role in preventing the client system from interrupting the problem sequence and/or a major role in the implementation of the solution sequence. In other words, he or she is a major part of the problem and/or the solution. Key clients usually have a significant degree of power within the client system. With a spouse presenting for therapy, IST assumes that his or her partner is a key client. With child and adolescent identified clients, the parents automatically fall into the key client role. In certain client systems siblings, grandparents, extended family members, friends (or enemies), and school or work personnel may have key client status by virtue of their role(s) within the client system. It is essential to include key clients directly or indirectly in planning interventions. Whether they become members of the direct client system depends on the collective judgment of the therapist and key clients. Sometimes a key client is best dealt with by keeping her or him in the indirect system, but planning for his or her role in the problem and/or solution sequence. For instance, a schizophrenic or borderline client may become dysregulated if present for a cathartic and empathic session with the other key clients. Like the client system concept, the key client concept is ineluctably ambiguous, a heuristic device to simplify the playing field.

Exceptions to the Interpersonal Guideline and the Alliance Priority Guideline

Of course, there are many exceptions to the interpersonal guideline that have to do with feasibility, appropriateness, and alliance. *Feasibility* concerns the availability of other members of the client system. If they are not geographically or physically available, the client can and should be seen individually (although it may be worthwhile to invite them to "visit" for several sessions). *Appropriateness* refers to whether a topic can and/or should be discussed in front of certain members of the client system. For instance, a husband wanting to explore whether to stay in his marriage or get divorced and marry the woman with whom he has been having an affair for 2 years could not fully explore his feelings and thoughts, at least initially, in the presence of his wife. Similarly, a couple in family therapy could not and should not explore their marital problems in any depth, particularly their sexual problems, in the presence of their children.

A critical exception to the interpersonal guideline concerns its interaction with the therapeutic alliance. To address this exception IST uses the *alliance priority guideline*, which asserts that growing, maintaining, and repairing the therapeutic alliance takes priority over other planning guidelines unless doing so fundamentally compromises the efficacy and integrity of the therapy. For instance, when an individual client refuses to be seen initially with "other" appropriate members of the client system after repeated attempts on the part of the therapist to include them, the therapist should see the client individually. The 16-year-old boy who refuses to be seen with other members of his family should be seen individually. The 43-year-old wife who refuses to be seen with her husband after the therapist has tried to convince her to include him in the initial session should be seen alone. However, if after time and work in an individual context it becomes apparent that the other members of the client system have to be involved, the therapist may have to insist that the client includes them or the therapy cannot continue.

Last, in regard to how to include other system members in the therapy, there are several important strategies. The first concerns who invites the other members. The operating principle is to start with the client inviting the other members to participate, and if that does not work, the therapist can then invite them in. Consistent with the IST strength guideline, this strategy—get the client to do the work, and if they cannot, show them how—assumes that the client has the skills and capacity to do what has to be done. If they demonstrate that they do not, the therapist can do it with the client as a coconsultant, model, and partner in the process.

The second strategy controls the message. This involves strategizing with the client about how he or she will ask the others to be involved. It is essential to avoid a "blaming" outreach that implies they have to come in because they are the cause of the client's problem. Rather, others have to be asked to come to help the therapist and client do their work. Invitees can provide an alternative perspective on what has been going on and what has to change. They can enrich the client's and therapist's understanding of the problem and the solution. We discourage using family and couples therapy language. The client or therapist should not say, "Please come in because this is family (or couples) therapy," rather, "Please come in because you and your perspective can help us understand what is going on and what can be done to improve things." Also, the invitation asks the others to come in for a session or two, not necessarily to join the therapy for the duration. If it makes sense for them to continue to be involved after the initial sessions, it usually will be obvious to everyone and will be a natural outgrowth of the session(s).

Temporal Guideline

This guideline, also reflected in the downward-pointing arrow in the matrix, asserts that therapy begins with a focus on the here and now and progresses to the past as more complex and remote constraints emerge. In other words, therapy focuses interventions on the past only as here-and-now interventions fail to transform the problem sequence. In the planning matrix, the top three planning metaframeworks—(a) action, (b) meaning/emotion, and (c) biobehavioral—are the here-and-now or contemporary planning metaframeworks. The bottom three metaframeworks—(a) family of origin, (b) internal representation, and (c) self—are the there-and-then or historical planning metaframeworks.

Cost-Effectiveness Guideline

The concept of cost-effectiveness is implicit in the large downward sloping arrow in Figure 6.1. The cost-effectiveness guideline asserts that therapy begins with less expensive (in terms of time or duration and money), more direct, and less complex interventions and moves to more expensive, indirect, and complex interventions, as needed. Stated simply, take the shortest, most direct, and simplest route before taking a longer, less direct, and more complex route. Consistent with the strength guideline, the cost-effectiveness guideline assumes that the client system possesses the resources to solve the problem and implement the solution sequence with minimal and direct intervention—until proven otherwise. Strategies and techniques within the upper three planning metaframeworks tend to be thought of as cost-effective. However, if feedback indicates they do not work, the therapist modifies hypotheses about the web and acknowledges the value of drawing strategies and interventions from lower on the matrix.

Small Arrow and the Problem-Centered Guideline

The small arrow in the matrix in Figure 6.1 links to the problem-centered guideline, which asserts that the process of therapy must always be linked, directly or indirectly, to presenting problems—the problems for which the clients are seeking help. Thus, as the therapeutic process moves down the matrix, as indicated by the large arrow, the process never loses its link to the presenting problem and the changes that have to occur in the action, meaning/emotion, or biobehavioral metaframeworks.

The small arrow gets at the question of how far down the matrix the therapy has to go. The therapy has to progress down the matrix to the point where the client system can implement an appropriate and effective solution sequence that solves or sufficiently ameliorates the presenting problem. In this sense, the progression down the matrix is not an ideal progression, but rather a necessary progression that occurs, as needed, until the solution sequence can be implemented. In IST, deeper or further down the matrix is not better. In regard to the "how far to go down the matrix" question, the answer is "as far as necessary."

Education Guideline

This last planning guideline pertains to the role of the therapist. The IST education guideline views therapy as an educational process in which therapists give away their skills, knowledge, and expertise as quickly as clients can integrate them. The IST therapist is a teacher who teaches clients more effective psychosocial problem-solving skills individually and collectively. The therapist's goal is to be just good enough. One consequence of the guideline is that at key points in therapy when solution sequences are falling into place, the therapist, like a good parent, will do less of the work to facilitate client growth. The therapist may interrupt and label a micro problem sequence in session several times and then sit passively as the clients play it out without therapist input. This planned passivity induces clients to be their own therapists as quickly as possible. Just as a good teacher expects his or her students to learn, the IST therapist expects change and sensitively communicates that expectation to clients.

One of the strongest messages that IST therapists want to get across to clients is the value of failure and the impossibility of perfection. When suggesting or encouraging certain solution sequences, the therapist is not sure they will work. If the suggested solution sequence does not work, it is an opportunity to understand the client system's web of constraints more fully and try again. Just as the therapist has to read the feedback from his or her interventions (see Chapter 8), clients have to try things, read the feedback, re-hypothesize about the constraints, and try again. The therapist is teaching the clients to internalize the essence of IST (Chapter 3) and the blueprint (Chapter 4) and, ultimately, to be able to use both on their own. In educating clients, a major hope and goal is that they will sustain and integrate their changes and learn to apply the new problem-solving principles they have learned to other problems in the future.

Flexible Arrows

In the matrix in Figure 6.1, both the large arrow and the smaller reverse arrow in it are depicted with dotted as opposed to continuous or solid lines. The dotted quality of these lines and the arrow figures connotes a light touch or flexibility in the application of the planning guidelines. The movement down the matrix, ideally in the face of failure, is not a rigid or absolute rule. The guidelines should be applied with flexibility and sensitivity to feedback. With certain clients, in the face of extraordinarily clear or overwhelming evidence (e.g., a terrible trauma history), it may make sense to move down the matrix more quickly. Similarly, following the matrix, IST therapists would recommend using psychotropic medication (from the biobehavioral planning metaframework) after giving action and meaning/emotion strategies a good try, but not before that. However, for certain overwhelmingly depressed, anxious, or psychotic clients who are prevented by depression or anxiety from being able to engage in the action or meaning/emotion strategies, medication may be an essential initial intervention. A final point regarding flexibility is that at certain points in therapy a skilled therapist will draw strategies or interventions from multiple planning metaframeworks at the same time. A therapist providing long-term individual psychotherapy to a client whose problem sequences contain both depressed mood and narcissistic vulnerability may use behavioral activation (action planning metaframework) to address the depressed mood while carefully monitoring and managing a client's intense affect and dependency to address deeply embedded constraints of mind (self-planning metaframework). The dotted arrows of the matrix and the guidelines (not rules) are meant to suggest their flexible, clinically responsible, and creative use.

Termination and the Problem-Centered Episode

IST conceptualizes therapy as occurring in episodes (sets of sessions) that address specific presenting problems. As depicted in the first chapter, these therapy episodes occur over the life course of individual members and at different stages in the life cycle of a family. The IST therapist is a primary health care professional available to the individual and families he or she has treated over the course of their lives. If he or she cannot provide the necessary therapeutic strategies, he or she will find and coordinate the professionals with the skills and knowledge to do so. The IST therapist is equivalent to a family physician who is available to the "system" to help with whatever psychosocial problem is being experienced.

An IST therapist may help a young newly partnered couple deal with the challenges of establishing healthy boundaries in relationship with their families of origin. Years later the therapist may help them deal with the loss of marital intimacy associated with the birth of their second child and the challenges of dual careers. Five years later, the therapist may help them find a neuropsychologist and educational therapist to help them with their second child's ADHD. Skipping ahead, 20 years later that child, now a 25-year-old adult living in another city, may ask the therapist to help find a therapist where he or she is living with his or her partner so they can decide whether they should get married or end their conflictual relationship.

The implication of this perspective in regard to ending therapy is that a therapy episode ends when the presenting problem has been addressed sufficiently to permit the client system to proceed as well as possible on their life course. Ideally, the presenting problems of the episode will be resolved completely, but frequently that may be impossible as originally conceptualized. The therapy may end when new solution sequences moderate the presenting problems sufficiently. The solution sequence for certain problems in certain episodes may entail acceptance of the presenting problem rather than trying to eradicate it. For instance, the pain of certain losses may never go away, but can be better lived with when the pain is shared with others, understood, and accepted. Termination is "goodbye for now." Essentially, this episode is closed, the learning from it consolidated as much as possible (learning inevitably continues after termination), regression planning is discussed, and goodbyes are said (Lebow, 1995).

THE IDIOSYNCRATIC AND IMPROVISATIONAL NATURE OF INTEGRATIVE SYSTEMIC THERAPY

The way in which an IST therapist negotiates moving down the matrix with a case will be unique to him or her as well as to the client system. Each client system has a unique set of constraints and will find, with the therapist's assistance, their own solution sequences. IST is not cookie cutter therapy. An IST episode is a structured and improvisational event that plays out over time.

A therapist's choice of strategies and techniques within a planning metaframework inevitably reflects that therapist's preferences, values, and sensibilities. A more affect-oriented therapist will tend to select more emotion-focused strategies and techniques from the meaning/emotion metaframework, whereas a more cognitively oriented therapist will select more cognitively focused strategies and techniques. That is expected and natural.

In addition, no therapist could ever master all the strategies in a planning metaframework and therefore must work collaboratively, developing alliances with other professionals to help the client system get what it needs to implement the "best possible" solution sequences to its problems. In addition, each planning metaframework is an open system, growing with the emergence of new knowledge and technologies. As such, the planning metaframeworks are evolving structures to help therapists grow and find the best resources for their clients.

7

CONVERSING

John and Dorothy, a married couple with no children, sought therapy to address an impasse that threatened their once stable 25-year marriage. The problem was that John, a partner in a law firm, had been offered a managing director position at a branch of the firm in another city. He viewed it as the chance of a lifetime and wanted to accept; moreover, his current job was highly stressful and was affecting his health. Dorothy, a psychotherapist, had a thriving private practice and did not want to move and have to rebuild her practice in a place where she had no reputation. She opposed the move. In a session, they had the following exchange.

> *John:*   This chance won't come along again, Dorothy. I know it's not good for your career, but we'll be financially secure, and I'll be able to get out before I drop dead from a heart attack.

> *Dorothy:*   Everything you say about this is absolutely correct, but I feel like I sacrificed for your career already. Now that I have a

http://dx.doi.org/10.1037/0000055-007
Integrative Systemic Therapy: Metaframeworks for Problem Solving With Individuals, Couples, and Families,
by W. M. Pinsof, D. C. Breunlin, W. P. Russell, J. L. Lebow, C. Rampage, and A. L. Chambers

good reputation that makes my practice thrive, I just don't want to leave it and have to start all over. You can go if you must, but I think I'll stay here.

John: Really, what would happen to us if we solved it that way? [Both turn and look expectantly at the therapist.]

Before reading further, imagine that you, the reader, are the therapist. What, if anything, would you say to this couple, and why would you choose that response? Some therapists might remain silent and wait for Dorothy and John to move the conversation forward. For some therapists, their preferred model of therapy would dictate what to say. This would be particularly true of manualized treatments. Other therapists would privilege the alliance and respond in a way that preserves it. Therapists who hold a radical common factors view of therapy would say that so long as attention is paid to the common factors (reviewed in Chapter 2, this volume), the therapist's behavior at any moment has little impact on the outcome of therapy.

Because integrative systemic therapy (IST) is an integrative therapy, the therapist has many conversational options. The chosen option emerges from considerations that are described in this chapter. We describe three possible responses. If the therapist reads the feedback and fears a split alliance might result if something is said that gives the impression the therapist is supporting one position over the other, the response might be an empathic statement intended to strengthen the alliance with both John and Dorothy—for example:

Therapist: I can see how terribly difficult this is for both of you.

If the therapist read the feedback from their interaction and hypothesized that gender imbalances might be constraining a resolution of the impasse, the therapist might say something to address the possible imbalance:

Therapist: Dorothy, you just said that in the past you have supported John's career. Throughout your marriage, when other hard choices had to be made, would you say that your voice was given equal consideration?

If the conversation between John and Dorothy happened as part of an enactment in which they had been directed to talk to each other about the impasse, the therapist might have requested they continue that conversation. Using statements and a directive, the therapist might say:

Therapist: This is a hard conversation, and I am wondering if you guys have ever gone beyond this point in it. Push ahead and see what you can uncover.

THE INTEGRATIVE SYSTEMIC THERAPY APPROACH
TO THERAPEUTIC CONVERSATION

As noted in Chapter 2, IST adopts a moderate common factors view of therapy. This view asserts that what therapists do in therapy does matter to the outcome; therefore, the therapeutic conversation becomes an important component of the change process. The conversation should be conducted with careful attention given to what the therapist says and how the therapist speaks. What the therapist says, however, should ideally arise strictly from what is said by the clients during the conversation. It is axiomatic, therefore, that IST therapists be skilled listeners because it is what they hear that guides what they say (Nichols, 2009).

IST therapists use the essence diagram (see Figure 3.1) and the blueprint (see Figure 4.1) to orient to the therapeutic conversation. The essence diagram described in Chapter 3 enables therapists to keep track of where they are in the problem-solving process. Recall that this process includes defining the problem, embedding it in a problem sequence, constructing and implementing a solution sequence, and identifying and lifting constraints. As we demonstrate, success with these components rests largely on the therapeutic conversation.

The therapist's contribution to the conversation also flows from information contained in the blueprint. Conversation is embedded in hypothesizing, planning, and reading feedback. The therapist always holds a hypothesis and uses conversation to confirm or disconfirm it. Hypotheses are coded with the hypothesizing metaframeworks, each of which has its own language: organization, development, culture, mind, gender, biology, and spirituality. For example, a therapist hypothesizing that a struggle the parents have with their daughter, Rebecca, involves a developmental oscillation might say, "It must be distressing that sometimes Rebecca acts like she is 2 and at other times like she is 22."

The therapist also draws on the planning metaframeworks when crafting a solution sequence. The previous chapter introduced the matrix that constitutes an integrative scheme for cataloging the plethora of strategies and interventions available to IST therapists. When IST therapists use an intervention originally associated with a particular model of therapy, they approximate the specific conversational requirements of that intervention. For example, if the therapist believes that client misattributions are part of the problem sequence, a cognitive restructuring exercise might be introduced as part of the solution sequence. This intervention relies on the conversational method of Socratic questioning that enables clients to discover other ways to think about what is distressing to them. In this instance, IST therapists must understand what is gained by approaching cognitive restructuring this way, but because Socratic questioning is but one of several ways questioning occurs in conversation, the IST therapist may never reach a level of expertise with Socratic questioning demanded by cognitive behavior therapy. In operating this way, IST therapists trade depth of expertise for range of expertise, believing this range enables a more flexible approach when therapy is not working.

Therapists are continually reading client and therapist feedback and sometimes sharing this with clients—for example, "Your facial expression made me wonder whether you are skeptical about what I just said." Feedback is the driver of the conversation because it anchors conversation to the clients and their needs, both globally with respect to goals and moment-to-moment as they reveal themselves in session. Feedback is so important that it occupies its own place in the blueprint and is the focus of the following chapter.

IST conversations are integrative in that they effectively blend conversational elements drawn from the models of psychotherapy. Just as hypothesizing and planning metaframeworks enable therapists to use both theories and interventions from the models without having to practice the model first, so too does an integrative conversation transcend specific model-driven conversations. An integrative conversation that is essentially a blend of conversational styles may seem fraught with challenges because so many conversational rules of the models seem at odds with each other. This is true from within the logic of the models, but not true once the conversational element has been lifted from the model. Some models of therapy hold that therapists should only ask open-ended questions—for example, "Please tell me more about your fears." Other models champion questions that are closed, such as circular questions—for example, "If you knew more about what happens when he visits his father, would you have fewer fears?" Depending on the circumstances, an open- or closed-ended question might be more appropriate for the therapeutic moment, and therefore, both should be part of therapists' integrative-conversational capability.

Clients and therapists both contribute to the conversation through their different roles. Clients seek therapy to get help in solving their problems. Therapists offer help by bringing their training, experience, and expertise to the problem-solving exercise. Help is mediated through the conversation. IST approaches these conversations as collaborative exercises. Clients are experts on the "local knowledge" that explains their experience and contextualizes their problems. For example, lesbian, gay, bisexual, transgender, and questioning or queer clients and ethnic minority clients have experiences of oppression that have shaped their way of being in the world. Therapists must welcome and embrace their stories of oppression to understand how oppression contextualizes their problems. IST therapists recognize, however, that the clients have sought their help; therefore, therapists openly offer their expertise. This expertise is conveyed respectfully through the therapeutic conversation that is guided by the essence diagram, the blueprint, and the alliance guideline.

For expertise to be introduced in the therapy, IST therapists assume a leadership role in the conversation. The therapist listens to the clients, but the conversation is not solely client driven. IST therapists exercise leadership by engaging actively in the conversation. They guide the conversation and interject themselves in ways that make the essence of IST possible. For IST therapists, the ongoing challenge is when and how to interject something of value into the conversation. We explain why and how therapists interject as we examine the anatomy of a therapeutic conversation.

Embedded in the IST approach to therapeutic conversation is the notion that leadership includes influence. Even though decisions are made with clients collaboratively, the therapist is always making suggestions about how clients focus on, think about, and change their system. To maximize the benefits of influence and to avoid damaging the alliance, IST therapists carefully measure their words so they are readily understood, resonate, and have an impact on clients. This is true regardless of the client system in the room; however, it is particularly relevant when two or more clients are present for therapy. The therapist's words influence the entire client system, both the direct and indirect parts of it. For example, each spouse in a marriage will feel the therapist's effort to influence a problem sequence. An obvious example is the structuring of high conflict interaction in which the therapist conspicuously uses conversation to de-escalate the conflict so a more constructive conversation can take place.

FUNCTIONS OF AN INTEGRATIVE SYSTEMIC THERAPY CONVERSATION

IST conversations serve four interlocking functions. The first is to develop and maintain therapeutic relationships. The second is to develop an understanding of the client system. The third is to engage clients in the process of change. Finally, the fourth is to structure the therapy. At times, the conversation completely privileges one of the functions. At other times, the functions are combined. For example, a structuring conversation may take place because the therapist is concerned that something about the structure is threatening the therapeutic relationship. The functions are embedded into the flow of a conversation that to a layperson sounds like any other conversation. What is different is the way IST therapists use conversation to skillfully weave the functions together as they pursue the goal of solving the problem.

Building Relationships

IST therapists build relationships through thoughtful consideration of the alliance. Knowing that the alliance grows out of three components— (a) bonds, (b) goals, and (c) tasks (Pinsof & Catherall, 1986)—IST therapists pay close attention to each. The therapeutic conversation is the vehicle through which therapists build bonds with their clients, using conversation to demonstrate their attunement to the clients. They use active listening skills to let the clients know they have been heard. They use accurate empathy, congruence, and positive regard to show acceptance of their clients (Truax & Carkhuff, 1967).

Building bonds is a necessary but not sufficient component of forming and maintaining an alliance. IST therapists also attend to the other two components of the alliance: goals and tasks. In IST, goal setting and task implementation are packaged through the goal of solving the problem and the tasks that are part of the solution sequence. The functions of building relationships and engaging clients in the process of change are both part of forming and maintaining the alliance. The alliance guideline stipulates that the preservation of the alliance takes priority over therapeutic interventions; hence, unless the therapist chooses to say something knowing it will tear the alliance, the therapist first calculates the impact on the alliance and either chooses not to say it or to say it with great care so as to preserve the alliance.

IST agrees that building and maintaining relationships inevitably includes transference and countertransference issues, here defined simply as the inappropriate repetition in the present of a relationship that historically was important to the clients or the therapist. Whereas psychodynamic therapies use the transference between therapist and client(s) to create change, in IST, the emphasis is more on monitoring transference issues so they do not negatively affect the alliance. The way a therapist presents himself or herself to clients in IST, therefore, is not the psychodynamic "opaque screen" but rather that of an authentic self that is transmitted through the therapeutic conversation. This authenticity sometimes encompasses issues of transference and countertransference, but authenticity is also created in the open process through which the therapist engages clients in problem solving and sometimes through a discrete use of self-disclosure.

Developing an Understanding of the Client System

Although it is a challenge to understand an individual who presents with a single problem (e.g., a single adult with generalized anxiety disorder), it is far more challenging to understand the client systems and their multiple problems treated in IST. To be successful, IST therapists use conversation to develop and test hypotheses that enable them to understand the client system.

Conversations use the language of problems, sequences (both problem and solution sequences), and constraints. Problems are rarely monolithic. Rather, clients often describe multiple interrelated problems that must be named and prioritized. Problems also exist in a context that is ultimately boiled down to a problem sequence. However, therapists must understand the interpersonal nature of the context. For each problem, the multiple perspectives held by the clients must be patiently heard and validated in the conversation. An additional complication is that often one or more people who are relevant to the problem are not in attendance at the outset of therapy, so the therapist must inquire about their contribution.

Ultimately, therapists are using conversations to extract the problem sequence out of the context. These sequences involve recursive chains of action, meaning, and emotion that must be meticulously pieced together. Clients rarely see the essential components of the chain, so therapists use conversation to patiently help them understand the relevance of any given component. For example, a couple presented with a relationship that had been distant for 5 years because the wife had had an affair. She complained that there was no warmth in the marriage and that when she and her husband did occasionally have sex, it was perfunctory. Finally, after much discussion, the husband revealed that he had made a vow to himself to punish his wife for the affair by never again passionately kissing her. Their exchanges of affection were, therefore, devoid of any erotic feeling. Once this behavior, the meaning of it, and the way it regulated emotion were understood, the couple was able to move forward to restore their relationship.

Understanding the client system also requires uncovering constraints to implementing the solution sequence. Constraints are embedded in the hypothesizing metaframeworks, so IST therapists use the language of these metaframeworks when asking constraint questions—for example, a constraint of organization: "What keeps you from telling your mother that it's not appropriate for you to share with her such intimate information about your marriage?"

Engaging Clients in the Process of Change

In IST, clients hire the therapist to help them solve one or more problems. This problem-solving endeavor overtly engages clients in a change process. This process requires that IST conversations include the function of "change talk" (Miller & Rollnick, 2012). The content of change talk in IST is straightforward and is described in detail in Chapter 3 in the essence diagram (Figure 3.1). The content includes conversations that elucidate the problem and the problem sequence as well as construct, implement, and monitor the solution sequence, including lifting constraints to its implementation.

The process of a change-talk conversation is not straightforward because of clients' ambivalence about change. Although change talk invites clients to change, it simultaneously puts pressure on them to do so: "Part of me chose therapy because I want to change, but another part of me fears or opposes change." Prochaska and DiClemente (1984) proposed a model of change that captures this ambivalence by placing readiness to change on a continuum involving five stages: precontemplative, contemplative, preparation, action, and maintenance. Change talk moves the client along this continuum. The client must recognize the need to change, commit to changing, and see a way to change and finally embrace and implement the change strategy. Prematurely forcing the client too far along the continuum can harm the alliance and/or lead to client drop out. How change talk is handled in conversations, therefore, can facilitate or impede change.

The change-talk function of conversations, therefore, is the most complex of the four functions. Although IST posits that change happens through a collaborative effort between the clients and therapist in which both participate, the actual impetus for change ultimately must come from the clients. Imposing change on clients engenders resistance. For example, a therapist working with Judy, a depressed woman, using cognitive behavior therapy (CBT) believed the depression was unchanged and decided to discuss a medication evaluation with the client. Consider two alternatives to presenting this idea to the client.

Alternative 1

> *Therapist:* Judy, your depression doesn't seem to be improving. I think it is time to consider getting a medication consult. I think an antidepressant might be needed.
>
> *Judy:* Are you sure this is what is needed? I thought CBT was the alternative to medication?

Alternative 2

> *Therapist:* Judy, today, I would like to review the progress we are making on your depression. How do you think things are going?
>
> *Judy:* I admit, I am getting frustrated, as I don't seem to be any less depressed.
>
> *Therapist:* I am sorry to hear that, but it does agree with my assessment of your progress. CBT is still the talk therapy of choice for depression, but I am wondering if we might add something.

> *Judy:* You are referring to medication?
>
> *Therapist:* Yes, and how do you feel about trying an antidepressant?
>
> *Judy:* I would prefer not to, but we have worked hard, and I have tried to do everything you suggested. I think it's time.

In the first alternative, the therapist took responsibility for medication and by suggesting the intervention inadvertently initiated a struggle. Rather than engaging the client in an episode of change-talk conversation, the therapist engendered a conversation of *sustain talk*—that is, talk that maintains the problem and the problem sequence (Miller & Rose, 2009). In the second alternative, the therapist invited the client to explore the possibility of medication, and the client responded with change talk. Although both alternatives took place in the context of a collaborative relationship, the first placed the impetus for change with the therapist as expert whereas the second placed the impetus with the client.

Studies of what makes change-talk conversations effective have largely been conducted with individual clients. These studies have found that change happens more readily when the therapist prompts the client to engage in change talk and then follows the client's leads in sustaining the conversation. In the end, the direction of change comes from the client rather than the therapist. Motivational interviewing (Miller & Rollnick, 2012), Socratic questioning in CBT (Padesky, 1993), and dialectical behavior therapy (Linehan, Heard, & Armstrong, 1993) have all shown that this client-centered change process is most effective.

The process of change-talk conversations is considerably more complex when the direct-client system has two or more clients. In these instances, several clients bring their perspectives about the problem, the problem sequence, and what constitutes a solution sequence. Not only must the therapist garner commitment to change from each client but she or he must also reach a consensus between or among the clients about what constitutes change. This must all happen as the therapist maintains an alliance with all clients. Lest the therapist become paralyzed by client processes of struggle and blame, the therapist must be more active than in conversations with individual clients. This means that sometimes the therapist must exercise overt leadership in the change-talk conversation while also seeking client consensus. Consider the following exchange in which a couple, Ralph and Loretta, are caught in a blame–defend problem sequence.

> *Loretta:* How many times have I asked that you discuss these things with me before you make a decision?
>
> *Ralph:* If I discuss anything with you, it ends up with you deciding what to do.

Loretta:	How would you know? You never give me a chance.
Therapist:	It looks to me like you are both caught in a sequence that takes you nowhere. Loretta, you can't demonstrate that you can engage in a collaborative decision-making process with Ralph because he preempts the decisions, and Ralph, you are getting a reputation of never bringing issues to the table. It seems like something needs to change here. What might each of you do?
Loretta:	He could start by talking to me.
Ralph:	Well, we have been there before.
Therapist:	Loretta, Ralph isn't convinced that you won't co-opt the decision. Can you tell him that you want to demonstrate that you won't co-opt the decision?

At this juncture, the therapist could engage in a line of Socratic questioning with both Ralph and Loretta to enable them to embrace the solution sequence, but this would be arduous, and the process could risk having the conversation getting stuck. Instead, the therapist encouraged Loretta to declare that she is ready to change. IST recognizes that the couple's effort to implement this solution sequence could fail. The failure would not be attributed to a faulty conversation, but rather to the presence of constraints that one or both of them have.

Structuring Therapy

Therapy is a contracted arrangement between the clients and therapist. The contract involves fees, sometimes insurance, a diagnosis, time of session, frequency of sessions, composition of clients attending sessions, and agreed-on actions of clients and therapist. Straightforward and transparent conversation around contractual matters strengthens the alliance. If the clients or therapist violate the contract, sometimes-challenging conversations have to take place. For example, if a client fails to attend a session without canceling, the therapist must decide whether to call the client and, if so, how to address the missed appointment. If a therapist consistently starts sessions late, the client may interpret this adversely unless a conversation takes place to explain it.

Currently, medical insurance requires that an *International Statistical Classification of Diseases and Related Health Problems* (10th Rev.; ICD–10; World Health Organization, 2016) diagnosis be given that is part of the medical record. The diagnosis should be shared with the client(s) using layperson language. Because insurance will not cover relational diagnoses, one of the clients must receive a diagnosis. The rationale for the decision must be shared with the clients lest this decision be construed as evidence that the diagnosed client is the source of the problem.

Moving clients in and out of the direct client system necessitates conversations about who will be attending subsequent sessions. Reaching agreements about who attends sessions and deciding how to invite clients to sessions who are in the indirect system necessitates thorough conversations. For example, if the therapist recommends that one or both spouses of a couple invite their parents to attend therapy, several sessions can be spent planning for this event. Failure to have these conversations can result in damage to the alliance.

In the remainder of this chapter, we present the anatomy of an integrative conversation used by IST therapists. We propose five elements of the therapeutic conversation. The first element is composed of the conversational building blocks that include questions, statements, directives, and silence. The second element is the language of action, meaning, and emotion. The third is the management of conversational turn taking in which a turn is defined as one contribution to the conversation. A turn can be as short as a single word or sentence or as long as a 5-minute monologue. The fourth element is nonverbal communication. Finally, the fifth element comprises alternatives to a talking conversation. We describe analogies and metaphors, visual images, and activities. For heuristic purposes, we first address each element on its own; in actual conversation, the elements blend to create a conversational moment. For example, in a turn, the therapist might focus on action and give a directive as part of an activity.

BUILDING BLOCKS OF CONVERSATION IN INTEGRATIVE SYSTEMIC THERAPY

The building blocks of any conversation are the sentence types used in everyday conversing: questions, statements, and directives. Such sentences can be used in isolation or in combinations we call *juxtapositions*. The sentence types can also be modulated by silence. When careful thought is given to the use of the building blocks, the conversation can be clearer, more efficient, and more impactful. Consider a moment from a classic consultation interview in which Salvador Minuchin interviewed a six-member family in which an 18-year-old son, Arthur, had been hospitalized (Minuchin, 1987). Early in the session, Minuchin read feedback from the family that led him to formulate a hypothesis that the family boundaries were enmeshed. At one point, he was talking to Arthur and his 16-year-old sister, Karen, about her boyfriend, Ricky. The following dialogue enabled him to confirm his hypothesis.

Minuchin: [To Arthur] How old is Ricky?

Karen: [Answering for Arthur] He's 17.

Minuchin: [To Karen] You are helpful?

Karen:	[Smiling] I guess so.
Minuchin:	[To Arthur] I asked you, Arthur, how old is Ricky, and you were thinking, and Karen said he's 17. She didn't wait for you. She volunteered. Is that something she does?
Arthur:	Yes.
Minuchin:	Anticipating you?
Arthur:	Yes.
Minuchin:	So she takes your memory?
Arthur:	I guess so.
Minuchin:	Who else in the family acts like that?
Mother:	We all act like that.

Through the use of several rhetorical questions (questions asked in such a manner that the answer is presumed) and a few statements, Minuchin (1987) built on a moment in the session to confirm his hypothesis that the family was, indeed, enmeshed. The point here is not that this is the only way to converse at that moment, but that Minuchin intentionally chose precise questions and statements to arrive at a place in the session in which he could work with the enmeshed boundaries of the family. Following this brief exchange, Minuchin created the main focus of the session by initiating an enactment in which he asked the son to talk with the father about changing the family boundaries.

A *question* is any sentence by the therapist designed to generate from the clients new information or examine existing information in the client system. A *statement* is any declarative sentence through which the therapist introduces new information or reinterprets existing information in the client system. A *directive* is any sentence whereby the therapist requests that the clients do something. *Silence* is the conspicuous withholding of therapist input to the conversation at some moment in therapy. Questions, statements, directives, and silence can also be juxtaposed to improve their effectiveness.

As we have noted, models of therapy sometimes privilege one building block over others, and some models explicitly eschew the use of other building blocks. Milan systemic therapy (Adams & Boscolo, 2003) holds that questions are always preferred over statements or directives. In integrative conversations, the rules of the models must be transcended to maximize conversational flexibility. IST, therefore, espouses the use of the conversational building block that appears most appropriate for a given therapeutic moment. Sometimes that is a question; at other times it is a statement or a directive.

Questions

We can think of questions simply as linguistic devices intended to gather the facts needed to understand our clients. Many conversational moments in therapy are just that simple—for example, "How many grandchildren do you have?" The use of questions, however, goes well beyond the facts. The skillful use of questions also uncovers heretofore-undisclosed aspects of a problem and reveals how certain behaviors, thoughts, and feelings come together to constitute a problem sequence. Questions are also central to the process of change. A line of questioning can guide a client to discover the need to or pathway of change (Padesky, 1993). Sometimes a single question serves as an intervention by creating an "aha" moment that leads to change (Tomm, 1987a, p. 5). Although it could be argued that any question designed to elicit the relevant information will do, IST contends that some questions are better than others. Consider, for example how the rhetorical questions used by Minuchin (1987) in the example quickly established his hypothesis. It is important, therefore, that IST therapists be able to draw on an array of questions in an integrative way.

To present the range of questions used by IST therapists, we summarize the following kinds of questions: Socratic questions, linear versus circular questions, open versus closed questions, scaling questions, and constraint questions.

Socratic Questions

Because therapy itself is a context of change, everything that happens in that context contains the element of change. All questions that are part of a therapeutic conversation, therefore, are somehow imbued with the notion of change. How the conversation is constructed with questions, however, can result in more or less movement toward change. Socratic questioning is used extensively in CBT, and many studies have demonstrated its effectiveness (Overholser, 1993; Padesky, 1993). The overall purpose of Socratic questioning is to invite clients to explore their thinking in a manner that moves them toward their goals. Socratic questions can be used to clarify concepts; to probe assumptions, rationales, reasons, and evidence; to question viewpoints and perspectives; and to probe implications and consequences. Although any single question could be labeled a Socratic question, what distinguishes Socratic questions is that they are systematic, sustained, and goal directed. Although Socratic questioning can be construed as a method to change clients' minds, it is better thought of as a conversational process by which clients discover a different way of thinking that contributes to the solution sequence (Padesky, 1993).

Socratic questioning is used by IST therapists, although not exclusively. Consider the following exchange cited in Padesky (1993, p. 3). The client (S), a depressed father, is reporting to the therapist feeling like a complete failure. This feeling became intensified after the client went to a family gathering and saw his brother interact with his children in a manner the client felt he himself could not. The therapist pursued the following line of Socratic questioning that created behavioral activation for a client who was stuck and feeling hopeless.

Therapist: You also indicated this was a change in your thinking. You've been depressed many times. And you've seen your brother and his family many times. How did you think about this in the past?

S: I guess I used to always think I was OK because I tried to be a good husband and father. But I see now that trying isn't enough.

Therapist: I'm not sure I understand. Why is trying not enough?

S: Because no matter how hard I try, they still are not as happy as they'd be with someone else.

Therapist: Is that what they say to you?

S: No, but I can see how happy my brother's kids are.

Therapist: And you'd like your kids to be happier?

S: Yes.

Therapist: What things would you do differently if you were less depressed or a better father in your own eyes?

S: I think I'd talk to them more, laugh more, encourage them like I see my brother do.

Therapist: Are these things you could do even when you are depressed?

S: Well, yes, I think I could.

Therapist: Would that feel better to you—trying some new things as a father, rather than simply doing the same thing?

S: Yes, I think I would. But I'm not sure it would be enough if I'm still depressed.

Therapist: How could you find that out?

S: I guess I could try it for a week or so.

In this exchange, the therapist engaged in change talk that moved the client away from his position of hopeless failure to one in which he is open to exploring what would happen if he related differently to his children. At that moment, an IST therapist would shift to planning on the blueprint and select from among the myriad strategies that could be adopted. The point here is that by using Socratic questioning, the therapeutic conversation created the opportunity for this planning to take place.

Linear Versus Circular Questions

IST therapists use both linear and circular questions. Questions are *linear* when they seek information that establishes a causal relationship between two variables—for example, "Did your headaches start after the car accident?" This question seeks to establish whether a head trauma has caused the headaches. Questions are *circular* when they explore a recursive relationship among variables—for example, "Who is most hurt when Dad cancels his visitation?" The answer to this question begins to establish the recursive relationship between feelings the children have and their father's inconsistent visitation.

A problem sequence is a collection of partial sequence arcs that together make up the whole pattern of interaction. Ultimately, IST therapists seek to understand the whole pattern—that is, the systemic relationship of all variables in a sequence. Because of the complexity of sequences, however, the therapist must sometimes ask questions that build the sequence one partial arc at a time. For some partial arcs, there is an obvious linear relationship between the two variables; hence, linear questions are needed. For other partial arcs, a recursive relationship might exist; hence, circular questions are called for. IST, therefore, uses both circular and linear questions. For example, if the therapist learns that a couple frequently gets into fights after going out to dinner and hypothesizes that alcohol fuels the intensity of the conflict, a linear question might be, "Did you have anything to drink before the fight started?" As part of the larger problem sequence that repeats over time, however, alcohol and conflict are recursively related to each other and to all other variables in the sequence. For example, if the drinker feels emotionally abused in a conflict, alcohol can be consumed as a protective strategy to cope with the anticipated conflict—for example, (to the drinker) "When you fear that you have to discuss something that might upset Joe to the point at which he becomes abusive, do you ever drink to calm your nerves?" It is, therefore, both appropriate and essential to use both linear and circular questions to gather the information needed to construct any sequence or understand a constraint.

Whenever a question is asked in which two variables are juxtaposed in an effort to understand the recursive relationship among them, a circular question is created (Selvini Palazzoli, Boscolo, Cecchin, & Prata, 1978; Tomm, 1987a, 1987b). For example, the variable of duration and emotion can be juxtaposed with this circular question: "If you could limit how long these arguments last, do you think you would feel more hopeful about the relationship?" Tomm (1988) presented an exhaustive analysis of circular questions and presented a figure showing the many variables that can be juxtaposed. It is beyond the scope of this chapter to cover all the variables, but among them, time, action, meaning, and emotion are often used. Time is important because it helps to create the temporal relationship between the variables. Action, meaning, and emotion are important because they are the domains of human experience that constitute sequences. The following are a few examples: "When she won't get out of bed, what do you do?" "When you think your relationship might be ending, how does that make you feel?" "When you feel your heart beginning to race, what do you do?" "Had you begun to question your trust in Rita before she discussed your relationship with her mother?" The use of circular questions engages the therapist and clients in a journey to establish a systemic understanding of the client system because the therapist is forced to think systemically when constructing the question, and the clients must think systemically when they answer.

Karl Tomm (1987b, p. 167) called circular questions that function as an intervention *reflexive questions*. The intent of a reflexive question is to get the client system members to reconsider how they experience something so they can come to a different conclusion on their own and without the therapist having to use a reframe to accomplish the same outcome.

Consider the following example. A therapist treated a 12-year-old African American girl who attempted suicide. He invited the whole family to attend a session to see whether a complex family dynamic was related to the suicide attempt. The family consisted of Laverne, a single mother; the patient, Lynette, 12; her sister, Latisha, 14; and younger brother, Kenny, 9. The dynamic of interest involved Kenny and his relationship with Lynette. Kenny spent most of his life in a hospital with muscular dystrophy. He had finally been allowed to come home, and the family was adjusting to both his presence and the enormous demands his physical condition placed on the mother. Lynette was described as angry and cruel to Kenny. She chided and made fun of him. The mother was constantly frustrated and angry with Lynette. Lynette constantly felt her mother's wrath. As the heretofore youngest child at home, Lynette must have felt displaced and, therefore, depressed and angry with Kenny. These circumstances would explain her despair and her consequent suicide attempt.

In the session, Lynette complained that Kenny often acted younger than his age by being incontinent and not properly chewing his food (something he had to do because he had a tracheotomy in his throat). The therapist hypothesized that the oscillation was related to the contrast between the demands of the hospital and home environments. Kenny was confused about his new role as a child in the family rather than being a star patient among the hospital staff.

Therapist: Is your mother easier on Kenny than she is on you and your sister?

Lynette: Yes, she never yells at him even if he sits for hours and doesn't swallow his food.

Therapist: What do you think keeps your mother from being firmer with Kenny?

Kenny looked upset and began to cry. Lynette noticed and began to snicker. Kenny looked furious with Lynette for embarrassing him. The therapist read Lynette's snicker as feedback and hypothesized that she did it to distract from the emotional intensity of the moment.

Therapist: [To mother] I wonder why Lynette finds this to be funny?

Laverne: I know that she does mean things, and I have told her that.

Therapist: I see. But let's say that Kenny's sadness gets Lynette really upset inside, and she wanted to stop him from being sad, stop him from crying. What could she do to stop him from crying?

Laverne: Well, sometimes she makes Kenny be strong and makes him stand up to what he's done.

The therapist's reflexive question served as a reframe of Lynette's behavior from "mean" to "making Kenny be strong." This shift allowed the therapist to begin to explore Lynette's motivation to make Kenny strong. She reported that the mother had been spoiling Kenny and that for Kenny to feel safe in his community without the immediate protection of his family, he would have to be more resilient. Thus, even though Lynette resented Kenny for the massive intrusion into her family, her behavior toward him was benevolently motivated. Using the biology, culture, organization, and development metaframeworks, the therapist initiated a conversation with the family about Kenny's transition from the hospital to home, the understanding of him that family members must have regarding his development and physical limitations, and the mother's role of leader to help Kenny succeed at home and in the community.

Open Versus Closed Questions

IST therapists use both open and closed questions. At each moment of therapy, the therapist's hypothesizing is moving in one of two directions: opening conceptual space to expand hypothesizing or limiting conceptual space so the clients and therapist can agree on a hypothesis. When Minuchin (1987) asked rhetorical questions, he wanted to limit the conceptual space because he was convinced the family was enmeshed. Open questions are more likely to expand conceptual space because the clients have greater scope from which to respond. Closed questions (e.g., "Is she right that you were feeling scared?") request specific information that can be used to evaluate the hypothesis of the moment.

Catastrophic expectation questions represent a special form of open questions often used in IST (Perls, 1971). These questions take the form of "What do you think would happen if . . . ?" For example, when a therapist asks a wife what would happen if she got angry at her husband, her answer could lead in many useful therapeutic directions. She might say he might hit her, which could lead the therapist to ask, "Has that ever happened?" If she says, "Yes," the therapist can follow up with "When?" "How?" and "Why?" If she says, "No," the therapist can ask, "Where does that fear come from?" which opens up other avenues to explore. Catastrophic expectation questions facilitate the determination of the extent to which constraints pertain primarily to the individual or the interpersonal context.

Scaling Questions

Scaling questions allow therapist and clients to calibrate the strength of some variable in a problem sequence. This calibration is crucial for two reasons. First, clients often have different experiences of that variable. Establishing these differences enables the therapist to judge how the differences function in the problem sequence. Second, changing that variable could be part of the solution sequence. Third, scaling a variable establishes a baseline from which change can be measured. Moreover, as is often the case, just paying attention to the variable often produces a shift in it. Finally, scaling the variable enables the therapist and clients to measure success not by a complete cessation of the variable, but rather by some change in it as measured by the scale. For any variable, three important scales are (a) frequency, (b) intensity, and (c) duration— for example, with regard to anxiety, how frequently do you feel anxious, how intense is the anxiety, and how long does an episode of anxiety last? Consider the following example. Sam and Roger had a problem sequence in which they argued about something. The arguments were fueled by cruel name-calling. When the arguments reached a certain point, Roger disengaged and then withdrew and showed his hurt by ignoring Sam, sometimes for days at a time. The therapist had the following exchange with the couple.

> *Therapist:* One way we can get a better grasp of these arguments is to scale them using three measures: their intensity, frequency, and duration. If we can get a consensus of

the measures, then we will have a better handle on whether you guys are making progress. So can I ask you a few questions about frequency, duration, and intensity?

Sam and Roger: Sure.

Therapist: How frequently do you have arguments that end with Roger disengaging?

Roger: I'd say at least once a week.

Sam: That sounds about right.

Therapist: What is the longest Roger has disengaged?

Sam: It can go on for days and sometimes up to a week.

Roger: Come on Sam, it's never been that long.

Therapist: So you have different experiences on duration?

Sam: Seems so.

Therapist: [To both Roger and Sam] On a scale of one to 10, with 10 being the most intense, how intense do these arguments have to be for Roger to feel enough hurt to disengage?

Sam: I'd say you are out of there at a six.

Roger: Not so, Sam, I hang in there until it gets to a nine.

After obtaining measures of frequency, intensity, and duration, the therapist worked with Roger and Sam first to gain a consensus between them and then to define a solution sequence in which they agreed to terminate the argument before it got to a six and for Roger to agree to speak to Sam, albeit tersely, within an hour after the argument. They returned the following week to report that only once did they have to stop the argument—it was far better than they thought it would be, but Roger found he could not speak to Sam until the next day. This was an improvement over several days, which constituted progress.

Constraint Questions

IST therapists do encounter instances in which the solution sequence works and the problem is solved. Far more often, though, the clients struggle to implement the solution sequence. At this point, the therapist must engage in conversation that explores the constraints to solving the problem. The portal to this conversation is the constraint question. Recall that the constraint pillar holds that something keeps the clients from being able to solve the problem.

Constraint questions, therefore, contain this logic. Versions of the language of constraints include: "What keeps you from . . . ?" "What is stopping you from . . . ?" "What prevents you from . . . ?"

In addition to the goal of uncovering constraints, implicit in constraint questions is the strength guideline purporting that clients would do what is necessary to solve the problem but for constraints to doing so. Clients are, therefore, far more receptive to constraint questions. Our often-used example about truthfulness makes this point. The constraint question "What keeps you from telling the truth?" is more palatable to a client than "Why are you lying?"

Clients are sometimes aware of their constraints and readily reveal them in response to a constraint question. In other instances, however, they are unaware of their constraints. The therapist does not take this feedback as confirmation that there are no constraints. Instead, the therapist will repackage clients' failure to perform the solution sequence and ask the constraint question again. Consider the following example. Johan and Ingrid were referred for couples therapy by Ingrid's individual therapist, who felt Ingrid's depression was associated with her complaint that Johan was never emotionally available. After several sessions, a solution sequence invited Johan to try to respond to Ingrid when she expressed her feelings to him. In a session, they discussed an episode in which they were unable to perform the solution sequence.

Ingrid: I received news from my mother that my grandmother, who is still in Austria, had a stroke, and no one knew the status of her medical condition. I was quite close to her as a child. The news filled me with fear and sadness. So I tried to talk to Johan, and I told him how I felt. He simply said, "Not to worry yet, Ingrid. It may have been a mild stroke, and she will be just fine."

Therapist: [To Johan] Is that how you remember what happened?

Johan: Pretty much. There was no need at that moment to jump to conclusions.

Therapist: I see. This seems to be a good episode where you were agreeing to work on being emotionally available to Ingrid. The news seems to have been so unsettling for Ingrid that she experienced some pretty intense emotions.

Johan: I agree, and I tried to calm her down.

Therapist: It sounds like you wanted Ingrid's feelings to stop, but she wanted to express them. What do you think kept you from recognizing that this was one of those moments where the two of you could have talked about her feelings as you had agreed to do?

Johan: I'm not sure what there was to discuss. It was premature, and I tried to point that out to Ingrid.

Therapist: Let's just say for the moment that part of your work in this therapy is to make a leap and just assume that Ingrid has feelings she wants to discuss with you and that you might think she shouldn't be having those feelings, but you know your job is to ask her about them and then see if you can discuss them. Is there something that might be keeping you from making that leap?

Johan: If I go there, it will get very messy.

In actuality, the therapist might have had to use multiple constraint questions to uncover the web of constraints that kept Johan from being able to perform the solution sequence. In addition to fearing the messiness of emotional connection, other constraints might have included his Austrian culture, his ideas about masculinity, his experience of emotion, and anger that he might have harbored toward Ingrid, to name just a few.

Statements

As a component of active listening and to be empathic, all therapists make statements to signal to the clients that they are being heard: "So I am hearing you say that it is hard for you to accept that your son wants to marry Melinda." Therapists also build the alliance by offering statements of praise and encouragement to clients: "I see you have really given this a lot of thought—that's great."

In IST, statements are used more broadly because of the education guideline that asserts that IST therapists pass their knowledge on to clients as soon as they are ready to embrace it. Moreover, this guideline holds that clients should acquire and retain the knowledge of how they solved their problems so that they can return to these strategies should the problems reoccur. Therapists make statements about the client's situation based on their clinical experience and research findings relevant to the client's situation—for example, "I've seen this situation many times in my practice, and from what you have told me today, I think we can work together to address your concern successfully," or "You know, some very good research has addressed this issue, and I'd like to share some of the findings with you."

Therapists must decide why they are choosing to make a statement and be clear about its content. They first mentally check the statement against the alliance primacy guideline and only make the statement if they deem either that the alliance will not be damaged or that the risk of damage is outweighed by the potential value or benefit of the statement with the knowledge that some alliance repair may be needed. This mental editing happens throughout the session, and many more statements are left unsaid than said.

IST therapists choose their words and delivery carefully. Depending on the words and delivery, two statements with the same content can be received very differently. Sometimes a statement can dramatically propel the conversation forward to the point at which the clients reveal crucial information that enriches the hypothesis or even suggests a pathway to change. Consider the following example. A Pakistani family attended a consultation session to address the problem of nocturnal enuresis experienced by Shira, a senior in high school. Shira's two older sisters were married and were out of the house. She had a younger brother, Hamed, who was described as a troublemaker. The family moved to the United States 5 years previously, and it was readily apparent that the children were more acculturated than the parents. In the conversation, both parents presented as quiet and reasonable people. Hamed was sullen. Josef, the father, described how he was a good observer but could detect nothing that would explain why Shira had this problem. As Shira described the nocturnal enuresis, her delivery was strident and combative.

> Shira: I do, I get up every night more than once, but the thing is I just don't feel it, and that's what I've been trying to explain to my parents and the doctor. [Emphatically] I don't feel it!

> Therapist: You know what I observe. I am a little bit of an observer too [joining with the father]. When I look at the family, you two [the parents] seem mild mannered, and you, Shira, seem fiery. [The therapist intentionally chooses a positive word to describe Shira's affect.]

> Mother: She is fiery. She used to be the angel of the house, the quiet one, but lately, 6, 7 months, when I talk to her, she snaps back.

> Therapist: She is getting more and more fiery.

> Shira: I was always the goody two-shoes of the house.

> Therapist: Can any of you identify what might have happened 6 months ago that could help us understand why Shira became so fiery?

The family revealed that the next-oldest daughter had gotten married and moved out of the house. This made Shira the "go-between" in the community for the parents. As a senior, Shira had dreams of going to college. Not only did this dream violate the cultural expectation that girls stay home until they got married but it also revealed the parents' belief that the younger son was not equipped to take over the job of go-between. As the conversation progressed, Shira admitted she felt trapped, and her fiery demeanor was a form of protest.

Directives

We have already established that IST therapists embrace their role as leaders of the therapy. The leader has the responsibility to facilitate the conversation both by guiding it and sometimes influencing its direction. This leadership role cannot be performed without the use of directives. This is true regardless of which clients are in the direct system. It is even more essential when there are two or more clients present because facilitation involves both the therapy conversation and the conversation among clients. For example, a high-conflict episode might erupt in a session necessitating that the therapist use directives to stop it. Directives are needed to move the conversation forward—for example, "Tell me more about how you felt." Directives are also essential for many of the strategies drawn from the planning metaframeworks. For example, enactments and sculpting require the use of directives.

In sessions, directives are used to start, stop, or redirect the conversation. Therapists use directives to start an interaction between clients—for example, "Tell Joe what you think of what he just said." Directives are also needed to start an activity such as a speaker–listener exercise. Directives are also used to stop an interaction—for example, "Hold on; you are getting into the weeds. Please refocus on trying to tell me what the problem is." Sometimes the therapist must be willing to be directive when a process is getting out of hand, even to the point of standing up and calling an abrupt stop to it—for example, standing up and saying, "Hold on; please stop. This interaction isn't getting you anywhere." If two people are talking and a third person keeps interrupting, the therapist may use a directive to draw a boundary around the clients: "Mom, I sense you are uneasy when your husband and daughter are talking. Let's both sit back and see whether they can do it." To father and daughter, "Go ahead, see whether you can work on this without Mom giving you help." If the interaction has to go in a different direction, a directive can be used—for example, "Excuse me, I hate to interrupt, but you are getting away from the topic. See whether you can stick to what you agreed to discuss." If one client begins to experience something and the other does not respond, a directive can be used to refocus the conversation—for example, the wife Sally began to tear up:

Therapist: Sally, something just happened to upset you? Bob, did you notice that?

Bob: No, what are you referring to?

Therapist: Sally, tell Bob what is making you tear up.

Directives are also an important conversation building block for creating and implementing between-session experiments. IST calls them *experiments* rather than *homework* for several reasons. First, labeling something as homework can engender resistance, and second, an experiment is a win–win exercise. Either the clients succeed, or if they do not, the failed outcome usually uncovers constraints that can be explored with questions such as, "I wonder what kept you from doing the experiment?"

There are an infinite number of between-session experiments. A couple with financial problems can be directed to work on making a budget. A couple that has not been out following the birth of their son can be directed to have a date night. Parents who disagree about how to handle an adolescent can be instructed to discuss what they will jointly agree to do the next time there is a transgression.

Between-session experiments must be thoroughly discussed with clients to garner buy-in from all clients to do the experiment and to assure that everyone knows how the experiment works. The *who, what, when, where,* and *how* of the experiment must be covered in the conversation. Failure to do so can leave a loophole that accounts for why the experiment was not implemented. If a client objects or acts lukewarm toward the experiment, it can be a sign of a constraint. The therapist can ask, "Is there something keeping you from being willing to do the experiment?" If the client reveals a constraint, it is sometimes best to postpone the experiment until the constraint is lifted. For example, a couple presenting with sexual problems could be asked to do a sensate focus exercise. When they demonstrate their discomfort, the therapist might ask what makes them feel uncomfortable. A subsequent conversation may reveal that the couple's sexual communication is poor; therefore, they both experienced high anxiety at having to tell their partner what they wanted in the exercise. At that point, the therapist might read the feedback and scale back the pace of solving the problem.

Silence

There are many moments when therapists decide to remain silent. By staying on the sideline of the conversation, therapists give clients space to advance the conversation on their own. They may be hesitant to say what is on their mind, and the silence allows them to reflect and then to take the risk of speaking. Silence in a conversation between spouses can interrupt old turn-taking patterns and encourage the quieter partner to take a risk by speaking up. When one client has been asked to take a turn and is hesitating, the therapist can use a directive to hold the silence as long as necessary— for example, "Look, you all challenged Bill to tell you how he feels. That may be hard for him, so let's sit tight and allow him to think it over until he's ready to say something." Last, in IST it is important in supporting clients' strengths to relinquish control in the face of adaptive behavior. Being silent and sitting back when clients are doing the right thing supports their growth and facilitates their internalization of the therapist's competence and confidence.

Juxtaposing Questions, Statements, and Directives

Thus far, we have discussed questions, statements, and directives independently, but as many of the clinical vignettes have illustrated, they are more effective when therapists juxtapose them in various combinations. Unless the therapist intentionally chooses to engender cognitive dissonance by saying something that catches the clients off guard or shocks or confuses them, the therapist wants the clients to follow the lead in the conversation offered by the therapist's contribution to it. Moreover, always following the alliance priority guideline, the therapist chooses words carefully to both make a point and preserve the alliance. Juxtaposing questions, statements, and directives facilitates these goals.

Depending on the circumstances, questions, statements, and directives can be juxtaposed in many ways. If the therapist wants to use a directive, preceding it with one or more statements is helpful. This is particularly true when initiating an enactment that may feel unfamiliar to the clients or involves some but not all clients present. Simply telling them to talk to each other can result in puzzled looks or even resistance: "I don't know why you are asking us to do this"—for example:

> *Therapist:* Excuse me, I see you are all eager to take part in this conversation, and that's really good, but I think we might get further if we have two of you at a time talk about this issue. Let's start with Mom and Dad. Can you turn your chairs toward one another and continue the same conversation, but this time just the two of you? Then we'll take a turn with the kids.

Sometimes the therapist wants to make a statement or ask a question knowing the clients may struggle with it. Softening the question with statements facilitates receptivity. For example, a couple presented as having drifted apart. In the third session with the therapist, they talked about the problem sequence, but still said nothing about sex. The therapist hypothesized that either their sexual relationship was not good or they had a hard time talking about it. Because they were not presenting with a sexual problem, but the therapist thought it important to establish how sex fit into the problem sequence, the following dialogue occurred:

> *Therapist:* You know, as I listen to your conversation about not feeling close, I find myself wanting to ask you a question, but I don't want you to think I am being too intrusive.
>
> *Clients:* That's OK; we can take it.

> Therapist: OK, thank you. In all of the conversations we have been having about the lack of closeness, neither of you have said anything about your sex life. Is it OK if I ask you how that's going?
>
> Husband: It's not going. We haven't had sex for over 2 years.
>
> Wife: Yeah, and look who's counting.

Juxtaposing is helpful in preserving alliances with clients. Sometimes the therapist has to ask one client a question that could end up hurting the alliance with another client, so the therapist makes a statement to anticipate this risk—for example:

> Therapist: Sandy, I need to ask Bob a question, but I am afraid you might take it the wrong way and think I am siding with him.
>
> Sandy: I doubt that would happen, but I appreciate that you thought of it.
>
> Therapist: So, Bob, when Sandy chose to go away with her friends on the date of your wedding anniversary, how did that make you feel?

MANAGING CONVERSATIONAL TURNS

Conversations unfold with participants taking turns talking. Person A says something, and then Person B says something. IST posits that therapeutic conversations are more efficient and impactful when therapists exercise leadership in the management of these turns. The management of turns varies depending on who is in the direct client system and what the goal of the therapy is at any given moment.

When one client is in the session, conversational turns are more straightforward but often still challenging. Some therapies allow for long turns, seldom interjecting. In IST, this style of managing turns can be limiting because achieving the steps of the essence diagram is limited by too few therapist contributions to the conversation. Every therapist has polite ways to slow or stop an unproductive client monologue: "I know what you are saying is very important, but I feel myself getting saturated. Can we pause a moment so I can see whether I have been following you?" IST cannot unfold unless the therapist gets sufficient turns. Sometimes the therapist has to ask several circular and/or Socratic questions.

When the direct client system involves more than one person, the management of turns is more complex because the conversation must be distributed between or among the clients and the interjection of turns by the therapist. If the client system is a couple, the management of turns has several options. One option is for client turns to be routed through the therapist. So one client takes a turn, and then the therapist responds, and so on. This option is useful when the therapist wants or has to limit the emotional reactivity between the couple. Another option is for the therapist to encourage the couple to talk to each other and to interject turns into their conversation. Finally, if the conversation is flowing between the couple, the therapist can sit back and simply observe. The following brief exchange is an example of managing conversational turns. Sally and Ben were in couples therapy because they had conflict over how to manage two careers and their three children.

Sally: I don't think you understand how abandoned I feel when you come and go as you please and I am left to do everything for the kids. It's crushing me.

Ben: Look, I am doing the best I can to do my part.

Therapist: Ben, I wonder what you think Sally meant when she said that having too much on her plate is crushing her.

Ben: I don't know. I guess it makes her sad.

Therapist: That's a good start, Ben, but can you ask her what she means when she says it is crushing her?

Ben: [To Sally] OK, so what does crushing mean to you?

There are many possible ways therapists could manage this moment. The point is not that the one described is the right way, but that the therapist was mindful of managing the conversation so that Sally and Ben were engaged in constructive work.

If the client system is a family with three or more members in the direct client system, the options for therapist turns is even more complex. To prevent a free-for-all, therapists must actively organize the conversation. When turns take place among family members, it should be clear to everyone why this is happening. For example, if two of three members engage in a conversation, the therapist should be explicit why the third member is not taking a turn. It is often useful to give an observing assignment to the nonparticipating member.

THE LANGUAGE OF ACTION, MEANING, AND EMOTION

All therapies seek change through the domains of human experience of action, meaning, and emotion. The language of action is about behavior, doing, and patterns of interaction—for example:

Wife: He said he would be home at 6:00. He even called, and then he shows up at 7:00.

Therapist: So what did you do when he got home?

The language of meaning is about cognition, thinking, narrative, and meaning making—for example:

> *Wife:* Clearly he doesn't care about me or he wouldn't say those things.
>
> *Therapist:* Can you explain what not caring about you means?

The language of emotion is about feeling and affect—for example:

> *Client:* Sometimes I feel so sad that I can't imagine ever getting out of this rut.
>
> *Therapist:* So it feels to you like you are going through a very tough time.

IST therapists attend to action, meaning, and emotion in both macro and micro ways. In macro ways, IST therapists apply the blueprint (see Figure 4.1) to guide the structure and direction of sessions. Their current hypotheses and plans signal them to privilege action, meaning, or emotion. Their use of conversation facilitates their plan. For example, consider the use of action language setting up an enactment between a single mother, Shayna, and her son, Brian:

> *Shayna:* He just walks right by the trash every day and won't take it out unless I yell at him.
>
> *Therapist:* That's a lot of extra effort for you and, Brian, I am sure you get tired of your mom yelling at you.
>
> *Brian:* Yelling is all she ever does.
>
> *Therapist:* Look, you both have a lot going on in your lives, and it's just the two of you. Talk to each other and see if you can agree on how to keep the trash from always being such a thorn of contention. So, Shayna, the next time Brian walks right past the trash, what are you going to do?

Micro attention to action, meaning, and emotion also occurs in the moment-to-moment conversation of the session. The therapist may be hypothesizing and planning in one domain, but cannot ignore feedback in another domain. To do so could tear the alliance or create a hypothesizing blind spot. Essentially, if the client says something in one domain, the therapist should respond in that domain. A decision must be made, then, whether to return to the domain driving the session or switch to the newly offered domain. For example, a therapist offered a reframe for part of the problem sequence when the client burst into tears.

> *Therapist:* Look, you both have a lot going on in your lives, and it's just the two of you. Talk to each other and see if you can agree

on how to keep the trash from always being such a thorn of contention. Wait a second. Shayna, something I just said seems to have triggered a strong feeling for you.

Shayna: What you are suggesting is all that I ever wanted.

At this juncture, the therapist could ask Shayna to explore her feelings or return to the reframe.

IST therapists must stay attuned to clients' preference for or need to converse more in one domain than another. For example, children who are at the preoperational level of development (some adults are stuck there too) think concretely; consequently, the language of action is most suitable for them (Piaget, 1952). Stereotypically, men often intellectualize their experience; therefore, it is important to converse in the language of meaning and not to press them prematurely to address emotion. This can be a challenge in couples therapy when part of the presenting problem is the wife's complaint that her husband is emotionally unavailable.

Every session has moments when it is vital to stay focused on one domain. For example, if the therapist reads feedback that a client is experiencing an emotion and the therapist wants that emotion to be available for work in the session, the conversation should stay within the domain of emotion. For example, a single mother, Janet, and her teenage daughter, Becky, were in therapy to address Becky's eating disorder. Janet was angry that Becky was compromising her health.

Janet: Becky, how many times do I have to tell you that your diet is putting you at risk?

Becky: I know what I have to eat. Just leave me alone.

Janet looked away, turned her head down, and swiped her hand across her face. The therapist read this feedback as Janet being both exasperated and fearful.

Therapist: Janet, you seem distressed.

Janet: I just don't know what to do. [Janet appears to be crying.]

Therapist: You are afraid.

Janet: Yes, she could die.

Therapist: I can feel your fear. Have you ever told Becky about your fear?

Janet: No.

Therapist: Listen to your tears, and tell her that you are afraid.

Janet: [To Becky] I am so scared. I don't know what I would do if I lost you.

Becky: [Begins to cry] I don't want to die.

NONVERBAL COMMUNICATION

Communication experts contend that most communication is nonverbal. Nonverbal communication consists of paralinguistic aspects of communication such as tone of voice and volume, facial expressions, and gestures of the hands and body (Breunlin, 1979). These nonverbal messages are being expressed and interpreted by clients throughout sessions. Often, nonverbal messages express the mood of the moment. If the therapist is not paying attention, something can shift in the conversation without the therapist's being aware of what caused it. For example, a therapist worked with Claudia, a single parent, and her two children, Latisha, a 6-year-old girl presenting with enuresis, and her 2-year-old sister, Monique. In the session, Monique lay on Claudia's lap (more like an infant than a 2-year-old), and Latisha sat by herself. This seating arrangement was a nonverbal communication about the organization of the family. In a brief sequence of just a few seconds, Monique appeared to play patty-cake with Latisha, who seemed to read the gesture as an invitation to play. Latisha leaned toward Monique and seemed to want to pick her up as if to signal, OK, let's play. As she reached for Monique, Monique whimpered and turned away from her. In one fell swoop, Claudia cuddled Monique and gave her a bottle. Latisha looked down, appeared sad, and began to suck her thumb. The therapist read this nonverbal feedback and formed a hypothesis that Latisha's enuresis was part of an oscillation (acting younger than her age) to be seen by Claudia, who seemed preoccupied with the younger Monique.

The therapist discussed the brief nonverbal sequence with Claudia, who came to see that Latisha was well intentioned when she reached for Monique. When asked whether something kept Claudia from letting them play, she said she did not want to be disrespectful to the therapist. The therapist set up a play experience for Latisha and Monique with the mother praising them for how well they played together.

As this example illustrates, the blueprint serves as a guide for whether and how to use nonverbal communication. If the therapist relates nonverbal feedback to the hypothesis being addressed and concludes it is consistent with the plan being implemented at the moment and it will not damage the alliance to make a note of it, it should be addressed. Discretion must be used with nonverbal communication, however, because clients sometimes are not aware of what they are communicating nonverbally and could be embarrassed or shamed when said nonverbal messages are noted. Sometimes a nonverbal communication serves as feedback that the therapist is on the wrong track and has to change directions.

Therapists must also be aware of their own nonverbal communication lest they "leak" something that offends the clients. An inadvertent smile can be taken as dismissive. A slight grimace can be interpreted as the therapist thinking the client's situation is hopeless. The next chapter on feedback further addresses nonverbal communication.

ALTERNATIVES TO TALK THERAPY

At times, the therapeutic conversation can become an impediment to change. This can happen for several reasons. The therapist is not clear enough. The clients have disparate ways to view the problem sequence. The ideas describing the problem sequence are too abstract for the clients. There is just too much verbiage in the conversation. When this happens, the therapist can take a step away from pure talk therapy and converse, instead, using alternative methods. By taking the problem outside the immediate intensity of clients' experience, it can be examined through new meaning and emotion, thus giving clients more options to make different choices. Next, we discuss analogies and metaphors, visual images, and activities as alternatives to talk therapy.

Analogies and Metaphors

There are some subtle differences between metaphors and analogies. A *metaphor* is a figure of speech in which an implied comparison is made between two different things that have something important in common. An *analogy* is a comparison of two things for the purposes of explanation and clarification. For use in therapy, analogies and metaphors serve the same function: They allow the therapist to heighten the significance of a client problem, process, or issue that clients are finding difficult to discuss and resolve. There is no catalog for analogies and metaphors, nor would a catalog be helpful because they must be organic to the situation. They largely emerge from the creativity of the therapist. Some therapists find it easy to generate analogies and metaphors, others not so much. To improve the art of using analogies and metaphors, however, therapists should cultivate the talent not just in sessions, but also in their day-to-day conversations. Consider the following example.

Rita and Bruce sought therapy to reinvigorate a marriage that had gone stale a decade earlier. The couple were now in their late 50s, and their three children were all grown and out of the house. When the children were young, Bruce worked and Rita stayed home to care for them. After the children had left home, Rita did not seek employment. Bruce had excelled in his career, but his promotions had required moving the family six times. With no promotions remaining, Bruce had slowed down at work, and he was anxious to spend more time with Rita. They talked about doing more together, but something always seemed to get in the way. The therapist elaborated this problem sequence and suggested a solution sequence in which the couple committed to one outing per week and daily time together. They both agreed.

For several weeks they did spend time together, but then for several subsequent weeks they did nothing. When the therapist explored the constraints to performing the solution sequence, Rita seemed to be the one who kept the outings from happening. Digging into her constraints, Rita owned that she held a long-standing resentment that Bruce's work had necessitated so many moves. She recalled the bitterness she felt each time they uprooted the children and left a house she was trying to make a home. She admitted that depriving Bruce of a better connection with her was a form of retribution. The couple talked about how they would lift the constraint of resentment. Bruce was empathic to Rita, admitted he had been selfish, and apologized. At the moment Rita felt better, but she could not let go of her resentment.

The therapist considered moving down the matrix to the family-of-origin planning metaframework but decided first to introduce a metaphor. She brought out a plastic knife and placed it on the coffee table. Rita and Bruce looked quizzical. Following seconds of silence, the therapist asked the couple what the significance of the knife might be. Neither Rita nor Bruce could come up with anything.

> *Therapist:* Making a marriage work for a lifetime is hard work. It's like crossing the Siberian tundra in a dogsled. It is arduous and challenging, and you have to do whatever you can to maximize the chance of success. To make such a journey, you have to have supplies stored in bags. Imagine that some of these bags fall off the sled and are being dragged behind the sled. You can't stop the sled, but you know the friction from the bags is tiring out the dogs. [Here the therapist pauses and hands Rita the knife.] So what do you do?
>
> *Rita:* I get it. I could reach back and cut the rope holding the bags. But what if the bags contain important supplies?
>
> *Therapist:* Of course, no metaphor is perfect, but let's say your choice is to cut and keep going and make it to the end or not to cut and thus to die on the tundra.
>
> *Rita:* That's easy, you cut.
>
> *Therapist:* Right, so let's go back to your marriage. Rita, what's in those bags?
>
> *Rita:* My resentment?
>
> *Therapist:* Of course. The question is: Do you want to cut the bags? [Rita looks hesitant. The therapist reads this feedback and

concludes she is not ready yet to cut the bags.] This has to be a difficult decision. Part of you deserves to be loyal to your feelings, and part of you knows your resentment is constraining the marriage. I suggest you go home and think about the sled, the bags, and the knife.

During the week, Rita was obsessed with the analogy. She and Bruce talked about it, and again he apologized. In the next session, she said the following:

Rita: [To the therapist] You made me realize that I do hold the knife, and I can cut the bags if I choose to do so. You also made me realize that holding on to my resentment keeps our marriage from growing, and I don't want that. Bruce, I hope you do something to atone for making us move so often, but even if you don't, I choose to cut the bags. She looks expectantly at Bruce.

Bruce: Believe me, Rita, I get it, and I promise I will do what it takes to make it up to you. I so want the sled to keep moving.

Visual Images

Recognizing that a picture can be worth a thousand words, the therapist can introduce a visual image to focus the client on important issues. The image can be a pie diagram to illustrate the way time or some other variable is distributed, a line representing a continuum of some variable, or a pictorial representation of some process. Whatever is selected, the image creates a common language and focus that makes a point and thus structures the conversation.

For example, a common element of a problem sequence is a polarization in which each party adopts positions that are mutually exclusive. So long as both clients hold their position, little progress can be made to create a workable solution sequence. A useful way to enable clients to grasp the insidious nature of a polarization is to show them a drawing of a sailboat in which balance is created by each sailor leaning out in opposite directions. This image allows clients to see that although they have balanced the sailboat, should one person abandon their position, the sailboat would capsize; therefore, the only workable solution is for each sailor to simultaneously lean in—that is, to soften and/or change their position.

In families, a frequent polarization is the splitting of parental functions so that one parent carries the nurturing functions and the other parent carries the limit-setting functions. This polarization creates a problem sequence in which the more the nurturing parent is perceived to be soft, and the more the limit-setting parent is perceived to be harsh. Both parents hold the perspective that the problem rests with the other parent: "I have to be harsh because you are spoiling them" and "I have to be soft because you are abusing them." Focusing the conversation on the visual image of the sailboat enables the therapist to keep the clients focused on the insidious nature of a polarization and incents them to adopt solution sequences that can eliminate the polarization. The solution sequence for the harsh–soft polarization is for these functions to be more equally distributed between the two parents. So, for example, the soft parent can no longer say "Wait till your father gets home," and the harsh parent must begin engaging in more nurturing behaviors.

Activities

Therapists can choose from a rich array of in-session activities that use action to structure conversation. When such activities are used, the focus of the session is on the experience generated by the activity. Behaviors or emotions not accessible through conversation are expressed, sometimes with greater intensity than would be shown as part of a conversation. The conversation is then used to process the activity. Time-tested activities include making a genogram; sculpting; using the "empty-chair" method; making a timeline, a drawing, or a collage; or playing a game. In-session activities are a sine qua non of family therapy with children because they provide vehicles for conversation that span the disparity between adult and child capabilities. Some activities are uniquely configured for specific client systems (such as working with children), but most can be adapted whether the direct client system involves an individual, a couple, or a family.

The following example illustrates how an activity can structure a conversation that addresses elements of the presenting problem, the problem sequence, and identifying and lifting constraints.

DeShawn, an 8-year-old African American boy, was referred because he was in danger of having to repeat second grade. The referral indicated that DeShawn was immature and passive and had difficulty completing work at school and homework. DeShawn attended the first session with his parents, Curtis and Angelica, and his 7-year-old sister, Moesha. Angelica had been an elementary school teacher for 10 years, and Curtis had been studying for years to obtain his undergraduate degree while working as an orderly in a hospital.

In the initial session, the therapist quickly used the development and organization metaframeworks to read several pieces of feedback that informed an initial hypothesis. Angelica spoke a lot, sharing many details and opinions, whereas Curtis seemed hesitant to speak, and what he did say was almost too quiet to hear. The behavior of the children seemed to mirror that of the parents. DeShawn spoke in a manner that seemed much younger than his age whereas Moesha had the same crisp tone as her mother. Moreover, whenever Moesha did something, DeShawn would mimic her. For instance, when she took off her jacket and placed in on the back of her chair, she did so methodically. DeShawn immediately removed his jacket and somewhat sloppily placed in on his chair only for it to fall off when he sat down. This prompted Moesha to giggle. Reading this feedback, the therapist formed a hypothesis that part of the problem for DeShawn was a hierarchal reversal in which he acted less competently than his younger sister. In the session, he seemed to have passively accepted this status in his family, and the parents seemed to tolerate it. The therapist discussed the hypothesis with the family, and the parents admitted they often turned to Moesha when they needed one of the children to do something at home such as take out the trash. This concerned the therapist because were DeShawn to be held back a grade, he would end up in the same grade as his sister.

The therapist thought DeShawn needed to experience more confidence so he could act in an age-appropriate way as a big brother. One solution sequence would be to restore DeShawn to his rightful status as the oldest of the siblings. To work on this, the therapist decided to engage the children in a mutual drawing activity. He also invited the parents to be observers of the activity.

Therapist:	DeShawn and Moesha, I'd like for you to do a drawing for your parents.
Moesha:	I love to draw. Where is my piece of paper?
Therapist:	Well, what I want you to do is to work with DeShawn so that the two of you make a drawing together. You can draw whatever you want so long as you each do some of the drawing.
Moesha:	But I want to do my own. DeShawn will mess up.
Therapist:	I understand that you are used to doing your own, but for this once I want you to do it together.

The therapist gave a large piece of paper and colored pencils to the children and organized them around a table. As they commenced, Moesha pulled the paper to her side of the table, leaving DeShawn to have to reach over to get at the paper.

Moesha:	[Emphatically] We're going to draw a house.
DeShawn:	OK.
Moesha:	I'll draw the house, and you can draw the sky. Put the sun and some birds in it.

DeShawn began to draw the sun hesitantly in a small corner of the paper while Moesha vigorously used most of the page to begin drawing the house.

Moesha: That's not where the sun goes.

DeShawn looked defeated and put his pencil down. Moesha took the paper, crossed out DeShawn's sun, and drew one in a different part of the sky. Moesha continued to draw, ignoring the fact that DeShawn was no longer participating.

Therapist: [To DeShawn] This is supposed to be a shared drawing. I want to see your part of the drawing.

DeShawn: Moesha won't let me.

The therapist decided to use an intervention drawn from structural family therapy whereby he would momentarily unbalance the sibling subsystem by encouraging DeShawn to stand up for himself (Minuchin & Fishman, 1981).

Therapist: Well, perhaps you should tell her where you want the sun to go. [DeShawn looks at the paper but does not do anything.] How am I going to see your part of the drawing if you don't do it?

DeShawn hesitated again and then reached over and took the paper from Moesha. As he began avidly to redraw the sun, Moesha appeared startled. She put her pencil down, pushed her chair back, and began to pout. DeShawn glanced toward his parents as if to ask permission for his behavior. The moment was pregnant with intense emotion. The therapist had myriad ways to use this activity to continue the conversation.

Therapist: [To the parents] What do you want to say to DeShawn and Moesha about what just happened?

Angelica: [To Moesha] Did it upset you when DeShawn took the drawing from you?

Moesha: It's not fair.

Angelica: Yes, it is. You were supposed to do the drawing together. It was good that DeShawn insisted that he was doing it with you. From now on, we all have to do a better job of helping DeShawn be a big brother.

Extending the art activity from this example to sum up this chapter, we wish to note that Fraenkel (2009) used the analogy of the artist's palette to discuss integrative therapy. This analogy can be applied to an IST conversation. On the palette are the building blocks of conversation (questions, statements, directives, and silence); how to manage conversational turns; the language of action, meaning, and emotion; nonverbal communication; and alternatives to straight talk therapy that include analogies and metaphors, visual images, and activities. To create the conversation, therapists combine elements just as artists combine colors. For example, the therapist might juxtapose a statement and a circular question to establish the relationship between a client's meaning and emotion leading up to a request to engage in a sculpting exercise. The combining of elements cannot be random or the conversation will feel false or stilted just as a painting would be ugly. Rather, when the elements are combined skillfully, the conversation is both elegant and effective. Earlier in this chapter, we mentioned that mastering the art of the therapeutic conversation is a lifelong journey; this is discussed more in Chapter 12.

8

FEEDBACK

In this chapter, we examine the fourth component of the integrative systemic therapy (IST) blueprint, feedback (see Figure 4.1). We present the way IST therapists read feedback and relate it to the other blueprint components: hypothesizing, planning, and conversing. Next, we address explicit feedback given by clients to the therapist and by the therapist to clients. Finally, we present the use of feedback instruments that can improve the outcome of therapy.

READING FEEDBACK

A couple entered therapy because their relationship had "gone stale." Both partners reported feeling invisible, taken for granted, and uncared for by the other. After using the blueprint in the first two sessions, the therapist's

http://dx.doi.org/10.1037/0000055-008
Integrative Systemic Therapy: Metaframeworks for Problem Solving With Individuals, Couples, and Families,
by W. M. Pinsof, D. C. Breunlin, W. P. Russell, J. L. Lebow, C. Rampage, and A. L. Chambers
Copyright © 2018 by the American Psychological Association. All rights reserved.

hypothesis was that the problem sequence involved an imbalance of positive to negative interactions that was skewed to the negative, thus increasing relational dissatisfaction and leading to discouragement. The therapist shared this hypothesis and invited the couple to create a solution sequence involving more positivity. The couple struggled to do this, so the therapist shifted to planning and suggested an experiment in which each partner did three small things daily to please the other and notice whether it made any difference in the relationship. They both agreed to the experiment.

In the next session, an important moment occurred when the wife pulled out a list and handed it to the therapist. In that instant, the therapist read the following feedback. The wife had an expression on her face that might have signaled pride or smugness. The expression on the husband's face seemed to be one of disdain. Then the wife announced, "I did my three things every day, just like you told us to, and you know what? It didn't even get noticed." At this point, the husband slumped in his chair, turned away, breaking eye contact with both therapist and partner, and muttered something that sounded like, "Just like you to turn even therapy into a competition that shows your superiority." Having read this feedback, the therapist leaned forward, looked interested and curious, and said,

> It seems like this exercise stimulated a troubling sequence in your relationship that I would like to understand. Can we talk about what you were communicating with each other by the way you responded to my suggestion and the way you are responding to each other right now?

This example demonstrates the importance of reading feedback in the context of the blueprint. The therapist began therapy with the problem of a "stale" relationship. The therapist hypothesized that the staleness was embedded in a problem sequence of negativity and conversed with the clients about a solution sequence that would bring more positivity into the relationship. The couple agreed to do the "three small things" intervention. In the next session, as they reported on how they handled the intervention, they revealed feedback about their relationship in the context of the intervention. The therapist's hypothesis about that feedback was that the intervention appeared not to have worked and pointed to possible constraints to positivity. For example, were they competitive about who was the "better" partner? Or was one partner unusually burdened during the week or in a depression? Was the wife using the task to prove how hopeless the relationship was? For positivity to flourish in their relationship, these and other constraints would have to be lifted. The therapist trusted that further conversation would point the way toward a new or modified hypothesis about the problem that could be tested out with subsequent interventions.

As this example illustrates, feedback is at the heart of IST. Indeed, feedback is so crucial to IST that it is incorporated as one of the four components of the blueprint (Figure 4.1) that also includes hypothesizing, planning, and conversing (Breunlin, Pinsof, Russell, & Lebow, 2011; Pinsof, Breunlin, Russell, & Lebow, 2011). It is feedback that stimulates hypothesizing that leads to planning that is implemented through the therapeutic conversation. Without feedback, it is impossible for therapists to know whether they are on or off course and, if the latter, to make course corrections.

Anything that happens in the course of therapy that provides information to the therapist about the client system and how to help it solve problems is a form of feedback. In its simplest, most easily intelligible form, feedback is a rational, verbal response:

Therapist: When you fight, I see that your emotional arousal gets high very quickly. I suggest you use a time-out to keep the fights from getting out of control.

Client: [The following session] We did that time-out thing you told us about last week, and it really worked!

If all feedback were as easily decoded, it would not take so long to learn how to be an effective therapist. In actual practice, however, feedback is far more subtle and complex. It goes in multiple directions (client to therapist, therapist to client, clients to each other) and is often neither verbal nor rational. For instance, in the first vignette, the therapist's initial feedback to the clients was offered as a fairly straightforward hypothesis and plan: "Your relationship is burdened by not having enough positive interaction, so try to do things to raise the frequency of that kind of interaction." The feedback, however, was far more complicated. First, the wife seemed to have completed and documented the task, whereas the husband had not. The wife seemed eager to convey a spirit of engagement and cooperation, which the husband seemed to interpret as some sort of "showing off." He appeared discouraged or possibly angry, but that was being conveyed in gesture and facial expression rather than words. What words are spoken convey a tone of criticism, but also sadness. At the heart of IST is the ability to track and make sense of feedback and to converse about it to move therapy forward. It is, however, no mean feat.

Reading feedback requires the therapist to pay close attention to what is happening during a session. When therapy involves multiple clients in the direct system, it is impossible to track all that is happening. Researchers in family process can work for hours coding brief snippets of family interaction (Gottman & Notarius, 2000). For a single therapist to listen, watch, and respond to several people in the course of an hour and then make sense of it all and figure out what to do next is truly formidable.

Although feedback occurs throughout a session, IST therapists attend most closely to feedback informed by their hypothesis. Think of watching a sports event on a split-screen television monitor. Having a view of the entire field as well as a close-up of a single player can add important information and context. But what would happen if the screen were divided into ten close-up shots, shown simultaneously? The viewer would quickly get both overstimulated and confused about the essence of what is happening. Having a hypothesis is a way of framing the scene and identifying what to watch for.

For example, a single mother entered therapy because her 12-year-old daughter suddenly showed a strong interest in contacting her biological father who had abandoned the family when she was an infant. The mother, a beautician, had a medical condition that threatened her employment. For her daughter to show interest in her father felt like a betrayal. The mother angrily told the daughter she should want nothing to do with him. The daughter, however, would not back down.

The therapist considered both the organizational and developmental metaframeworks in regard to hypothesizing. Was the daughter trying to exercise leadership (organization), and was she manifesting a developmental oscillation (i.e., acting older than her age)? The therapist hypothesized that the daughter, sensing that the mother's health issues were making the family's stability precarious, concluded that more adult support was needed and decided her father was the prime candidate. This hypothesis would allow the therapist to reframe the daughter's wish in a way that might not be so hurtful to the mother—that is, by suggesting that it is a father, not her particular father, that was being wished for.

If the hypothesis were valid, the therapist would expect the mother to soften and be less angry and the daughter to confirm the hypothesis. The hypothesis directed the therapist's attention to notice evidence of those shifts. If the mother relaxed in her chair, sat back, took a breath, unfurrowed her brow, looked directly at her daughter, or said something such as, "I never thought of it that way," the therapist would read the feedback to mean that the hypothesis had some merit and should be further developed. However, a blank stare from the mother, an averted gaze, a sigh of exasperation, or a verbal exclamation communicating disbelief were all feedback signals indicating that the hypothesis was not being accepted and more conversation was needed. Simultaneously, the daughter had also to be observed. Was she slouching, leaning forward, looking perplexed, or shrugging her shoulders? Although the list of behaviors to be observed was not short, having a hypothesis guided the therapist to read relevant feedback.

Feedback, therefore, is the link between the hypothesis and the intervention designed to build a solution sequence. This link is built through conversing, possibly resulting in modification, elaboration, or rejection of a therapeutic hypothesis. Once IST has commenced, the therapist works to understand the web of constraints that is keeping the client system from solving its problem. Conversation about the problem allows the therapist to develop a hypothesis about the web of constraints that can be tested with an intervention. Sometimes the intervention can be suggested and enacted during a session, but other times the therapist asks the clients to try something new between sessions. It is extremely important that the therapist asks for feedback about the solution sequence early in the following session. This inquiry signals to the clients that therapy continues between sessions and that the therapist values feedback about the results. If the solution sequence has been successful, at least a part of the problem may have been resolved. The clients are complimented on their good work. If not, the therapist will begin using the hypothesizing metaframeworks to investigate constraints holding the problem in place.

As noted in the initial example, not all feedback is verbal. Indeed, scholars who study the topic (Birdwhistell, 1962) believe that most feedback is nonverbal and is conveyed by facial expression, gesture, body posture, and nonverbal vocalizations. The study of emotion contained in facial expression is a discipline with a substantial literature that has established that basic facial expressions of emotions are universal. They can be decoded by infants as young as 5 months (Gopnik & Seiver, 2009). There are, however, cultural rules regarding the display of these emotions (Ekman, 2003).

Humans speak the same language of facial emotion, and the brain recognizes and responds to expression of emotion before the emotion is put into words (Fishbane, 2013). The speed of this feedback loop far outpaces a therapist's capacity to intervene. For example, one partner can simply raise a dubious eyebrow that the other partner responds to with a scowl, setting off a cascade of negative affect (and possibly harsh words). Hence, therapists are often playing "catch-up" with client feedback: "Something just happened here. Help me understand why your mood has suddenly shifted."

In addition to facial expression, feedback may be conveyed by body posture. Picture the arms-crossed, slouching body of the adolescent client eloquently yet wordlessly conveying, "I am here under protest, and there is zero chance you will get me to participate." Leaning forward, leaning back, turning away, turning toward, crossing the arms—all these postures can convey important feedback. In a similar vein, a nonverbal utterance such as a sigh, tongue cluck, throat-clearing, or a chuckle may also communicate feedback.

It is inherent in any interpretation of behavior that some meanings are privileged, whereas others are suppressed or rejected. Scheflen (1978) beautifully illustrated the complexity of interpretation in family therapy in a classic article about the multiple and contradictory meanings a group of therapists attributed to a single moment of therapy in which a daughter smiled at her father. Although meaning making is inevitable in therapy, it is also vulnerable to error and must, therefore, always be presented and understood as conditional.

The feedback in family therapy often presents as a choreographed dance with several moves. Consider the following example. A family of five consisting of two parents and three daughters—Angel, 15; Juanita, 12; and Carmen, 9—came to therapy to work on problems presented by Carmen. At one point in the session, the therapist took a break to discuss the session with the supervision team behind the mirror. Left alone in the therapy room, the team observed the family engage in the following interaction. First, the father raised his head and looked at Carmen, who was sitting across the room from him. Then Carmen stood up, crossed the room and climbed into her father's lap and received a big hug. As she crossed the room, the middle sister, Juanita, also stood up and moved behind the mother. The oldest sister, Angel, was already sitting next to the mother. The family froze in this position with the two older daughters giving Carmen "dirty looks." All family members seemed to recognize this choreographed dance. The supervisor noted this feedback and asked the team to read it. They hypothesized that the final positioning of the family revealed two subsystems: the mother and the two oldest daughters and the father and Carmen. Using the organization metaframework, multiple hypotheses were generated, and one was chosen to guide the plan when the therapist returned to the session.

GIVING AND RECEIVING FEEDBACK

As one of the four components of the blueprint, reading feedback is central to the therapeutic conversation and how it facilitates hypothesizing and planning. As the conversation unfolds, however, the clients and therapist frequently give each other feedback. To manage all alliances, therapists must be skilled at managing this feedback, which goes in both directions. Next, we address giving and receiving feedback. We begin this section with a discussion of the types of feedback that can be exchanged between clients and therapist.

Types of Feedback

Feedback has several purposes (Claiborn & Goodyear, 2005). The simplest kind of feedback is *descriptive*. For example, a client comes into the office and says to the therapist, "It's 10 after the hour. You're running late today." The client has just given the therapist descriptive feedback. It may or may not be important to address the matter any more than by saying, "Yes, I'm sorry about that." Silently, the therapist may make a mental note to be more careful about being on time for this particular client.

Although descriptive feedback is relatively easy to receive and to understand, it is less important than other kinds of feedback. Therapists must also give and receive *evaluative* feedback. For example, the client might say to the therapist, "I don't like it when you run late. It makes you seem sloppy and disorganized." Such evaluative feedback would require a more elaborate response than a simple apology.

Feedback may also be *emotionally disclosing*. The client might open the session by saying, "When you run late, it makes me anxious." Such a direct statement of feeling would require careful attention from the therapist because it demonstrates the emotional vulnerability of the client and may signal a rupture in the therapeutic alliance.

Finally, feedback may be *interpretive*. Again, using the example of the therapist running late, the client might say, "I think your lateness is a sign that I bore you." In this instance, the therapist must address the client's feedback: "Tell me more about this. Have you noticed other behaviors of mine that convey to you that you bore me?" This conversation might reveal a rupture in the alliance that must be repaired so the client believes the therapist is fully engaged in the therapy.

Another important aspect of feedback is its *valence*—that is, whether it is positive or negative. In therapy, positive feedback connotes approval, support, or validation, as in "You did a really good job of explaining why you felt the way you did." Conversely, negative feedback has a critical tone, as in "When you speak in such a harsh tone, it's difficult to keep listening to you." Humans have a strong, instinctive tendency to be receptive to positive feedback and rejecting of negative feedback (Claiborn, Goodyear, & Horner, 2001). When the therapist is giving feedback to clients, therefore, it is useful to start with the positive, describing aspects of the clients or the problem sequence that show strength or health, and then follow with the negative—for example, a constraint or a conflict.

Unexpected Feedback

Feedback can spontaneously emerge and not in response to the interaction of the session. Such feedback can be triggered by a misperception of the client, by something that happened earlier or perhaps outside the therapy context altogether, or by an association to a traumatic event. At such times, therapy requires improvisation in which the therapist steps aside from the direction of the session and attends solely to the feedback.

For example, Bob and Carol are a heterosexual couple in the early stages of working on "communication issues." From the outset, the therapy agenda was driven by Carol, whereas Bob was a reluctant participant. Carol offered a lot of encouragement and support to Bob, acknowledging that it was not an easy process for him. The therapist joined this endeavor by working to building an alliance with Bob, encouraging his conversation, using his metaphors, and affirming his observations. Out of nowhere, as it seemed to the therapist, Carol accused the therapist of siding more with Bob, of assuming she should do all the heavy lifting in the therapy, whereas all he had to do was show up.

The therapist then had to do several things at once: control emotional reactivity, be curious about and open to what Carol was saying, note how this development was being observed and coded by Bob, find out what triggered Carol's reaction, and repair the alliance so therapy could get back on track. Controlling the therapist's emotional reactivity is essential because, without it, she would not be able to process all the feedback, much less formulate a plan.

When unexpected feedback has temporarily derailed the therapist and disrupted the session, the therapist should slow everything down. For example, she might say, "Something just happened here, and I want to slow us down so I can be sure I get it." In a single sentence, the therapist has signaled interest in the clients and willingness to consider a therapeutic mistake as well as conveyed a belief that it can be sorted out. This is encouraging to the clients and models good communication.

Returning to the example, once the process is slowed down, the therapist can hypothesize (perhaps using the gender metaframework) to formulate questions to guide conversation about the client's experience. For example, she might acknowledge focusing on the alliance with Bob, having judged that Carol was more fully engaged. The therapist could then explicitly assess with both clients their level of engagement and their alliance to the therapist. Further conversation could return therapy to the current goal of the work on good communication.

Delayed Feedback

For both clients and therapists, thinking about therapy often occurs outside therapy sessions. Sometimes a specific context such as consultation or supervision stimulates the therapist to think about a particular client and develop new hypotheses. At times, clients randomly show up in the therapist's thoughts in a replay of a moment from a past session or in the form of a new hypothesis or plan. In a similar vein, the therapist is also the subject of clients' thoughts between sessions.

Between-session feedback can and should be brought to session by either client or therapist: "I was thinking about what you said last week." Such a sentence usually rivets the listener's attention. For the therapist, the client's referring to a previous session means that something the therapist said has been meaningful enough to be revisited. This is a good sign for the therapy in general and the alliance specifically. For the client, the idea that one's therapist continues to work on one's problems even outside the session is deeply gratifying.

As therapy progresses, the likelihood of delayed feedback increases. Both client and therapist have more experiences that connect them to each other and create new awareness, feelings, or ideas. The therapist is increasingly able to see the nuances of pattern in the problem sequence and give the clients feedback on it. If the alliance is good enough, clients are more willing to receive that feedback and, in turn, more willing to give the therapist feedback about their dissatisfaction or disappointment him or her.

Contradictory or Split Feedback

Doing systemic therapy with multiple clients in the room creates the probability that at some point they will disagree with each other and give the therapist different, even contradictory, feedback. "Things were better this week," one partner may say. "Better? What do you mean better? We had a huge fight on Sunday," the other might respond. Sometimes such a discrepancy is easily explained. In this example, the Sunday fight, the focus of one partner's report, might have been followed by 3 good days, the focus of the other partner.

More challenging to the therapist are situations in which partners have significant, clearly stated, and firmly held opinions that are mutually exclusive. For example, one parent may be convinced that an intervention directed toward changing a child's behavior is having an effect, whereas the other thinks the child is worse. One spouse may believe that an attempt to repair some rift with an in-law was met with rejection and disdain, while the other spouse thinks the in-law in question was just being cautious or confused. When there is split feedback, the therapist must acknowledge it while conveying confidence that the difference can eventually be sorted out or bridged by the partners. Subsequent work must find the common ground in clients' experiences.

Indirect Feedback

Feedback can be given indirectly. Examples of negative indirect feedback could include clients chronically showing up late for sessions, canceling at the last minute, forgetting to do between-session work, failing to pay their bill on time, not maintaining a regular therapy schedule, or forgetting their therapist's name. Such behaviors might signal problems of managing life effectively; however, the therapist should also consider that they signal a problem with the alliance—for example, clients are not engaged in the work, do not see the connection between the problem and the solution sequence, or do not have a strong bond with the therapist. The therapist should ask whether there is some meaning to such behaviors. On the therapist's part, forgetting the client's name or part of the story, missing a scheduled appointment, or drifting off during a session are all examples of indirect feedback that will have meaning for clients.

Indirect feedback may also be unexpectedly positive. A compliment on how the therapist looks, a comment on the quality of the university from which the therapist graduated, a small gift of appreciation at holiday time, a nod of the head as the therapist speaks, might all be indirect feedback to the therapist, signaling either a generally positive regard by the client or specific approval of something the therapist just said.

GUIDELINES FOR GIVING CLIENTS FEEDBACK

There are several guidelines for giving feedback. First, at the outset of therapy, clients should be told that although feedback from them is always welcome, they too will receive feedback from the therapist. This lets clients know that therapy is a process of developing and checking out hypotheses. The therapist expects that clients will evaluate some hypotheses as incorrect or incomplete. The statement "I expect I will make some mistakes along the way, and I hope you will let me know when you think that is the case" conveys the message that therapy is a collaborative process that sometimes involves mistakes and false starts and that by using the iterative process of conversing, hypothesizing, trying out solutions, and getting and giving feedback the problem can eventually be resolved.

The timing of feedback can dictate its utility. Too much too soon risks making the clients think the therapist is jumping to conclusions without an adequate understanding of the complexity of the problem. This can result in clients losing confidence in the therapist. However, clients want to know what their therapist thinks, so some feedback early on is usually advisable. By the end of the first session, the therapist should be able to give clients at least some descriptive feedback, such as, "Here's what stands out for me from our time together today." Such feedback may summarize what the clients said with the possible addition of something to think about in the coming week. The feedback should also include a compliment and a statement of hope to the clients, such as, "I appreciate how open you both were about the problems you have. That's a great sign that we are going to be able to work well together."

As the alliance grows stronger, the therapist gives more evaluative or interpretive feedback. For example, a couple entered therapy because the husband had had an affair. Early on, the therapist explained that recovery depends on the rebuilding of trust. Transparency and rigorous honesty with the betrayed spouse, therefore, were essential, an idea readily endorsed by both partners. If a small breach in that honesty occurred in the first few weeks of therapy, the therapist would certainly give some feedback regarding the breach in terms of rebuilding trust. The therapist may not yet have had sufficient understanding of the client's constraints to honesty to evaluate or offer a hypothesis. However, if the same breach occurred after several months of successful work in which there had been real progress in repairing the marriage and a strong alliance had been built, the therapist may give strong feedback to the client about how this dishonesty puts the marriage at risk and how the client seemed to be demonstrating the same pattern of withholding information that he developed in his family of origin.

Because positive feedback is easier to absorb than negative feedback, it should always accompany negative feedback and be offered first—for example, "I can see that both of you are working hard to control your reactivity to each other, but there are still too many times when both of you are triggered by old hurts." Such statements create hope and encouragement for clients who may be feeling discouraged. Sequencing feedback so it begins with the positive and then moves to the negative also makes it easier for clients to absorb.

A final guideline is that feedback should incorporate the client's language and metaphors rather than be expressed in purely technical or clinical terms. If a client thinks her problem is "having a bad temper," there is little to be gained by telling her she is "easily dysregulated." Similarly, if a client is a basketball fan (and the therapist is familiar enough with the sport to adapt its vocabulary to the problem at hand), it might be useful to frame an intervention as a variant of the "man-on-man defense."

GUIDELINES FOR RECEIVING CLIENT FEEDBACK

Therapists must practice care and skill in giving clients feedback, but clients are under no such obligation; therefore, receiving client feedback requires that the therapist have good emotional regulation, intellectual curiosity, and a firm belief that even critical feedback provides an opportunity for growth and learning. In IST, the alliance between the therapist and each client and the client system is regarded as the foundation for all change. Receiving feedback from clients is one of the mechanisms through which the alliance is developed, sustained, and repaired.

The therapist's stance regarding feedback from clients is crucial. He or she must be open and welcoming of feedback, particularly if it is critical, and yet must also reserve judgment about whether the feedback is valid and should alter the course of the therapy. For example, in the first phone contact with the client, the therapist is setting up norms and expectations about how the treatment will proceed. He or she says, "The problem you are describing clearly involves both you and your partner. I would like to see both of you in the first session." If the client agrees, the therapist sets up the initial appointment. But, an alternative response from the client might be, "I think it would be better if I see you alone first to explain some things about what's going on. After that, we can bring in my partner."

The client has just given the therapist some challenging feedback, demonstrating an unwillingness to simply defer to the therapist's judgment about who should attend the first session. Without the benefit of an established relationship, an understanding of the nature of the problem, or even the ability to read the facial expression of the client, the therapist has to make a decision about how to respond. Whatever response is offered will be feedback to the client. A response that simply allows the client to make the choice of who comes may convey to the client that this therapist can be easily influenced and all future directives may be taken merely as suggestions. However, the therapist might respond with further conversation, attempting to understand why the client wants to come in alone: "That's not how I generally operate. I'm curious about your reasoning. Tell me why you think it will go better if I meet alone with you first." This response gives the client the following feedback: "I am taking your request seriously, but I am reserving the right to decide the question depending on your explanation." A third alternative might be for the therapist to say, "It is my policy and practice never to begin couples therapy with an individual appointment. I'll be happy to explain my thinking on this, and then you can decide whether you still want to see me." These examples demonstrate that the early moment of engagement with a prospective client involves feedback from the client that will influence the therapy process.

Conveying Openness to Feedback

The most important element in receiving client feedback is openness to it. Were the therapist in the earlier example to get defensive or immediately insistent that "it's my way or the highway," the client may feel unheard or even disrespected, experiences that could keep the therapy from going forward or impair the formation of a strong alliance if it did. Throughout the course of any therapy, a steady willingness to hear what the client has to say about the accuracy and usefulness of the therapist's questions, statements, and directives and their link to hypotheses is an important ingredient of the treatment. Openness facilitates trust and candor, qualities that, in turn, encourage clients to accept the therapist's various attempts to be helpful.

Openness is conveyed in words such as, "Tell me more about that," "How did you feel when I said that?" or "Did that suggestion make sense to you?" A truly open therapist will invite feedback from the beginning of therapy, making it clear that all feedback will be taken as the client's effort to provide useful information. Openness is also conveyed nonverbally. A therapist who makes eye contact, leans slightly forward, and sits in an open position (i.e., not crossing the arms and legs) facing the client, with a neutral to positive facial expression is likely to be experienced as "open" by the client, in contrast to a therapist who is facing slightly away, looking out the window, with a grimace on the face and arms folded across the torso. Typically, IST does not encourage therapists to take notes during therapy because that tends to diminish the client's sense of the therapist's openness and transparency.

Recalling that the alliance is composed of tasks, goals, and bonds, it is crucial that therapists attend to clients' reservations about an intervention. Openness will be communicated by the therapist's willingness to be told that the intervention did not work, was unhelpful, confusing, or too complicated. For example, a therapist worked with parents trying to establish a regular bedtime ritual with a 5-year-old child who had spent most nights sleeping in her parents' bed since she outgrew her crib. Starting with the action planning metaframework, the therapist developed a behavioral procedure for the parents to use, involving the creation of a set of bedtime rituals (getting into pajamas, brushing teeth, reading a story, drinking water, saying good night, etc.) followed by a procedure to use when the child got out of bed and came into the parents' room. In the following session, the parents entered the office looking both weary and wary, sat down as far from each other as possible, and began the conversation by announcing that their little girl was still spending every night in their bed. Each accused the other of not following the plan. They looked to the therapist for confirmation that it was the other partner who had "messed up."

Note that in this example the parents did not blame the therapist for being unclear, overly ambitious, or naive about 5-year-old children. Instead, they turned against each other, which was feedback to the therapist suggesting that at least one constraint holding the problem in place was that the parents' alliance (at least about this issue) was weak and would need strengthening. Following the principle that positive feedback is easier to hear and should be given before negative feedback, the therapist complimented the parents on taking the task seriously and for being so observant about each other's participation. He also conveyed interest in exactly what went awry, as well as confidence that the three of them together could solve the problem. This feedback was given in words, of course, but also by the calm, unperturbed, receptive demeanor that the therapist conveyed in vocal tone, facial expression, and body posture.

Accepting Critical Feedback

Feedback that is critical of the therapist is by far the most challenging. Imagine the parents in the earlier example starting a session by attacking the intervention for "just addressing the symptom, not the real problem." Or it would be harder still if one of them bluntly asked whether the therapist had children. This kind of feedback can challenge even an experienced therapist. At such a moment, openness requires the therapist to manage her or his emotional response, be empathic to the frustration of the clients, convey a willingness to hear what went wrong, and still be able to think about what to try next.

It is a tall order never to be defensive in the face of what may feel like an attack from a client. In fact, there are moments in the life of all therapists when it is impossible. At such a moment, the therapist may stammer, get defensive, or blame the client. Depending on the context, such a blunder can rupture the alliance. If the rupture is not repaired, the clients might terminate therapy. When such alliance ruptures are addressed and successfully repaired, powerful shifts occur in the therapy, and the alliance becomes even stronger (Goldsmith, 2012). For example, a session ended shortly after a client's feedback provoked a defensive response from the therapist. In the next session, the therapist began the conversation by saying,

> I want to revisit our last conversation. You were trying to tell me something about our work, about me as your therapist, that I was having trouble taking in. I am sorry about that, and if you are willing, I'd like to try again to hear what you have to say.

Many clients are unaccustomed to such openness and validation and respond positively. Such an admission usually has the effect of not only repairing the tear in the alliance but also strengthening it.

SYSTEMATIC AND EMPIRICAL FEEDBACK

The epistemological foundation of IST holds empirical (quantitative) and experiential (qualitative) information as equivalent. From this perspective, science is not different from human perception or experience. It is just another form of knowing. In fact, our definition of science as a set of rules to minimize the likelihood of our lying to each other places science not on a different knowledge continuum but toward the systematic pole of that continuum. Direct perception and experience (thinking and feeling) are just less systematic ways of knowing. All ways of knowing in IST are equally valuable, appreciated, and used. This section addresses forms of feedback on a continuum from less to more systematic. The more systematic forms of feedback are also more empirically based, relying significantly on quantified data.

Patient-Focused Research and Empirically Informed Therapy

Over the last 30 years there has been a strong movement in all fields of psychotherapy to enlarge and enhance its scientific foundation. The primary manifestation of this movement has been the development and proliferation of *empirically supported treatments* (ESTs). These are typically specific models that have been developed to treat specific problems (e.g., anxiety, depression, addiction) in specific populations (e.g., adults, children). These treatments have been manualized and tested in randomized clinical trials, which have demonstrated their superiority over no treatment (waiting list control) or some form of alternative treatment.

The findings of this line of research provide an array of clinical strategies and techniques valuable to IST, many of which were presented in Chapter 6 on planning. However, for a variety of reasons, we do not advocate the doctrinaire use of manualized treatments. The primary reason behind this position is that ESTs derive from therapist-focused research, which emphasizes how therapists act during the course of treatment. The lack of flexibility of ESTs and the belief that only particular types of therapist behaviors lead to particular outcomes or effects contradict the systemic principle of *equifinality* (von Bertalanffy, 1968; Watzlawick, Bavelas, & Jackson, 1967). This principle asserts that in open systems, different pathways, causes, or inputs can and do lead to similar outcomes. In other words, in psychotherapy "many roads lead to Rome."

The alternative that we favor to enlarge and enhance the scientific foundation of IST and more generally the practice of psychotherapy is what has come to be called *patient-focused research*, which focuses on the behavior and experience of patients over the course of therapy. A branch of patient-focused research that we have called *empirically informed therapy* collects data from patients over the course of therapy and feeds the data back systematically to therapists, who are free to integrate their clients' data and adjust their behavior accordingly. In fact, we advocate collaborative, empirically informed therapy in which quantitative data from clients are used collaboratively by therapists and clients together to partner their way through the blueprint. We advocate collaborative, empirically informed hypothesizing, planning, conversing, and (reading) feedback. From this perspective, client data are used through all phases of therapy.

Measurement and Feedback Systems in Couple
and Family Research and Practice

Toward the goal of providing therapists (and clients) with empirical data to inform practice, a number of measurement and feedback systems have been developed over the past 20 years. Pinsof, Tilden, and Goldsmith (2016) compared and reviewed all these systems. There have also been a number of studies in individual and/or couples therapy, including one meta-analysis that compared treatment with a measurement and feedback system to treatment as usual, all of which showed that the treatment with empirical feedback was more effective than treatment as usual. Pinsof et al. (2016) also reviewed these studies.

The extant treatment systems can be organized in regard to complexity, sophistication, technology, and breadth. The most complex, technologically and clinically sophisticated, and broadest system that has been developed to date is the Systemic Therapy Inventory of Change (STIC; Pinsof, 2017; Pinsof, Goldsmith, & Latta, 2012; Pinsof, Zinbarg, et al., 2015). It is briefly described next.

Systemic Therapy Inventory of Change

The STIC was designed as an integrative and multisystemic measurement and feedback system to be used with IST. The STIC is completely online—it is filled out by clients at the office or at home before every session, and therapists immediately receive a feedback report by e-mail as well as a link to the STIC website if they want more information. The feedback report was designed to provide a snapshot of client progress since the first and last session that therapists can digest in 90 seconds before a session. It gives them a picture of what is improving, deteriorating, or staying the same.

The STIC consists of an extensive demographic questionnaire that was designed to be used to help situate the client and the client system in regard to many of the hypothesizing metaframeworks (especially development, organization, gender, spirituality, and culture). The STIC also consists of six system scales that ask responding clients about how they are doing individually regarding their family of origin, their partnership (if partnered), their current nuclear family, and their children. It also contains a scale to measure the therapeutic alliance from a multisystemic perspective. The STIC was normed with a nationally representative sample from the United States so that each client's score on each dimension of each scale is shown in regard to where it is located in the normal or clinical range for that dimension or scale.

The STIC was designed to inform hypothesizing by providing an empirical assessment of clients and their systems that could be integrated with the other information provided by the clients. It was designed to be used in planning by showing therapists and clients a number of potential problem targets (the "big six"—the six dimensions furthest into the clinical range for that client). It was also designed to inform conversing by providing therapists with information about the current status of the therapeutic alliance with each client (particularly any ruptures). Last, it was designed to provide therapists and clients with feedback about their progress that could be used to inform any of the other blueprint components. In addition, STIC data are displayed graphically so that each client's data in the case are displayed alongside the data from the other clients. More information about the STIC is available in an online chapter for this book (Bonus Chapter 2), which can be found online (http://pubs.apa.org/books/supp/pinsof).

Other Measurement and Feedback Systems

Although the STIC was designed to be used with IST, it can also be used with virtually any kind of therapy. In addition, IST can also use other measurement and feedback instead that can be helpful in bringing more scientific and systematic data into treatment. The important takeaway from this chapter is that we believe IST should use some form of empirical feedback to inform how practitioners apply the four components of the blueprint when working with clients. The specific system is less important than the fact that a measurement and feedback system is being used to bring science into practice.

9

THE INTEGRATIVE SYSTEMIC THERAPY APPROACH TO WORKING WITH FAMILIES

Throughout this book, we have emphasized the systemic underpinnings of integrative systemic therapy (IST). Everything is related to everything all the time (Russell, 2005). IST therapists, therefore, hypothesize systemically about the role of family in problem formation, maintenance, and resolution. Accordingly, the family is seen as one, albeit important, level of the multi-leveled biopsychosocial system. Also of importance are the relational and individual subsystems nested within the family. The family is also a subsystem within its community and the larger society. Because the problem sequence can manifest in myriad ways across all these levels, IST therapists are mindful of the role of the family but not focused exclusively on it. The family and/or its subsystems are brought into the direct client system to empower those clients to participate in the creation of solution sequences.

It is also important to note that the creators of the IST perspective have long-standing and deep roots in the family therapy movement dating

http://dx.doi.org/10.1037/0000055-009
Integrative Systemic Therapy: Metaframeworks for Problem Solving With Individuals, Couples, and Families,
by W. M. Pinsof, D. C. Breunlin, W. P. Russell, J. L. Lebow, C. Rampage, and A. L. Chambers
Copyright © 2018 by the American Psychological Association. All rights reserved.

back as far as 4 decades when family therapy was in its heyday and offering a true paradigm shift to the mental health establishment. Deeply schooled in and influenced by this movement and the many models of family therapy it spawned, IST recognizes the central role played by the family in problem maintenance and resolution. Family therapists understand that potential for change emerges by just bringing the family together to grapple with their problems. This potential is contained in the systemic axiom that the whole is greater than the sum of its parts. Commit the family to address their problems, and magic often happens as they access unused resources to solve them. For IST therapists, this recognition is operationalized in the planning matrix through which they are advised to begin therapy with the family. This preference is predicated on two considerations: first, that the problem sequence is most visible and more thoroughly understood when articulated and revealed by most, if not all, of the members who participate in it and, second, that the resources needed to create and implement a solution sequence are more readily identified and harnessed when the therapist works with the family.

Family therapy theory and practice as embodied by the classic family therapy models and their derivatives (Lebow & Sexton, 2015) become relevant to IST through the application of the hypothesizing and planning metaframeworks. Hence, the conceptual understanding of family as rendered by the models is lifted from them and placed in the hypothesizing metaframeworks. This makes it possible to hypothesize using the family therapy models' theories without having to practice the model. For example, Minuchin's (1974) ideas about family structure are part of the organization metaframework, and the theory of object relations underpinning object relations family therapy is part of the mind metaframework.

Likewise, established family therapy models' planning strategies are housed among the planning metaframeworks in IST. For example, the practices of structural family therapy (e.g., enactment) fit within the action planning metaframework (Minuchin, 1974) and Bowenian therapy (e.g., coaching) within the family-of-origin planning metaframework (Bowen, 1974). The decision tree for deciding which family therapy strategies to use is operationalized by the arrow on the IST planning matrix (see Figure 6.1). For example, enactments would precede coaching.

Working with the family in IST is a more fluid process than is typical of classic family therapy models. For example, some classic family therapy models locate the problem in the family system and call for the family to always be present for all sessions. Some family therapy models espouse one path to clinical outcome. For example, solution-focused therapy single-mindedly works with the family to identify exceptions when the problem is not being experienced (de Shazer, 1985). IST makes a distinction between whole family therapy, in which all relevant family members attend sessions, and relational family therapy, in which just key clients are present (Breunlin & Jacobsen, 2014).

This style of working with the family is best illustrated with a case example. Our case example in this chapter tracks the course of therapy from the initial phone call to the follow-up a year after therapy was finished. Although every therapy is complex and involves a number of steps, the description of the therapy here focuses on key episodes when the family work was deemed essential to the success of the case.

CASE EXAMPLE: THE PRITCHARD FAMILY

The Pritchards were a Caucasian family consisting of a heterosexual couple, Sarah, 45, and Jordan, 46. This was the second marriage for Sarah. She was married for 6 years to Burt and had two children from that marriage, Ethan, 18, a freshman away at college, and Andrea, 17, a junior in high school. Sarah was the primary parent for these children, although they did sporadically see Burt. Sarah and Jordan had a son, Tim, who was 11. Sarah was the eldest of five siblings. Her parents were poor, and Sarah acted in a parent-like role growing up. She completed high school and worked as the office manager for a general medicine practice. Jordan was an only child of working-class parents. He completed high school and an associate's degree. He was an assistant manager of a grocery store.

Sarah initiated therapy because of the constant arguments with Andrea that were creating a corrosive atmosphere in the family. Other presenting problems included Tim's Type 1 diabetes that was poorly managed, school problems for both Andrea and Tim, and Jordan's growing frustration with the toxic atmosphere created by the fighting between Sarah and Andrea. During the course of therapy, which lasted 25 sessions, all these presenting problems were addressed. In addition, the relationship that Ethan and Andrea had with Burt was identified as a problem, as was the fact that Burt and Sarah had sparse contact with each other. Both problems were addressed in the therapy.

Therapy began with Sarah, Jordan, Andrea, and Tim (Ethan was away at college). In the early sessions, the therapist identified two problem sequences, one a face-to-face sequence of high conflict (referred to as "the war") and the other a sequence involving the family routine. The former sequence was embedded in the latter. The routine of relevance occurred after school when Andrea and Tim were expected to come home to help with chores and do their homework. Andrea was also expected to monitor Tim's food intake. Andrea resented that the routine took time away from her social life. Conflict between Sarah and Andrea erupted when Sarah arrived home to find the routine had not been followed.

The therapist chose to focus on the routine sequence first because the presenting problem of high conflict and the other problems were part of it. He focused first on the problem of poor management of Tim's diabetes, externalizing it and the fear it generated, and used a number of interventions to put Tim in charge of managing the disease. This included working with the medical team treating Tim. The second problem addressed was performance at school. As this problem was explored, Andrea revealed another problem, debilitating anxiety that impaired her school performance. The therapist provided Andrea with a workbook that contained basic strategies for managing school-related anxieties and taught Jordan and Sarah how to help her use it. This solution sequence resulted in Sarah relaxing the after-school routine so that Andrea had more time for her social life. Changing the after-school routine eliminated several constraints and softened the relationship between Sarah and Andrea; consequently, the high-conflict sequence improved. The therapist also worked to create solution sequences that promoted better communication between Sarah and Andrea.

The therapist believed that organizational constraints in the client system could prevent the solution sequences from stabilizing. These constraints included a weakened marital subsystem for Sarah and Jordan, insufficient leadership collaboration between Sarah and Burt, a disengaged relationship between Burt and his children, and the loss of Ethan's stabilizing role brought about by his departure for college. The therapist pursued a series of subsystem sessions and interventions to lift these constraints.

THE INITIAL PHONE CALL

The following description of the initial phone call illustrates how IST therapists secure clients' commitment to family therapy. This work at the outset pays huge dividends throughout the course of the therapy.

Sarah made the initial call to request therapy. She said she was desperate to resolve what she called the constant war between her and her daughter, Andrea. When the therapist responded that it must be difficult to live in a war zone, Andrea's tone of voice softened as she acknowledged that she was exhausted and that her husband, Jordan, was hinting that he could not take the tension in the home for much longer. The therapist responded, "So this war is taking a toll on everyone. Is there anyone else living in the home?" Sarah mentioned Tim and added that her eldest, Ethan, was away at college. The therapist asked how Tim coped with the war. Sarah replied that he was reclusive and spent most of his time at home in his room. She added that Tim had Type 1 diabetes.

With just a few questions and statements, the therapist acknowledged the presenting problem—the war—but also spread the problem description to include both Jordan and Tim. The development, organization, and biology hypothesizing metaframeworks quickly opened, and the therapist wondered what impact Ethan's departure for college might have had on the war, whether the family had successfully blended, and what impact Tim's diabetes had on the family. None of this, however, was shared with Sarah, because she wanted help with the war.

The therapist asked Sarah to elaborate on what the war looked like to her. She stated that every day when she arrived home from work, she and Andrea got into an argument over the latter's responsibilities, including her schoolwork and chores. Within a few seconds, Andrea would become tense and tell her mother not to hassle her. Unless Andrea dropped the issue, the war would then quickly escalate to the point at which Andrea would be screaming at her mother and hurling angry barbs; this usually ended with Andrea saying she hated her mother and storming off to her room. Sarah was saddened by the breakdown of her relationship with Andrea and concerned that she could not communicate with her. She added that Andrea was also doing poorly in her junior year of high school, thus jeopardizing her chances of graduating, let alone going to a good college. Sarah was hoping to set up an appointment with a therapist so Andrea could talk about her feelings toward her mother. When asked whether she had spoken with Andrea about therapy, Sarah acknowledged that she had and added that Andrea said she would not go.

This is a typical call from a parent seeking help for a problem involving a child or adolescent. The default request is for individual therapy, with the calling parent expecting, at most, to bring the child to therapy and perhaps provide some information to the therapist. In this modern world, engaging families requires most callers to shift their perspective from the assumption that therapy means individual therapy to agreeing to bring in the family (Breunlin & Jacobsen, 2014). There are various approaches to making this argument. The following exchange between the therapist and the mother ended with the mother agreeing to invite Andrea, Jordan, and Tim to the first session.

Therapist: So you are thinking that I should see Andrea alone?

Sarah: Yes, isn't that how it works?

Therapist: Well, yes, sometimes it works that way, but I have found that another way might work better in the long run. Can I share it with you?

Sarah: Sure.

Therapist:	So hear me out on my idea because your first reaction is likely to be negative.
Sarah:	OK.
Therapist:	I know you want to end the war, but even supposing Andrea would agree to go to therapy, she would arrive believing she is being blamed for the problem, and that will make her guarded about therapy. If we make the problem a family problem, say that there is too much tension in the family, then Andrea doesn't get singled out, and other members have something to gain by coming to therapy. How does that sound to you?
Sarah:	It makes sense, but I seriously doubt whether you could ever make something like that happen. Jordan would say he's too busy, and besides, Andrea is my daughter, and it's my relationship with her that's the problem. Tim would say that Andrea is crazy and needs help, so it's a waste of his time to go to therapy.
Therapist:	I get all that, Sarah. I just need you to deliver them to me for one session, and I'll do the rest. All you have to do is make an authentic appeal to them to come to see me for at least one session because what is happening in the family shouldn't continue.
Sarah:	OK, I'll make a leap of faith here, but I still don't know what to say.

For the next 5 minutes, the therapist coached Sarah on how to approach family members with the invitation, encouraging her to take some ownership of the problem. Sarah admitted that one component of the problem was work–life balance. She admitted that she was often tired and preoccupied and knew she sometimes approached interactions with Andrea with a "shoot-from-the-hip" style of communication. Having thanked her for this disclosure, the therapist further coached her in how to get all family members to agree they hated the atmosphere in the home and wanted it to change. Finally, the therapist instructed her to encourage all of them to call and talk with him. If they declined to make the phone call, they were still invited to a session all together.

Once Sarah was on board with bringing the family to the first session, one other negotiation had to take place. The therapist thought about clients who might be in the indirect system, particularly Andrea's father, Burt. He asked Sarah about the relationship between Andrea and Ethan and their father. The groan from the phone was audible.

Sarah:	You aren't suggesting that I have to involve Burt, too, are you?
Therapist:	It sounds like there might be some bad feelings between you and the kids' father?
Sarah:	That's putting it mildly. If you get me started, you won't get home for supper.
Therapist:	Look, I sense this is complicated, but I don't want to set us up for failure before we even get started. We don't need to go into great detail, so maybe I can just explain why I am bringing up Burt now?
Sarah:	OK.
Therapist:	OK, do you and Burt share custody?
Sarah:	Yes, but that's about it. He hasn't been consistent with visits since the kids became teenagers, and they have come to not depend on him. It's a waste of time to try to get him involved.
Therapist:	I see. How would Burt feel about the kids being in therapy?
Sarah:	He'd hate it because he'd be certain he's being blamed for Andrea's attitude.
Therapist:	Exactly, and I don't want to get off on the wrong foot with him because he could sabotage the therapy. So here's what I propose doing. He doesn't have to be involved now, but we may need him at some point down the road. I think most custodial parents appreciate the courtesy of a call from the therapist. So I suggest giving him a call just to introduce myself, explain the purpose of the family therapy, let him know that his perspective about his kids is incredibly valuable, and ask whether I can talk to him once I understand the situation better.
Sarah:	Knock yourself out, but don't expect much.

WORK BEFORE THE FIRST SESSION

After the phone call with Sarah, the therapist took a few notes that reflected systemic hypothesizing about the family. This was a postdivorce blended family with two hardworking adults who had one sick child and one angry and underperforming adolescent. Even without the war, those factors alone put great strain on the family. In terms of leadership, what organizational issues kept Sarah from being a more effective leader? There were also questions about development. The leaving home transition of Ethan's departure to college could be important. What about Tim's diabetes? How was it being managed, and was there, as is often the case, an oscillation going on with him? What was going on between Sarah and Burt, and was there more to her anger toward him? What else was involved in the problem sequence besides repetitive and escalating hostility? How should the therapist manage the intensity in the upcoming session? What if the war broke out right in the session? The initial solution sequence had to involve calling a truce, but how would that be accomplished? Without a truce, necessary conversations about the web of constraints would be difficult if not impossible.

Before the initial session, the therapist also called Burt. At first, Burt was guarded, but when the therapist explained that the goal of the call was simply to inform him that some family therapy was being planned that would involve his children, he became more open. The therapist complimented Burt by saying he was an expert on his children and expressed interest in any insights he might have about them. Burt praised both kids. He added that Ethan's departure for college had been hard on everyone because Ethan had always been the levelheaded one who often mediated disputes between Sarah and Andrea. He added that Sarah was a control freak and a workaholic and that Andrea resented how Sarah prioritized her work over the family, something he said Sarah would never admit. Asked what his contact was like with his children, he said that, like most teenagers, they preferred flexibility, so he saw them when it was convenient for them. That translated into a dinner once every couple of weeks. It also meant that Sarah was responsible for Ethan and Andrea 24/7, so she never got a break. After the call, the therapist e-mailed Sarah to let her know the call to Burt had been made.

THE INITIAL SESSION

The therapist was relieved to see that all family members came to the first session. They filed into the office with glum looks and, except for Sarah, stared blankly at the therapist. He first greeted each member, learned their names and something about each of them. He then discussed ground rules for the therapy, emphasizing the importance of the sessions' being a safe place to talk. The therapist also acknowledged that for some sessions only some of the family members would be present and that, occasionally, he might speak with a family member between sessions. In these conversations, members could express their opinions, and the therapist would, if asked, keep these opinions confidential. The therapist would not, however, keep secrets because this would ultimately do harm to the outcome of the therapy. He then turned to Sarah.

> *Therapist:* Congratulations, Sarah, you managed to get everyone here. How did you make that happen?
>
> *Sarah:* I just did what you recommended. We sat down, and I told them that we all know that it feels like a war zone at home and that I knew we are all unhappy and we should do something to change that.
>
> *Therapist:* Do you all agree with what Sarah just said?
>
> *Andrea:* I'm here, but I don't have anything to say.
>
> *Therapist:* OK, Andrea, I'm glad you came today. I respect your reluctance to talk. It's OK; you can just observe for now. So who can tell me why communication turns into a war?

Jordan began by saying the war was between Sarah and Andrea. He stayed out of it because he was the stepparent. He added that Tim was reclusive and seldom came out of his room. Recognizing that a mother–daughter dyad can be volatile, the therapist wondered whether Jordan or Tim ever tried to be influential behind the scenes. Jordan said that in private he tried to tell Sarah not to "take the bait," but she always replied that she would not let her daughter be disrespectful. Tim said he told his sister she should not make such a big deal out of their mom's demands. The therapist asked Tim what he meant by "demands," and Tim shared that Sarah always had a list of chores for Andrea and him to do when they got home from school. He said he viewed it as no big deal, so he just did them, but Andrea frequently did not comply. When Sarah got home and saw something had not been done, she asked Andrea why not, and that started the war. Here Sarah chimed in to offer her explanation for wanting the kids to help. Andrea sat up in her chair and glared at Sarah; the therapist read this feedback as evidence that she wanted to enter the conversation. Not wanting to shut her down by overtly inviting her into the conversation, the therapist allowed a small silence to build and then glanced toward Andrea.

> *Andrea:* This stuff about helping out is pure crap. None of my friends have to come home and do chores.
>
> *Sarah:* We're a family. It's important that both of you participate.
>
> *Andrea:* [Screaming] Just because you had to take care of your brothers and sisters doesn't mean that it's fair for you to expect the same of me.
>
> *Sarah:* [With tears in her eyes] I'm your mother. I decide what you do.

Reading the feedback that the war had been engaged with just a few turns between Sarah and Andrea and that further turns might end in Andrea bolting, the therapist decided to interrupt the escalation.

Therapist: Hold on. So this is the war. Let's stop for a second. That really happened so fast! Please, let's all just take a few deep breaths and gather our composure.

During these few moments, the therapist shifted to hypothesizing on the blueprint (Figure 4.1) to consider what had just transpired. An experienced IST therapist can do this efficiently because the hypothesizing metaframeworks are easily accessible and offer hypotheses for most of what had just transpired. The face-to-face interaction was an example of the war and a key problem sequence. Andrea's anger escalated rapidly, and neither participant listened to the other. Sarah seemed entrenched in her views about helping out and viewed the problem sequence as being about respect. The silence of Jordan and Tim was also noteworthy.

The face-to-face sequence, however, was also embedded in a sequence of the family's routine. The routine sequence looked something like this. Andrea wanted to hang out with friends and resented having to come home after school, and she acted out by not doing her chores. Sarah worked long hours and arrived home late and tired. They were both in bad moods. Sarah confronted Andrea about the chores. They engaged in the war and then disengaged having settled nothing. Andrea then ate her dinner in the family room while Jordan, Sarah, and Tim had an uncomfortable meal in the kitchen. The therapist also hypothesized that the routine sequence was further embedded in a transgenerational sequence in which Sarah was replicating the routine of her family of origin.

Shifting to the planning component of the blueprint, the therapist knew that the first order of business was to de-escalate the war; however, attempting to address the high level of expressed emotion directly without stronger alliances seemed risky. He decided to address some of the issues associated with the routine that seemed to fuel the war, including respect, leadership, illness, and loss of a social life. He then shifted his attention to the conversing component of the blueprint. In the following dialogue, descriptions of the use of the conversational palette discussed in Chapter 7 are placed in brackets.

Therapist: [Gesturing to Sarah and Andrea] Excuse me, look, this is our first meeting, and I don't want it to end in failure because you have the war just like at home and nothing changes. I'm glad I got to see the war. It's easy to see how it goes, but I need to interrupt it now. I'm sure it's painful for Sarah and Andrea to be part of it and also painful for Jordan and Tim to have to witness it. So let's call a truce for a moment. I need to say a few things, and then you can continue the conversation. [To stop the escalation, the therapist juxtaposes statements and a directive.]

Andrea, I am glad that you chose to join the conversation. We won't accomplish much without your voice being heard. [The therapist compliments Andrea.] Sarah, I know these moments must feel excruciatingly painful to you, and you want to find a way to communicate with Sarah differently, but we have to figure out how to do that. [The therapist assures Sarah that her primary goal is not going to be ignored.]

Jordan, you looked shocked to see two people you love go at each other that way, and Tim, if I had a rock for you to crawl under, that's where you would have gone. Look, this is family therapy. You bring problems here, and my job is to get all of you participating in finding solutions to them. [The therapist sets the stage for engaging the whole family in the work.] Look, the conflict seems, at least in part, to be about how this family uses its resources to function on a day-to-day basis. Is that what is meant by everyone helping out? [The therapist uses a statement and a directive to redirect the session.]

Sarah:	Exactly, and that's what Andrea refuses to acknowledge.
Therapist:	Wait. Let's not start up the war. We need to find a way to use the truce. [Fearing that the conflict will just ignite again, the therapist uses a directive and a statement to keep the focus on the truce.] So look, you are a dual career couple raising teenagers who have lives and school, so it's going to be a challenge no matter how you go about it. So can we take a moment and look more closely at how your routine works? Sarah, is it OK if I ask Jordan about the routine?
Sarah:	Sure. I know he's not Andrea's father, but he has a pretty good relationship with all of my children and is totally committed to them. I wish he would be more involved. [The therapist builds the alliance with Sarah by gaining her approval to bring Jordan into the conversation.]
Therapist:	Great. So, Jordan, let me ask you. What else is driving the routine? [The therapist normalizes the struggle for routine and decides to give Jordan a turn to expand the conversation to the whole family.]
Jordan:	OK, so here are a couple of things they didn't talk about. First, I should say that Sarah and I aren't on the same page

about this issue. She believes that schoolwork and family are the most important and social life comes after that. So she wants the kids home by 5:00 so they can do their chores and start their homework.

Andrea: [Interrupting] Yeah, so if I want to hang out with my friends or be in an activity, it's not possible.

Sarah: You have the weekends, and you sometimes go out after I get home.

Therapist: Excuse me. Let's let Jordan finish what he's saying. Andrea and then Sarah can jump into the conversation when he's done, taking turns. [The therapist uses a directive to give the turn back to Jordan.] So, Jordan, you have added some important information. What else do you have to say about the after-school routine?

Jordan: I agree that school is most important, and quite frankly, both of them are struggling in school, but I also believe it is shortsighted to restrict an adolescent's social life. I would vote to let them come home later.

Sarah: I might be persuaded to adopt that plan so long as we address their poor school performance, but Jordan, how can you forget that this plan is also in place because of Tim's diabetes. We know he doesn't control his eating well. He has had attacks, even recently, that have put us in the emergency room. I can't get my job done if all I do is worry that Tim is having an attack.

Andrea: Yeah, so there you go. My life sucks because I have to cover for my kid brother who is old enough to take care of his diabetes but won't do it. Neither of you do a damn thing to make him grow up and face the fact that he has to deal with a chronic illness for the rest of his life. [Shifting the conversation to include Jordan and to focus on the routine has brought forth news of important constraints that provide clues to Andrea's anger and disdain for Sarah that keep the war from changing.]

The therapist read the feedback and recognized that two important constraints had been revealed that explained the routine: poor school performance and mismanagement of Tim's diabetes. Sarah has fears, perhaps catastrophic expectations, that Tim could die. She seemed to have had a lot of responsibility as the eldest sibling in her family of origin. She designated Andrea as the person to monitor this situation, and her fear made her rigid about her expectations. The therapist wondered whether this had been Ethan's job before he left for college. When the job fell to Andrea, was she upset because it interfered with her social life but she could not refuse to do it?

The therapist was in the midst of a classic IST moment: being faced with a plethora of hypotheses that revealed the systemic underpinnings of the presenting problem and the problem sequences. To hold these hypotheses, he opened several metaframeworks, including organization, development, mind, and biology. The therapist wanted to confirm or refute these hypotheses and also to collaborate with the family to begin finding a solution sequence.

The therapist envisioned a solution sequence that involved several strategies. The first was easing the rigidity of the after-school routine. Doing this, however, required finding out what was constraining success in school and keeping Tim from managing his diabetes. How family resources were used to handle domestic demands had to be explored and modified. Finding a solution sequence for the routine might have improved the relationship between Sarah and Andrea, thereby draining intensity from the war. Having done this hypothesizing and planning, the therapist continued the conversation.

> Therapist: Andrea, is your job to be at home in case Tim's blood sugar puts him at risk, or are you also supposed to monitor what he eats?
>
> Andrea: [Softening a bit] Mainly the first, but I know he is sneaky, and if I don't pay attention, he'll be hitting the carbs.
>
> Therapist: That's a tough assignment. Did Ethan have that job before he went to college?
>
> Andrea: Yes, and Ethan—no offense, Mom—is a nerd. All he did was study, so he didn't mind being home.
>
> Therapist: Now that you have the job, are you fearful that something might go wrong?
>
> Andrea: Yes, of course. He's my brother. I just wish my mom would understand that it's too much to ask of me.
>
> Therapist: [To Tim] Tim, how does it make you feel to have your sister police your diabetes?
>
> Tim: I hate it. They should just let me do it on my own.
>
> Sarah: We've been there and then in the emergency room. Right now we can't take that chance.
>
> Therapist: [To Tim] It sounds like you want another chance to show that you can manage your diabetes?
>
> Tim: If they'll let me.

Therapist: [To the family] I bet all of you share the same fear about Tim's welfare. There are a lot of moving parts to this situation in addition to managing the diabetes: school challenges, having a social life, demanding jobs, and relationships. We can't tackle all of them at the same time. It seems to me that job one is for the family to defeat the fear you all have about Tim's welfare. That entails coming up with a better plan for managing the diabetes. How do you all feel about making Tim's diabetes management our first order of business?

Sarah: I admit that every day is a nightmare for me because I can't be sure my son is safe. [Sarah begins to cry.]

The therapist indicated to Jordan where the tissue box was, and he handed it to Sarah. The therapist nodded at Jordan, and he moved closer to Sarah. He sat silently looking at her. The therapist used silence to let the moment build. Sarah looked at Jordan, but it soon became apparent that Jordan did not know what to say. The therapist read this feedback and decided to rescue him.

Therapist: It can be hard to know what to say when the stakes are so high. We will be working on communication as one of the tools you all use to defeat the fear.

The remainder of the session was spent gathering information about the diabetes and sharing ideas about what a solution sequence might look like. Everyone participated, and the war did not continue. The therapist opened the biology metaframework and listened to the family. Through her job, Sarah was able to locate competent providers for Tim, but she felt they were assuming Tim could be more autonomous than she believed he could. It seemed the treatment team and Sarah were not on the same page. Jordan had deferred to Sarah. The therapist secured permission and signed consents from Sarah and Tim to talk to the treatment team. The therapist noted that the after-school routine was also predicated on poor school performance. Both Andrea and Tim acknowledged they were struggling. Andrea contended that she did not want to go to college, so what difference did it make that she had average grades? Hearing this, Sarah bristled. Andrea compared herself with Ethan, who loved school. Tim had been a good student until he was diagnosed. Since then his grades had fallen off, in part because he missed a great deal of school and was chronically behind in his work. The therapist acknowledged that the school issues must also be addressed.

The therapist knew the plan would fail if Sarah and Andrea kept fighting and wondered how they could avoid the war until the next session. He risked damaging his alliance with Sarah by telling Andrea the family should work to create a routine that better enabled her to have a social life and that this would be discussed in the next session. He then got Sarah and Andrea to commit to a truce. Andrea agreed to be more cooperative, and Sarah committed not to lose it if she found that something had not been done. Recognizing that the mother–daughter conflict seemed deep and entrenched and probably involved other issues, the therapist wondered whether it might have been a mistake not to focus first on the war. At the outset, IST inevitably involves making difficult choices because every systemic consideration cannot get equal treatment.

WORK BETWEEN THE FIRST AND SECOND SESSIONS

Between sessions, IST therapists revisit their hypotheses, plan for upcoming sessions, and manage the therapy system. In regard to hypothesizing, the therapist wondered just how much Ethan's departure for college had affected the seemingly beleaguered Pritchard family. In regard to other resources, so far there had been no mention of any extended family help. Finally, what kept Burt from serving as a better resource for Ethan and Andrea? As part of the work ahead, the therapist decided to invite Ethan to a session when he came home for an upcoming holiday, to meet with Burt to see whether he could be enlisted as a resource for his children, and to find out whether grandparents, adult siblings, or cousins lived in the area.

The therapist also contacted Tim's treatment team. The nurse returned the call. Fortunately, the nurse possessed a high level of psychosocial sophistication, making it easy for her and the therapist to be on the same page regarding the biobehavioral aspects of Tim's diabetes management. She said that the family had reacted normally to learning of the diagnosis but that Sarah had focused primarily on safety issues. The nurse said that is always the parent's first concern but that a chronic illness, especially one as complicated to manage as diabetes, also affects emotional, social, and behavioral aspects of a child's development. First, she noted that the diabetes diagnosis causes children of Tim's age to be set apart from their peers. For example, although a healthier child of this age thinks little about food, a child with diabetes must do so continually. These children can also be singled out at birthdays and other social events because either they are not eating the same food as everybody else or they need to check their glucose levels, both of which call unwanted attention to them as "different." It would also be important to assess whether Tim ever deliberately acted against medical advice regarding his diabetes in an effort to reject his parents' values and assert his independence.

If the whole family is not committed to understanding and facilitating every aspect of a child's psychosocial development, the child also acts younger than his or her age. This shows up in emotional and behavioral delays such as poor school performance. Opening the development metaframework, the therapist hypothesized that Tim was in a developmental oscillation that had to be dampened. The nurse indicated that psychoeducation groups were offered but the family had not availed itself of them and that only Sarah usually brought Tim to his appointments. The therapist recognized that a lot of work had to be done for the family to be able to handle the diabetes differently, but most important, control over the management of the disease had to begin with Tim.

THE NEXT FEW SESSIONS

Therapy is rarely a tidy affair that proceeds exactly to plan. In the interest of space limitations, therefore, what follows is a highlight of the main themes addressed in the second through seventh sessions.

Addressing the Diabetes

At the outset of the second session, the therapist greeted the family and asked how things had gone at home. Sarah volunteered that she had tried not to react when she got home, and she appreciated that Andrea seemed to be trying to control her temper. Only one conflict episode had occurred, but Andrea had approached Sarah later that evening to apologize for snapping at her. The therapist congratulated Andrea and asked how she had managed to do that. Andrea replied that although she knew she could be mean, she was not a monster. She had just decided to try to control herself and felt mad at herself when she failed. The therapist reiterated that Sarah and Andrea had some issues that still had to be addressed but congratulated them for managing the conflict better so the family could focus its attention on the after-school routine. Jordan added that it felt better to come home and find that an explosion had not occurred. Next, the therapist set the stage for the work of the session.

> Therapist: OK, so today we are going to see if there is another way to manage the routine after school. From last week, we learned that two obstacles are how the kids are performing at school and how Tim manages his diabetes. I think we said we would tackle the diabetes first. Before we proceed, I just want to ask you, Andrea, whether focusing on this issue is a problem for you because Tim has already been a big focus of this family.

> Andrea: Thanks. The diabetes dominates this family, but look, if working on it allows me to get my life back, I'm all in.

Therapist: That's great to hear. So, look, as we all agreed, I had a chance to talk with the nurse on Tim's treatment team, and here's the big takeaway. They believe an 11-year-old child is capable of being largely responsible for the management of his diabetes on a day-to-day basis. That includes both knowing what can be eaten and eating in a responsible way and being able to test for blood sugar levels and recognize when it is necessary to take insulin. Will there be mistakes? Yes, of course, but if there is a backup plan, the risk is negligible. The nurse reported that Tim has already demonstrated interest in his own care as he asks questions in appointments and clearly understands the answers. Something is getting in the way, and when that happens, the diabetes ends up tyrannizing all of you. My question to all of you is, what's keeping Tim from being that 11-year-old who can manage his disease?

This is a classic moment in IST in which the therapist asks a constraint question that organizes the family regarding the quest to address an important issue (management of diabetes) in a more constructive way. The question invites everyone to participate both in identifying the constraints and figuring out how to lift them. Sarah opened the conversation by saying, no offense to the treatment team, but she should know what her son is capable of. She added that if Tim could not turn in an assignment for school, how could he be expected to be on top of a life-threatening illness? Jordan countered that Tim's decline in school performance came after the diagnosis of his illness. Andrea added that Tim had just lost his mojo. Using "mojo" as a metaphor for the solution sequence of diabetes management, the therapist proceeded.

Therapist: So, Tim, do you agree that you have lost your mojo?

Tim: I guess so. What's the use? I'm just 11, and I have a disease that will never go away, and besides, someday it might make me blind or make me have to have a leg cut off.

Therapist: Whew! That's a mojo-killing way to look at this! Of the family members, who most shares this mojo-killing view?

Tim: Mom is the most like that because she works with doctors, and they taught her how to Google things on the Internet.

Therapist: Is that right, Sarah?

Sarah: I guess, but I didn't realize it would kill your mojo.

Therapist: Tim, do you want your mojo back?

Tim: Yeah, but how?

A conversation followed in which the family members contributed ideas about how Tim could get his mojo back. Jordan admitted he had allowed Sarah to set the tone for how the family dealt with the diabetes and added that Sarah was a big-time worrier. Jordan volunteered that he had to have more of an opinion. Sarah said she would welcome that; however, when Jordan said all of them should attend the education sessions offered by the treatment team, Sarah said they were just too busy to commit to that. After some back-and-forth, they all agreed to go. Sarah then added that even if Tim got his mojo back, there were still things that could be done to back him up. She said she and Jordan would have to do a better job of grocery shopping. They would also have to be sure Tim understood how to control his blood sugar levels through the foods he ate and the insulin he had to take.

Continuing to externalize the diabetes, the therapist pointed out how it had cast a cloud of fear over the family that was keeping members from risking that Tim could use his mojo. He asked how they could defeat the fear. When there was silence, he turned to Sarah and asked how physicians assess and manage risk. He wondered how a doctor would determine the risk to a child who managed his diabetes well. Sarah said the doctors she worked with would let Tim do it, but Tim was not their son. The therapist noted that Sarah's maternal fear was defeating her. When the maternal fear was named and discussed, Sarah declared she would have to overcome it.

Over the course of several sessions, a plan emerged for Tim to get his mojo back. Food entering the house was more closely monitored. Because the blood sugar reading was a tangible measure of risk, the parents agreed that Tim would test and text the number to both parents. In the event a crisis emerged, they developed a plan to respond. Andrea was no longer in that loop. Tim embraced the job of being responsible. He recorded a string of days with no missed school. Jordan visited the school and worked with teachers to create a plan so Tim could turn in missed assignments. Tim's grades showed improvement. Tim joined a support group at the hospital for kids with a chronic illness. He made friends with other children who faced similar challenges. He learned about a summer camp for children with diabetes and asked whether he could go. He reported that his mojo was back.

Work on the War

The therapist knew that the war remained to be addressed. Although it had not erupted for a few weeks, the only solution sequence had been to address the after-school routine. At the outset of a session, the therapist first addressed Jordan and Tim by forewarning them that Sarah and Andrea were going to do the heavy lifting in this session, but that their roles as observers were important. Deciding to focus on the sequence before uncovering the psychological pain that fueled the high-intensity emotions, the therapist invited them to provide an anatomy of the sequence. What was going on before the sequence? How was the conversation initiated? What were some of the triggers that escalated the argument? Were there any ways the argument could be aborted before it got out of hand? What sustained the intensity once it was reached? The therapist also pointed out that although anger seemed to be the prevailing emotion at the height of the argument, perhaps there were other feelings involved that had to be explored.

Andrea started by noting she was usually hanging out with friends after school. Just when things seemed to jell, and the group decided to go somewhere, Andrea realized she had to go home. She hated being the only one who had to leave and always stewed about it on the way home. Sarah said that work was always one hassle after another, and she left for home exhausted and frustrated. She hated the drive home because she always thought about the things that Andrea would not have done, so she entered the house on edge. She said she tried not to go looking for evidence but could not help herself, and as soon as she saw it, she felt compelled to seek out Andrea to point it out. Inevitably, Andrea was in her room texting, and Sarah would say, "Andrea, can I have a minute?" For Sarah, that was code for "you are in trouble." Andrea said her mom always began the conversation with a guilt trip such as, "Why haven't you cut up the vegetables?" Andrea admitted this would trigger her to feel guilty, and she would immediately attack Sarah, saying something snotty such as, "If you didn't care so much about your job, maybe you would once in a while get home in time to cut up the vegetables." This old dance then became predictable, and Andrea said the argument quickly reached a point at which she just unloaded on Sarah, who would always indignantly respond by playing the respect card.

The therapist invited them to consider moments in the sequence when something different could happen. What if Sarah first came to Andrea's room and said "hi" even before looking to see what had been done? What if they spent a few minutes talking and then Sarah asked what had to be done to get the dinner going? What if Sarah invited Andrea to work with her to prepare the meal? The therapist asked whether they would practice this solution sequence in the session, and they agreed.

> *Therapist:* So just pretend that Sarah has arrived home from work and goes up to Andrea's room to say hello.
>
> *Sarah:* OK. Andrea, I'm home. Are you in your room? Hi, Andrea.
>
> *Andrea:* Hi, Mom.
>
> *Sarah:* So how was your day?

> *Andrea:* Ugh, I hate Dr. Roberts. He's such a dork. We had to write this ridiculous essay on whether Jane Austen is a feminist. The guys didn't even know what he meant.
>
> *Sarah:* Dr. Roberts is respected in the English department. I am sure his assignment was carefully selected. So did you do it?
>
> *Andrea:* [Raising her voice] Why wouldn't I?
>
> *Therapist:* OK, let's stop there for just a second. Andrea, why did you raise your voice?
>
> *Andrea:* My mom just cares whether I did the assignment. She doesn't give a damn how I felt about it.
>
> *Therapist:* Sarah, can you see where Andrea was trying to express feelings?
>
> *Sarah:* Sure, she disrespected her teacher.
>
> *Therapist:* Sarah, are you being hooked by your issues regarding respect?
>
> *Sarah:* How is she going to learn if she doesn't respect her teachers?

Here the therapist experienced something similar to Andrea's frustration. Sarah did not seem able to step into the perspective of an adolescent and translate the word *dork* into a feeling. Not wanting to shame her, the therapist gently led her back to that moment by evoking her expertise as an office manager to express interest in Andrea's world.

> *Therapist:* Sarah, we are trying to create a conversation between the two of you that doesn't escalate. Even though you might not quite see where Andrea is going with her comments about Dr. Roberts, Jane Austen, and feminism, what if you use your office manager skills to see if you can get to the bottom of what Andrea is concerned about?
>
> *Sarah:* OK, so, Andrea, why does asking you to write about Jane Austen and feminism make your teacher a dork?
>
> *Andrea:* Because he just is.
>
> *Sarah:* Hold on, feminism didn't exist when Jane Austen was writing, so what do you think Dr. Roberts was getting at?

From there the conversation picked up, and Andrea and Sarah connected. It took a lot of repetition, but eventually they executed the solution sequence without any escalation. At the end of the session, the therapist suggested they try the solution sequence for a week and return for a mother–daughter session. This time Andrea agreed.

When they returned, they both reported some success but also acknowledged that some tension still permeated their relationship. The therapist invited them to identify the source of the tension. Sarah hesitated and then offered that it constantly shocked her that Andrea seemed to have so little drive. She noted that at Andrea's age, as the eldest child, she, Sarah, was expected to help her parents but still had dreams of being successful in life.

Therapist: You certainly know hard work.

Andrea: Actually, Mom, that is all you know. Did you even have any friends in high school?

Sarah: Well, not real friends. There just wasn't time for them.

Therapist: So what do you experience when you see Andrea so passionate about being with her friends?

Sarah: Hmm. I want to say that friends are just a luxury, but honestly, I'd have to say I feel jealousy.

Andrea: So I am good with friends, and you are good with work.

This first glimpse of a primary emotion seemed to put Andrea at ease. Perhaps she had never seen her mother be vulnerable. As they continued to discuss the feelings under the anger, Andrea said she was in awe of her mother and knew that only Ethan had the right stuff to come even close to what she had accomplished. She admitted she felt destined to be mediocre. Sarah mused that as a little girl, Andrea was immensely talented, and she reminded Andrea of her precocious drawings. Andrea then commented that that was all before the divorce. A long silence followed as everyone squirmed in discomfort.

Therapist: [To Sarah] Ask Andrea what it was about the divorce that might have changed something.

Sarah: [Sighing] Do we have to go there?

Therapist: I know you don't want to go there, but Andrea has a connection to make. Help her make it.

Sarah: OK, Andrea, I know you sometimes think I don't listen, but this time I am really listening.

Then Andrea revealed something she had always hidden from her parents. She talked about how the divorce process had been terrifying for her. She knew her father had done something bad for which her mother could not or would not forgive him. She recalled the ugly scenes and hiding in the bedroom clinging to Ethan. She remembered her father moving out and the long period when Sarah refused to let the kids see him. She remembered a series of caregivers, some of whom seemed mean and rigid. She remembered wondering when her mom would get home and too often being told she would be late because of some emergency. She said she once liked school, but gradually she faced each day of school with dread because she was always caught in a haze of anxiety. Eventually, school made her anxious.

Sarah: Andrea, I am so sorry. Why didn't you tell us?

Andrea: I tried, but you didn't seem to hear me. I guess I just got angry, so eventually, that's the only way I could express how upset I was.

Sarah: What else are you upset about?

Andrea: You don't really want to know.

Sarah: Trust me, I really do.

Andrea: OK, you asked. I didn't want you to marry Jordan. When you guys married, I slipped from second to third (work was always first), and then when Tim came along I slipped to fourth. When Tim got sick, it was like the divorce all over because you were so obsessed and didn't see Ethan or me.

Sarah: I guess I have been asleep at the wheel. I am sorry. What can we do?

The therapist summarized the conversation and noted its importance. Andrea's anxiety seemed to be a major constraint keeping her from realizing her potential in school. The therapist arranged to meet with her to assess her level of anxiety. Identifying the presence of anxiety served as a reframe for Sarah, who acknowledged she now understood that Andrea was not lazy or unmotivated but that something was keeping her from succeeding in school. By the end of the session, both Sarah and Andrea seemed more relaxed and connected.

Stabilizing Andrea's and Tim's Academics

Both Andrea and Tim needed solution sequences. In this section, we focus only on the work with Andrea. The solution sequences needed to address her problems of school performance involved multiple steps. First, the therapist met with Andrea and through a clinical assessment confirmed she met the criteria for the diagnosis of generalized anxiety disorder. In a subsequent session with Andrea, Jordan, and Sarah, the finding was presented. The therapist gave Andrea a workbook containing strategies based on cognitive behavior principles for managing school-related anxiety. The parents and Andrea agreed to read a chapter a week and apply the strategies. The therapist noted that if this self-help approach did not work, individual therapy for Andrea could be tried.

In a subsequent session with Andrea, Sarah, and Jordan, a plan to address the constraint of anxiety was created. The three of them also met with Andrea's counselor to share the diagnosis and secure help from the school. Andrea did not need an individualized education plan, but the counselor arranged for her to meet with her teachers when needed and secured tutors for her most challenging subjects.

In addition, a solution sequence was needed to replace the problem sequence of dealing with school performance by having Andrea come home to do her homework. This problem sequence only bred resentment from Andrea, whose social life was affected by it. The therapist said it would take time for Andrea's anxiety to be addressed, so in the interim could another solution sequence be designed? When the therapist asked Andrea, "If you were given more autonomy over your use of time, would that have any impact on your approach to school?" she replied that having such control would help to address her resentment, and she would be more motivated to take greater responsibility for her schoolwork. The therapist complimented Andrea and suggested an experiment be implemented between sessions. All members expressed interest in hearing more details. The therapist first asked whether Sarah monitored Andrea's courses through the school's online system that tracked her grades and assignments for each of her courses. When Sarah said that was Andrea's job, the therapist countered that until Andrea took better ownership of her schoolwork, checking online would be a way for Sarah to give Andrea more autonomy while also monitoring her progress. The monitoring would replace coming home after school. In the session, the therapist went online, and the family looked at the current state of Andrea's courses. The therapist proposed that Sarah contact the teachers to find out whether Andrea could still turn in some overdue assignments. If so, a plan would be made for her to do so. Meanwhile, the experiment would specify that so long as Andrea did not accumulate any further missed assignments, she was free to be home by suppertime. If the online report revealed a missed assignment, she agreed to come home after school and do it.

Andrea and Sarah agreed to the experiment. Over the course of the next 2 months, the frequency of missed assignments steadily decreased. Andrea received all B's on her quarter report card. She was clearly pleased, and Sarah praised her (following some coaching from the therapist). Andrea reported being more connected with her friends and had joined an after-school club. The online monitoring was reduced to once a week.

Other Subsystem Work

Problems and problem sequences can appear to take on a life of their own, but they are always embedded in a context. That context includes the organization of the family, consisting of its leadership and particularly how authority is handled and resources are allocated. In the service of shoring up a solution sequence, IST therapists, therefore, address organizational issues. Doing so usually necessitates bringing relevant subsystems of the family into the direct system. In the case of the Pritchard family, the therapist formed the following hypotheses, each one of which suggested a threat to the solution sequences. First, Sarah and Jordan's marriage could be at risk. Were it to deteriorate and/or end in divorce, both Andrea and Tim would be affected. Second, in regard to parenting styles, although Sarah was on top of parenting through an autocratic parenting style, she had little contact time with the children, who probably regarded her as unavailable. Jordan's style of parenting began as a peripheral stepparent to Andrea and Ethan, and this style seemed to have carried over to how he dealt with Tim. Third, the postdivorce family functioned in a somewhat disengaged way. Ethan and Andrea had little contact with Burt, and Burt and Sarah seemed to do little coparenting. The net effect was to increase the parenting burden on Sarah.

Finally, the therapist hypothesized that the organization of the family had been weakened when Ethan left for college. As the oldest sibling, he may have been parentified or may have served as a resource for Andrea and Tim. As the two biological siblings living in a blended family, Ethan and Andrea may have formed a close relationship. If he disappeared into his college experience, Andrea and Tim might have been experiencing a huge loss. By addressing these organizational issues, the therapist believed that solution sequences would be more stable.

The following presentation of the Pritchard family's therapy highlights this work. The therapist devoted three sessions to shore up Jordan and Sarah's marriage, their coparenting, and the relationship between Sarah and Burt. To further strengthen Burt's relationship with Ethan and Andrea, sessions were held alone with Burt; then with Burt and Sarah; with Andrea and Ethan; and with Andrea, Ethan, Burt, and Sarah. The therapist had an individual session with Ethan and a family session that included Ethan.

SESSIONS WITH JORDAN AND SARAH

The therapist had four goals in mind for sessions with Sarah and Jordan. The first was to assess and discuss their marital health. Beginning with the intake call, the therapist was concerned about Sarah and Jordan's marriage. Sarah had commented that Jordan had signaled his waning resilience and in the early family meetings he seemed somewhat remote. The second goal was to discuss their leadership style and, if necessary, to adjust it so that parenting would become more harmonious. Sarah seemed to have an autocratic style of leadership, and Jordan seemed prone to defer to her; consequently, there was little that could buffer the tendency of conflicts to escalate. The third goal was to raise the issue of Sarah's coparenting relationship with Burt. By having such a casual and limited relationship with his children, Burt eliminated a resource that could simultaneously deepen his relationship with them and provide relief and support for Sarah and Jordan's family. The fourth goal was to discuss work–life balance. Both Sarah and Jordan worked long hours. Their work narratives were syntonic with their identities, so they saw no need to question them. The therapist hypothesized that the resulting limited contact time they had with their children had to affect family life. Although Ethan had seemed to thrive with sparse parental contact, Andrea and Tim seemed to struggle.

In the first session with Sarah and Jordan, the therapist noted their disengagement and felt worried about the strength of their marriage; consequently, it was important to find out how they were doing. Jordan assured Sarah that he was not thinking about divorce. His signals about leaving were the product of frustration because the war drained him of what little energy he had after working long hours. Surprisingly, Sarah had little reaction to this news. When asked to describe their marriage, both Sarah and Jordan concurred that from the outset they both had but modest expectations of the marriage. They both wanted a reliable partner with similar values who provided financial security and respected their strong work ethic. When asked, they both reported that, though infrequent, sex was mutually satisfying. Neither seemed to want anything more from the marriage. The therapist hypothesized about their relational development and concluded that they would not welcome an invitation to work toward greater intimacy. The therapist did point out they had embarked on the transition of emptying their nest; Ethan was in college, and Andrea was a year from graduating from high school. In 6 more years, they would be empty nesters. Highlighting research that showed couples often struggled to renegotiate their marriage at that time, the therapist suggested they consider developing some shared activities.

To address the second goal, the therapist opened the organization metaframework to hypothesize about the couple's leadership style. Working backward chronologically, Sarah went from coparenting Ethan and Andrea with Burt to being a single parent for a time, to introducing Jordan into her children's lives as a stepparent, to finally having a family structure in which Jordan was a stepparent and the biological parent for Tim. If she functioned as the dominant parent with Burt and the only parent after the divorce, chances were that she would have emerged naturally as the dominant parent in the current family structure. The couple confirmed this leadership hypothesis, and when asked whether they saw any downside to the arrangement, Jordan sheepishly offered that Sarah could become autocratic and strident, and he felt powerless to influence her. The therapist noted that one benefit of coparenting is the ability of each parent to offset lovingly the negative tendencies of the other parent. At first, Sarah bristled at the notion of a negative tendency, but when Jordan challenged her, she admitted that she sometimes lost it and did not know how to prevent that from happening. She said her father had been a dictator and, for her as a child, compliance had been a survival strategy. She admitted she wished Andrea could just be that way too. Asked how it would feel to her to share more leadership with Jordan, she acknowledged it could be a positive experience. This work unfolded over several sessions. They discussed the shift to more balanced parenting in a family session. They were clear that Sarah would remain the disciplinarian for Ethan and Andrea and that she and Jordan would share that role more equally with regard to Tim. Several times Sarah undermined Jordan, and it took a session in which the therapist helped Jordan stand up to Sarah for her to finally recognize what she was doing. The therapist knew the alliance with Sarah had been torn and worked hard to repair it.

The third goal addressed Burt's involvement with Ethan and Andrea. The therapist hoped to set the stage for Burt to strengthen his connection with Ethan and Andrea. For this conversation, he considered asking Sarah to come in alone but decided that having Jordan's support would help her make some necessary changes. The hypothesizing about this goal potentially covered many issues, such as how had the marriage failed, what the divorce process was like, what was in the parenting agreement, how Burt had become peripheral, and what the relationship between Sarah and Burt was like. To the extent that the aforementioned kept Burt from being more involved, they would have to be addressed.

Sarah reported that Burt had had an affair that devastated her. Burt wanted to repair the damage, but Sarah could not forgive him, so she filed for divorce. Because Ethan and Andrea had been young at the time, they did not know the full extent of these details. Initially, she had been angry and had tried to keep the children from seeing Burt, but the divorce had not been particularly ugly or lengthy. The parenting agreement was standard. They had joint custody; Sarah was the primary parent, and Burt had visitation 1 night a week and every other weekend. The visitation schedule worked when the children were young, but as they became teenagers, they objected to giving up their weekends to be with their dad. Burt did not object, so the kids only saw him sporadically, and when Ethan departed for college, Andrea saw him even less. Sarah confessed that she was all right with this decline in visitation because Andrea did not seem to mind, and it eliminated the hassle of communicating with Burt. The therapist acknowledged how Sarah's feelings drove her stance, but he also pointed out that it inadvertently eliminated a valuable resource—time when she and Jordan did not have responsibility for

Andrea. The emotional terrain of the family was also confounded because Andrea's feelings about her father bled into her feelings about Jordan. Sarah accepted all this but doubted anything could be done to alter the situation. The therapist asked permission to try to engage Burt in an individual session that, if successful, could lead to sessions between him and the children and maybe a session with the four of them. Sarah said, "Knock yourself out, but I'll be shocked if that gets us anywhere."

The work–life balance goal targeted both the personal welfare of Sarah, Jordan, and their marriage and the vulnerability of Andrea and Tim. Altering work–life balance would be challenging because work constituted such a significant part of their identities. Both Sarah and Jordan had been stable introverts growing up. Neither had dated in high school nor pursued any activities. In this sense they were "two peas in a pod," so neither recognized the impact of their extreme work ethic on those around them. Recognizing the rigidity of their work narratives, the therapist decided to see whether they might modify them by recognizing that Tim's chronic illness and Andrea's anxiety disorder were big risk factors that constrained their development. They would both benefit from more hands-on parenting, which could only be achieved by Sarah and Jordan altering their work schedules. With gentle encouragement from the therapist, they both agreed to find ways to be home more often. The therapist assured them that although this seemed like an enormous sacrifice to both of them, their children would certainly notice and benefit from their efforts. As these changes were implemented, the contact time between parents and children gradually increased, and both children began to seek out the parents for emotional and practical support.

THE SESSIONS INVOLVING BURT

The therapist called Burt to inform him about Andrea's diagnosis and invited him to attend a session alone. The therapist began the session by asking Burt to describe his children and his relationship with them. Burt provided valuable insights that had not been provided by anyone else. The conversation then shifted to how Andrea might benefit from more contact with him. Burt said he would be open to that but did not think it was something Andrea would want. The therapist asked whether Burt would be open to meeting with Andrea to discuss how this might work. He agreed.

Burt and Andrea attended the next session. They were both awkward and guarded, and it was clear that the relationship was strained. The therapist searched for common ground and discovered they both followed a popular band. They began to talk about musicians, and Andrea complimented Burt for being in the know about contemporary music. Asked how special events were handled, Andrea reported that when Ethan graduated from high school, Burt took him out to dinner but did not attend the family party. When asked whether Andrea might want him to be more involved when she graduated, she said yes, but she did not think her mother would favor that idea. The therapist asked Burt whether he would meet with Sarah to discuss ways the original family could be created from time to time. Burt said he would.

The therapist next met with Sarah and Burt. The therapist used psychoeducation to discuss best practice for postdivorce families and stressed the value of their being together for special events. The therapist read the feedback that venting of old feelings would be counterproductive and instead asked them to negotiate how they could celebrate their children's accomplishments together. In the next session, the therapist learned that Burt had been a high school teacher before starting a small business. After much conversation and some resistance from Sarah, Burt agreed to take over the coordination of tutoring for Andrea. She would meet the tutor at his house, and Burt would monitor her academic progress. At first, Andrea was opposed to this plan, but because Burt lived close to the school, it allowed Andrea more time to hang out with friends before meeting the tutor and took some pressure off Sarah to be responsible for every aspect of Andrea's life.

Finally, Burt, Sarah, Ethan, and Andrea attended a session. The therapist's primary goal for this session was to demonstrate that they could all be in the same room together. After some awkward exchanges, Ethan took the lead and said it felt good to have this gathering and asked what would keep it from happening outside therapy. Andrea supported this idea, and the therapist saw how Andrea fed off Ethan's self-confidence. Whatever internal turmoil was present for Burt and Sarah, they chose not to express it and agreed to support the idea.

The subsystem work described was intended to create organizational changes that would stabilize the solution sequences. Sarah and Jordan agreed to increase their contact time and be more hands-on as parents. Ethan recognized the need to not disengage from the family and strengthened his connection with Andrea through regular Skype time. Burt's commitment to strengthening his relationship with Andrea turned out to be disappointing. Although he did handle the tutoring, he and Andrea could not seem to improve their relationship.

CONSOLIDATING THE WORK AND MOVING TOWARD TERMINATION

As the family stabilized, sessions were held less frequently. Both children performed well in school. Tim managed his diabetes well. The infrequent conflicts between Sarah and Andrea no longer felt like wars. In the fall of Andrea's senior year, she began to discuss wanting to go to college. She had two sessions with the therapist to discuss her options and organize how she would work with her school counselor to find a good college fit. All members of the family agreed that further sessions were not needed, but they agreed to contact the therapist should a new problem arise. Not long after starting college, Andrea had one high-anxiety episode that was addressed successfully in a Skype session with the therapist.

FOLLOW-UP

The Pritchards attended a follow-up session when Andrea was home for winter break. Her first-semester grades were good. Tim was doing better in school. He occasionally cheated on his food choices but had become knowledgeable enough not to have a blood sugar crisis. About a year later, the therapist bumped into Jordan on the street. He reported that everyone was doing well. Tim had become more outgoing and had joined the chess team. He and Jordan often played, and Tim usually won. Andrea had pledged a sorority and had decided to major in art. The talent she had evidenced long ago had returned. Jordan said Sarah had been diagnosed with hypertension. She made a commitment to her health, and she and Jordan joined a gym and worked out together regularly.

FAMILIES IN INTEGRATIVE SYSTEMIC THERAPY: INTERLOCKING SOLUTION SEQUENCES

In this chapter, using the treatment of the Pritchard family as a case example, we demonstrated how IST therapists involve the family in therapy. The therapist started with the presenting problem of the "war" between Sarah and Andrea and identified two problem sequences in which the problem was embedded: the face-to-face sequence of the war and the after-school routine. The former was embedded in the latter, and the latter included three additional problems: (a) the mismanagement of Tim's diabetes, (b) poor school performance, and (c) Andrea's resentment over her restricted social life. Over the course of therapy, solution sequences were developed to solve the presenting problems. To generate and implement these solution sequences, the therapist sometimes worked with the whole family and sometimes with appropriate subsystems. The family was expanded from the blended family consisting of Sarah, Jordan, Ethan, Andrea, and Tim to include the postdivorce family that included Sarah, Burt, Ethan, and Andrea.

Constraints to implementing the solution sequences were identified, and strategies and interventions were adopted to lift them. For example, the strategy for Tim to get back his mojo included the following interventions: form an alliance with the diabetes treatment team, engage the family and Tim in psychoeducation groups, send Tim to diabetes camp, have a contingency plan if Tim got an aberrant reading, and remove Andrea from the monitoring role.

A major constraint to Andrea's school performance was her anxiety. The therapist used a self-help workbook to structure her handling of her anxiety and coordinated with the school to provide support that included increased teacher contact and tutoring. Sarah and Jordan also became more available as a result of adjustments to their work schedules.

The therapy included strategies designed to strengthen the family organization to better buffer against the return of problem sequences. Examples of these strategies were addressing Sarah and Jordan's marriage, balancing their coparenting and increasing their contact time in the family, reconnecting Ethan with the family, and strengthening the relationship that Ethan and Andrea had with their father.

Because this therapy was a multisystemic effort involving work with combinations of clients using a range of strategies and interventions, it is not possible nor even desirable to argue what the mechanism of change was other than to say the presenting problems were solved using interlocking solution sequences and lifting constraints. The therapy did include the use of common factors and some empirically validated interventions. The case exemplifies an assumption core to IST that no single empirically supported treatment could have achieved this outcome. IST's integrative and systemic approach facilitated the expansion and development of the family as well as the resolution of the presenting problems. It left the Pritchards happier, stronger, and smarter.

10

THE INTEGRATIVE SYSTEMIC THERAPY APPROACH TO WORKING WITH COUPLES

In this chapter, we present a case study that illustrates how integrative systemic therapy (IST) manages the complexity of couple relationships and attends to aspects of confidentiality and the therapeutic alliance that pertain to couples therapy. We describe a methodology for integrating individual and conjoint sessions during the initial phase of therapy. This methodology is optional within IST, but we believe that many therapists, particularly graduate students and less experienced therapists, will find it helpful in managing the onslaught of information and emotion that therapists face when they begin work with couples in distress.

When a couple has a relationship challenge, couples therapy is usually the best context in which to facilitate change. Seeing the couple facilitates a more complete understanding of the couple system and is the most effective way to delineate the problem sequence and search for solutions. If John has a

http://dx.doi.org/10.1037/0000055-010
Integrative Systemic Therapy: Metaframeworks for Problem Solving With Individuals, Couples, and Families,
by W. M. Pinsof, D. C. Breunlin, W. P. Russell, J. L. Lebow, C. Rampage, and A. L. Chambers
Copyright © 2018 by the American Psychological Association. All rights reserved.

relationship problem with Jane, it behooves the therapist to hear from both of them. There are exceptions to this preference for seeing couples conjointly (i.e., both partners present), which include serious violence, fears of violence or retribution, and conditions that require treatment (e.g., severe addiction issues) for couples therapy to be effective.

The IST couple therapist seeks to understand each individual, the relationship, the environmental context in which the individuals and the relationship operate, and the mutual causality among these systemic levels. Though this can be overwhelming for any therapist, and especially for therapists in training, remember that IST has a foundational logic that provides therapists with a blueprint for how to proceed in a thoughtful and effective manner. With that in mind, in this chapter, we provide a "how-to" guide for using the blueprint with couples to sift through the complexity of their lives such that problem sequences are crystallized and the inevitable web of constraints is revealed. We also address common issues and challenges germane to conducting couples therapy.

WHAT IS A COUPLE, AND WHAT IS COUPLES THERAPY?

As a starting point, IST defines a *couple* as any two people who consider themselves to have a committed relationship—a relationship with a past and potentially a future. This inclusive definition covers married couples in monogamous relationships, dating couples, unmarried cohabiting couples, and unmarried cohabiting coparents. Couple partners may be straight, gay, lesbian, or transgender (Pinsof, Breunlin, Chambers, Solomon, & Russell, 2015).

Couples therapy typically occurs when a couple seeks the assistance of a licensed mental health professional (or professional-in-training) to address problems the partners have with each other and/or their relationship. It may also begin when a person seeks help for what he or she sees as an individual problem but is seen with a partner by a therapist who construes the problem in relational terms. Couples therapy usually involves conjoint sessions with the therapist, but it may also involve individual sessions adjunctively. Couples therapy can be used with couples in nonsexual relationships and couples in explicitly open or nonmonogamous relationships. We see both partners as deserving the same fundamental rights, privileges, and opportunities, knowing full well that this may not operationally be the case with some couples. We see couple relationships as politically and socially symmetrical, without denying that couples may have satisfying complementary role relationships in different domains of their lives (Pinsof, Breunlin, et al., 2015).

AN INTEGRATIVE SYSTEMIC THERAPY APPROACH
TO STARTING COUPLES THERAPY

In IST, we unequivocally believe that assessment is an ongoing, iterative process that occurs throughout therapy. Therefore, the traditional distinction between assessment and therapy is artificial. Consistent with the epistemological pillar of partial and progressive knowing (discussed in Chapter 2, this volume), the therapist continually formulates and tests hypotheses about the couple's problems and the constraints that prevent their resolution. Because knowledge is progressive, starting therapy with a couple can be more overwhelming at the beginning of therapy than later because there is a mountain of information to gather and organize. Thus, it is useful to have a format that helps therapists manage this challenge.

THE FOUR-SESSION EVALUATION AND INTRODUCTION
TO COUPLES THERAPY

The four-session evaluation (Chambers, 2012) is one IST-friendly approach to starting couples therapy that many therapists, especially beginning therapists, find useful. Although this approach includes an individual session with each partner at the beginning of therapy, it is equally valid from an IST perspective to commence couples therapy without the individual sessions.

In the four-session evaluation format, the therapist initially meets conjointly with both members of the couple and then meets with each member separately. Then in the fourth session, they come back together as a group to discuss the therapist's impressions and the couple's reactions to them, as well as to establish an initial plan for the therapy. Throughout this introduction, questions are asked to identify problem sequences, solution sequences, and some of the constraints facing the couple. Additional goals of the conjoint sessions are to build balanced alliances, garner basic information about the couple's life, and explore the presenting problem in detail. The goals of the individual session are to strengthen individual alliances with each partner, assess each partner's feelings about their own and their partner's level of commitment to the relationship, rule out domestic violence and other risk issues, and acquire brief individual and family-of-origin histories as well as any significant history of previous romantic relationships.

Advantages to the Four-Session Evaluation Format

The advantages for the four-session introduction are multiple. First, it provides a systematic method for collecting and organizing complex information about a couple's problems while maintaining the integrity and richness of each partner's story. Consistent with systemic thinking, IST embraces the complexity that may be required to change a system and encourages therapists to pay attention to a broad range of variables. Thus, having a format for navigating that complexity can be helpful. Second, using a systematic approach can create a sense of expertise and consequently hope that one will be able to help with the couple's problems. In fact, couples frequently report being comforted by this structure and appreciate its thoroughness. Third, consistent with one of the core competencies in couple and family psychology (Stanton & Welsh, 2012), it is important for systemic therapists to have a case formulation, which is best formulated with careful attention to the numerous sequences described by the couple and observed by the therapist. Thus, the initial four sessions can help slow down a couple's understandable sense of urgency and help the therapist develop and present a more comprehensive understanding of the couple's problem sequences.

An additional advantage of the four-session format is that the couple is invited to make only an initial, limited commitment to therapy. It is not uncommon for one member of the couple to call a therapist saying, "My partner will not come to therapy." This leaves the therapist with the challenge of persuading the ambivalent partner to give couples therapy a chance. Having a discrete number of sessions can allow the ambivalent member of the couple an opportunity to try couples therapy without having to "sign up for life." In fact, once they complete the four-session evaluation, the vast majority continue with treatment. Finally, the four sessions can help clarify the motivation of each partner and tease apart when couples therapy is contraindicated and when a treatment program or individual, group, or no therapy is recommended.

Advantages of Individual Sessions

There are several advantages to conducting the individual sessions. First, individual sessions can help the therapist like a person better than when that person is seen with their partner. Concentrating on one person's experience can facilitate an understanding of current circumstances, personal history, and point of view, any of which can help increase empathy for him or her. It is also noteworthy that the dynamic between conflictual couples in conjoint sessions can bring out their defensive, less likable parts. Second, consistent with IST's guideline of privileging the alliance, individual sessions allow the opportunity to build stronger alliances with each partner. It is not uncommon for partners to vehemently disagree with their partner's view of the problem(s). Thus, any sympathy the therapist may express to one partner may inadvertently hurt the other and may consequently strain the alliance. Moreover, when there is extreme conflict in the initial conjoint session, individual sessions allow the therapist to give the client undivided attention without having to manage interference from the other. Third, when there is ambiguity about one partner's feelings and level of commitment to the relationship, individual sessions can allow a more accurate assessment of that ambivalence. Finally, an important reason for conducting the individual session is that it allows for a thorough assessment of any intimate partner violence (IPV). If there is any IPV, individual sessions allow for the creation of a safety plan and an assessment as to whether couples therapy is currently appropriate. It is contraindicated in cases of severe abuse.

When Not to Conduct Individual Sessions

Despite the many advantages of the four-session evaluation model, there are times when the individual sessions are contraindicated. For example, in some cases involving infidelity, the injured partner feels especially uncomfortable with the therapist meeting individually with the partner who has been unfaithful. It can create a sense of secrecy and transfer some of the injured partner's distrust to the therapist, which will constrain the development of a therapeutic alliance. In such cases, the therapist should conduct only conjoint sessions at the outset of therapy. In a more general sense, whenever a couple has a strong preference not to have individual sessions, IST's alliance predominance guideline suggests that the therapist respects their preference. In such cases, the therapist would conduct all the beginning sessions with both parties present and cover much of the same ground as would be covered by the formal four-session evaluation.

Confidentiality

When meeting with a partner individually, the therapist must be cognizant of confidentiality concerns. Individual sessions always carry the risk that a partner will disclose "secret" information the other partner is not privy to (Chambers & Lebow, 2008). Therapists vary significantly in their level of comfort with being the keeper of secrets. Some therapists understandably believe therapy can be enhanced when they have all the secret knowledge because it places them in a better position to be helpful. Although we appreciate the benefits of such a position and under particular circumstances may temporarily establish an agreement to proceed as such (see Chapter 1), we believe the risks outweigh the benefits of keeping secrets because it can be particularly damaging to the alliance. Moreover, keeping a secret, such as infidelity, potentially places the therapist in an ethically compromising position of attempting to be an equal advocate for both members of the couple while maintaining a secret that disadvantages one partner. This can be particularly problematic for certain racial and ethnic minority couples who, understandably, may already have a hard time trusting in general (Chambers & Kravitz, 2011) and may especially struggle to trust a mental health professional. The IST perspective encourages therapists to explicitly tell the couple the parameters of confidentiality for the individual sessions. Please see Chambers (2012) for a more detailed description of the process along with sample questions.

CASE EXAMPLE: ADAM AND JANE

To illustrate both the structure and flexibility of IST couple work and to show how the four-session evaluation works, we present the case of Adam and Jane. Their case demonstrates the diversity and richness of hypotheses and interventions that IST therapists can use to help couples.

Adam, a 35-year-old fiancé (to Jane, 34), called to set up an appointment to get help with their relationship.

> *Adam:* Hello. My name is Adam. My previous individual therapist referred me to you for couples therapy. My partner and I have been fighting more, and I think it is time for us to get some help.
>
> *Therapist:* Is your partner also willing to come in?
>
> *Adam:* Yes.
>
> *Therapist:* That's good. Let me tell you how I work. I would meet with the two of you together for the first session, and then I would set up an individual session with each of you and then meet with the two of you together for the fourth session. In that fourth session, I will give you some feedback about what I think is going on and what I think will be a good plan moving forward. And we would discuss your reactions and feedback as well. After that, most of our sessions would be together. How does that sound?
>
> *Adam:* That sounds good. I appreciate knowing you will do more than just listen—that you will give us your point of view.
>
> *Therapist:* I'm glad that works for you, and yes, my style is to be fairly active. I also have an online questionnaire that I would like the two of you to fill out before each session so I can track our progress. Would the two of you be willing to complete the questionnaire?
>
> *Adam:* We would be happy to do that—anything that helps with the process.

Therapist: Excellent! I look forward to meeting the two of you, and please tell Jane that if she has any questions, she can feel free to contact me.

In this dialogue, the therapist intentionally asked whether the partner was willing to come in because it is not uncommon for one member of the couple to be ambivalent. He was also mindful that the alliance started with the phone call and thus was transparent about the process of getting started. He also invited the partner to call in advance of the session as an attempt to keep the alliance balanced. Successful IST rests on building a good alliance with both parties.

The First Session

Before the first session, the therapist examined the questionnaires that Jane and Adam had completed. Both partners reported feeling depressed and anxious. Adam's questionnaire showed him having low trust in Jane, and both partners reported significant difficulties in their families of origin. The questionnaire also revealed that they were both highly educated. The therapist kept the information about their families of origin in mind in case it proved useful in hypothesizing about the case, but the next step was to hear directly from the clients about how they saw their problems and what they wanted to do about them.

The therapist began the first session by asking Jane whether Adam had told her about the initial four sessions. The IST therapist is constantly "collecting data" to form hypotheses about the constraints facing the couple. In this case, the therapist was wondering about their communication.

Therapist: Jane, did Adam tell you about the initial four sessions?

Jane: Yes, he did. After today you are going to meet with each of us individually, and then we'll meet back as a group, and most of the future sessions will be together. Is that right?

Therapist: Yes, that's spot on! I appreciate the clarity of your communication on this. OK, so I'd like to talk with you briefly about confidentiality. Everything we say here is completely confidential in regard to the rest of the world, but everything we say here is shared by the three of us. In terms of the individual sessions, whatever we discuss in them I would like the freedom to share when we come back as a group. Second, if either of you gives me a phone call or sends me an e-mail, I will want to share the contents of that communication when we come back together as a group. So basically it's an open book policy with no secrets between us. In fact, if you are going to send me an e-mail, it is best to go ahead and copy your partner on the e-mail. How does that sound?

Adam: That sounds reasonable.

Jane: Yes, I agree. I really like that. Secrets can get you in trouble. [Given the tone of Jane's voice, the therapist briefly wonders about her prior experience with secrets.]

Therapist: So before we jump into what brings you here, let me get to know you a little bit. I've looked at your answers on the questionnaire you filled out, but I'd like to hear directly from you. Tell me a little about yourselves, your work, schooling, hobbies. Jane, do you want to go first? [The therapist starts with Jane to balance the alliance because he has already spoken with Adam on the phone.]

Jane: Sure. I'm 34 years old. I was a copywriter for a number of years, but I'm currently unemployed and considering a career change. I plan to take some classes to explore options for graduate school. When I met Adam in college, I was a liberal arts major. In terms of hobbies, I enjoy music, reading, and the arts.

Hobbies can be a great source for developing metaphors that have personal meaning to clients. Couples therapy aims to help the couple move from an independent, right–wrong framework to an interdependent framework. Metaphors can help achieve that goal. For instance, an individual who plays tennis provides the opportunity to discuss the difference between playing singles and doubles. Or the individual who loves basketball provides the opportunity to illustrate how an individual can be a great player (e.g., Michael Jordan) but still lose the championship if he does not think about how he fits in with the rest of his players. See Chapter 7 for more examples of using metaphor as part of therapeutic conversations.

Therapist: How about you, Adam?

Adam: I am 35 years old, and I work as an electrical engineer. I majored in math and engineering with a minor in chemistry.

Therapist: How do you like your job? And can you tell me about the demands of the job in terms of hours and travel? [Given the number of hours many professionals work, it can be helpful to know how much the job is a potential constraint for connection in terms of number of hours spent at work as well as how satisfied the client is with the job. Job dissatisfaction can be a significant contributor to relationship distress. Moreover, asking about travel is helpful in determining whether there is any correlation between their problem sequence and travel.]

Adam: I mostly enjoy my job. Sometimes it's pretty stressful. You know, when there is a deadline. I generally work a 40-hour week, though, and only have to travel once or twice a year for work.

Therapist: Can the two of you tell me about any recent life changes? [Given the research demonstrating the negative impact of environmental stressors on relationship satisfaction (Neff & Karney, 2004, 2009), asking couples about such stressors can be helpful in identifying additional constraints.]

Adam: Well, we got engaged 2 months ago. Since then we have heard that my parents have filed for divorce and my sister is pregnant and about to get married. These things have contributed to our fighting. [Following this exchange, the therapist asks questions to further understand these important contextual issues. The couple shares further background information and their views of these circumstances. Then the therapist acknowledges the impact of what they have shared and moves on to other areas of inquiry.]

Therapist: Well, you really have a lot on your plate. I want to hear more about these things, especially if you think they are important to our work, but I have one more question before we get into the concerns that bring you here. How do the two of you feel about being here and getting started with couples therapy? [This question can be particularly helpful in assessing motivation for therapy as well as possible split agendas.]

Jane: I'm glad to be here. I like therapy. [Jane and Adam look at each other and laugh.]

Adam: I'm also happy to be here. I think we need to be here. But I am a little nervous about being judged. [The therapist wonders about shame, which can be a powerful constraint to being open and vulnerable in therapy.]

Therapist: Adam, I appreciate your candor. Please know that my job is not to judge but to help identify what is keeping the two of you from having the kind of relationship you want. Also, know that you do not have to share anything that makes you feel very uncomfortable.

Adam: I appreciate that.

Therapist: So let's jump in. What brings you to therapy at this time?

Jane: We need to be able to fight less and fight better. Lately, we have been fighting more and more, and our fighting is getting more charged. We fight about big topics like our future, do we want kids, and what our marriage will look like. [Jane gets teary-eyed, whereas Adam hangs his head.]

Therapist: Jane, you sound sad.

Jane: I am sad. Sad that we are struggling with each other. I'm anxious about our future and frustrated that we can't seem to get on the same page.

Therapist: Adam, what are your thoughts?

Adam: I completely agree with Jane.

Therapist: It sounds like the fighting is a big problem. It would help me if you could give me an example of a recent fight.

Adam: We are both bisexual. Although I am attracted to men, I have never had sex with a man. The idea of getting married and having to suppress that part of myself is hard to accept, especially since Jane has been with other women. I need to talk about this, and Jane refuses.

Jane: Well, I am certainly not going to be in an open relationship where we can hook up sexually with other people! I was promiscuous in my early 20s and did a lot of drugs and drinking. I have been sober for 10 years, and I associate an open relationship with drugs and alcohol. I want us to be exclusive.

Therapist: Adam, what do you do with your sexual thoughts about men?

Adam: I look at gay porn. I look at it pretty much daily.

Therapist: Jane, how do you feel about Adam looking at porn or gay porn?

Jane: I don't have a problem with him looking at porn as long as it stays just porn.

Therapist: Tell me about your sexual relationship.

Adam: We have a very satisfying sexual relationship. We have a lot of gender fluidity in our sex life.

Jane: I agree that we have a good sex life. We have sex five to six times a week. I initiate because I used to reject him in the past. I am OK with initiating because it allows me to be in control.

Adam: You know, I think I can accept not being with a man, but she needs to appreciate that and realize that it is a sacrifice.

Jane:	Being monogamous shouldn't be viewed as a sacrifice if you love me!
Adam:	You see—she doesn't get it!
Therapist:	There is a lot wrapped into a couple's sexual relationship. It can represent things like commitment, love, security, trust, identity, and vulnerability. So, we should definitely talk more about what monogamy and sacrifice mean to you in the context of your relationship. For now, though, I would like to get back to a more general discussion of the patterns in your relationship. Have your fights escalated to the point where your commitment has diminished?
Jane:	I absolutely love him, and my commitment to him is strong.
Adam:	I am also very committed to our relationship. [The therapist notes that this is consistent with their responses to the questionnaire.]
Therapist:	It is great that the two of you are so committed! Not all couples who come into my office can say that. It also sounds like the two of you have been able to get your sexual needs met in the relationship by being flexible with each other, which is also quite good. I know we are running short on time, but I would like to ask about your financial situation. Jane, you indicated that you are unemployed, and so I wanted to know how the two of you handle finances and whether that has been a source of conflict.
Jane:	Right now, I am financially dependent on Adam, which I do not like. I value my independence, and so having to depend on him is not comfortable.
Adam:	I can cover most of our expenses, but I do ask my dad for help from time to time.
Therapist:	I want to learn more about this part of your life, but we're running out of time, and so I would like to schedule our individual sessions.
Adam:	That sounds good.
Jane:	I agree. So who should go first?
Therapist:	It doesn't really matter who goes first; that's primarily a pragmatic decision based on schedules.

The therapist looked toward the individual sessions to further delineate the problem sequences as well as the more obvious constraints to implementing an initial solution sequence. He suspected that information about their families of origin would help contextualize the constraints. He also planned to rule out IPV given their mutual reports about escalating fights.

Individual Session With Jane

Therapist: Jane, it's good to see you! Before we get started, I just want to remind you that whatever we talk about today I would like to be able to share when we come back together as a group.

Jane: OK.

Therapist: To start with, I am interested in your thoughts and feelings about the first session.

Jane: Although I was nervous about starting to address our issues, I felt relieved to finally be addressing them. We briefly talked after our session, and we both felt good about it, and we both felt comfortable with you.

Therapist: I am glad to hear that! One of the areas I wanted to follow up on was the escalating conflicts. I understand that both of you are concerned about this. Can you tell me more about what starts the fights and how bad they get?

Jane: There is no one thing that starts our fights, and so I am not sure. We are fighting more, and the fights are getting worse.

Therapist: When you say more, how often?

Jane: It feels like almost daily, but at least several times a week.

Therapist: Can you say more about "worse"?

Jane: Now there's name calling, cursing at each other, and some-times he gets in my face. Our fights can last a couple of hours and result in ultimatums!

Therapist: Has he ever hit you or hurt you?

Jane: No, but he has punched a wall.

Therapist: Have you ever been scared of his anger? Have you ever called the police?

Jane: No, nothing like that; I have never called the police. I don't fear for my safety, but his anger can be intimidating.

Therapist: Have you ever hit him?

Jane: [In a sheepish voice] Yes, I have hit him but not since I stopped drinking, which was 10 years ago.

> *Therapist:* Are the two of you more likely to fight if he has been drinking?
>
> *Jane:* Honestly, the fighting seems to happen independent of drinking.

The therapist worked to clarify several things about this conversation. First, he wanted to understand whether there had been any physical injury or psychological abuse. Second, if there had been physical aggression, the therapist was interested in understanding whether it had been committed by one or both parties. It is unequivocally true that women are at an increased risk of injury by men; however, a systemic perspective acknowledges that both parties can be contributors to that sequence. Finally, the therapist asked about the role alcohol played given the high comorbidity between alcohol and IPV.

After this exploration of IPV, the therapist spent some time carefully eliciting further details about various aspects of the problem sequence (the escalating conflict) before returning to Jane's earlier statement about ultimatums.

> *Therapist:* You stated earlier that the fights can result in ultimatums. Do you mean that the fights make you question whether you want to stay in the relationship?
>
> *Jane:* Sort of. In that moment we say things like "I can't keep doing this," but we quickly rebound from that. We never mean it.
>
> *Therapist:* So the only time your commitment is low is when you are both upset from fighting?
>
> *Jane:* Yes!
>
> *Therapist:* OK, that's helpful to know. I would like to switch gears and talk a little about your past. The questionnaire stated that you had some difficulty in your family when you were growing up. Can you tell me about your family, especially anything that you feel may help me understand your struggles with Adam? [The therapist introduces the idea of linking the past to the present to understand any intergenerational sequences that may be constraining.]
>
> *Jane:* Wow! Well, how much time do you have? Let's just say that my family was really messed up! My parents never loved me, because I was a girl! They wanted a boy, and from an early age, my dad would say things like "You are not attractive! You are dumb! You look like a boy. No one will ever want you! I wish I had a son!" [Tears flow down her cheek.] In addition to the emotional abuse, my father

frequently touched me inappropriately, and no one in the family acknowledged it! I tried to talk to my mom, and she would change the subject and tell me how wonderful my father is. My dad also never acknowledged it and to this day acts like he never did anything wrong! [Pausing to catch her breath] I went to therapy years back and worked on this a lot. Despite all these tears, I'm OK with it now.

Therapist: I'm so sorry you had to go through that!

Jane: My mom never protected me. She was scared of my father, who was emotionally and physically abusive to all of us. I realized very early that I could not depend on anyone.

Therapist: Given your background, I am particularly struck by your resilience to achieve all that you have. Can I ask you a few more questions?

Jane: Thank you. Yes, go ahead.

Therapist: Have you ever been in any other uncomfortable sexual situations? [Assessing for abuse or trauma history can be helpful in understanding issues of dependency, attachment injury, and sensitivity to power and control.]

Jane: In college, I was very promiscuous, and given my drinking problem, I put myself in a lot of dangerous situations. A boyfriend assaulted me, and I filed a report with the college police. They took it seriously.

Therapist: I am glad that you took action, which I think took a lot of courage!

Jane: Thank you. I guess it did.

Therapist: You're welcome! Before we conclude, I would like to ask what your goals for therapy are. What are you hoping to achieve, and how would you know that therapy has been a success?

Jane: I want us to learn how to fight better. I want to feel less anxious. And I want us to be able to have a shared vision for our relationship.

Therapist: Those are all reasonable goals. Finally, let me ask if there is anything else that you feel is important for me to know that we haven't discussed. [The therapist conveys to the client that this is a collaborative process and that her voice and opinion matter.]

Jane: No, we have covered a lot.

Therapist:	OK, I am going to meet with Adam next, and then when we come back together as a group I will give you my feedback about what I think is going on, and we can work together to develop a good plan for moving forward.

Individual Session With Adam

Therapist:	Adam, it is good to see you! Before we get started, I just want to remind you that whatever we talk about today I would like the freedom to share when we come back together as a group.
Adam:	Got it.
Therapist:	To start with, what were your thoughts and feelings about the first session?
Adam:	Although I am still a little nervous about being judged, I feel like I can open up to you.
Therapist:	I am glad to hear that. If at any point you are feeling judged, I hope that you will let me know as that is never my intention.
Adam:	Will do.
Therapist:	One of the areas I wanted to follow up on was the escalating fighting that you both report. Can you tell me more about what starts the fights and how bad they get?
Adam:	When we fight, things rapidly escalate to ultimatums. A big trigger is her anxiety. She can get anxious or reactive, which makes me angry and judgmental. My biggest fear is that Jane can't manage her anxiety, and that means I can't trust that she can be there for me because I always have to be there for her. I really need her to take care of her anxieties as a commitment to me and the relationship!
Therapist:	You seem to be saying that her anxiety feels like a burden for you, one which you don't want to carry. Is that right?
Adam:	Yes. That's exactly it.

Following this exchange, Adam shared an example of the problem sequence of escalating conflict. The therapist then asked about IPV, and Adam confirmed the information Jane had provided on this topic. Adam went on to further clarify his views of their conflict and emphasized that Jane's anxiety sometimes "made" him feel anxious and reactive.

Therapist:	You mentioned that you were in CBT [cognitive behavior therapy] before for anxiety. Do you feel you are still too anxious or that you have it under control?

Adam: I can still get anxious, but the CBT was helpful in being able to manage it. [Adam then talks in some detail about his struggle with anxiety, the nature of his therapy, and the coping skills he learned.]

Therapist: I'm glad to hear that the therapy was helpful. I would like to hear a little about your family of origin, especially since that seemed to be a big trigger for starting therapy. Can you describe your parents' relationship?

Adam: My dad made all of the money, while my mom was a stay-at-home mom. My mom always had to be the center of attention, especially when she drank. My mom was a violent drunk. From a young age, I had to console her when she was drunk, and I had to be her caretaker. [The therapist realizes why Jane's anxiety is a particularly powerful trigger for Adam.] To this day, I have a hard time relating to either parent. My dad uses money as a method of control, and my mom can be very manipulative, and so I never trust either to have my best interests at heart.

Therapist: That must be difficult for you. I can see you are feeling something just thinking about it.

Adam: Yes, it still affects me.

Therapist: I do want to ask you a routine question that I ask as part of my process of getting to know couples. Have you ever been sexually abused or in any uncomfortable sexual situations? [The therapist normalizes the question and wants to test out a hypothesis from the first session in connection with his pornography use.]

Adam: No, I have not been sexually abused, but I remember as early as 8 years old and really up to my teenage years that my mom would walk around with her robe open. She would also talk about sex a lot. It always made me feel uncomfortable! [The therapist begins to wonder about the connection between his high libido and being oversexualized as a child.]

Therapist: She was not respectful of your boundaries or your sexuality.

Adam: Absolutely. That's why even talking about her or talking to her can be a trigger for me.

Therapist: I understand. This is a very difficult and painful subject that we will get back to. Can we move on to some of the other issues? [Adam nods and says yes.] Going back to the relationship and what brings you to therapy, I am interested in hearing about your goals for this therapy. How will you know that the therapy is helping?

Adam: I have given this a lot of thought, and I have several goals. First, I want us to be able to manage our conflict better. Second, I want to have a safe place to talk about my sexuality and our future, especially as it pertains to things like planning a wedding and whether or not to have kids. Third, I want Jane to be able to better manage her anxiety. If you can help us with all of those, you are a godsend!

Therapist: Well, I am going to do the best I can, and I have some ideas of how to help. Before we stop, is there anything else that you feel is important that we have not discussed or that I did not ask you about?

Adam: No, I think we have covered a lot of ground, and I appreciate just being able to get this off my chest.

Therapist: I'm glad to hear it. The next step is that I am going to meet with the two of you and share what I have come to understand about your relationship. Then we will develop a plan for moving forward.

Adam: That sounds good. I look forward to hearing what you've learned.

Understanding the Problem Sequence and Constraints

An important and sometimes overwhelming part of doing couples therapy is trying to sort out and make sense of all the data. IST is a useful heuristic toward that end. Simply stated, the therapist seeks to understand the problem sequence and the constraints that prevent implementation of the solution sequences. In the case of Adam and Jane, the presenting problem was the increase in the frequency and intensity of their conflict because of their inability to discuss hard topics. The immediate problem sequence involved the escalating pattern of their conflict. Although the problem sequence seemed straightforward, the complexity was quickly elucidated as the therapist gave initial consideration to possible constraints by opening various hypothesizing metaframeworks. Immediately prominent was the development metaframework. The therapist noticed that their fights often revolved around the themes of commitment and the future (i.e., marriage and kids). He hypothesized that they were struggling with trying to figure out the next stage of their lives. This overlapped with their different levels of independence from their families of origin. Jane was fairly independent of her parents, but Adam was dependent on his father for money, which the therapist believed could be a constraint to shifting Adam's allegiance to Jane.

The therapist also opened the organization metaframework because there were issues with power and decision making. The couple struggled with decisions about their future, and neither of them was able to take the lead to help sort it out. Moreover, the couple struggled with power, as evidenced by their escalating arguments that were often inappropriately intense, which suggested a lack of flexibility in their conversations.

The culture and gender metaframeworks were particularly salient as both partners identified as bisexual and saw gender fluidity as a factor in their relationship. However, the therapist learned that Jane was further along on accepting her sexual identity than Adam, who reported more shame. This difference was a source of many conflicts because Adam already had a difficult time expressing himself and had to be able to share his journey with Jane. (Adam's difficulty expressing himself was also supported by the questionnaire, which showed he was a standard deviation into the clinical range on that particular scale.) However, when he shared his desire for men, it triggered Jane's anxiety that he wanted an open relationship. Although Jane identified as bisexual, she was committed to having a monogamous relationship with Adam, and even the remote prospect that he might want to have a sexual relationship with a man was unacceptable and thus triggered the problem sequence of escalating conflict.

The therapist also opened the biology metaframework because of the couple's mutual reports of anxiety. Adam reported a history and propensity toward anxiety, for which he had sought CBT a few years ago, which had helped. This was supported by the questionnaire, which did not indicate clinical levels of anxiety. Jane's questionnaire, however, did suggest clinical levels of anxiety. The therapist posited that productive communication about hard topics was constrained by their propensity to get anxious, especially Jane, who, by her own admission, had few strategies for reducing her anxiety.

Another salient metaframework was mind. On the questionnaire they completed, there is a scale that asks about each person's family of origin, which is further divided into several subscales. Both Adam and Jane were two to three standard deviations into the clinical range on each subscale of family of origin. The therapist speculated that current feelings and thoughts might be linked to early family-of-origin experiences. Moreover, because of their childhood traumas, their feelings and thoughts may have reflected rigid internalizations of early family relationships. Thus, the therapist considered that projective identification (M2 hypothesis) and perhaps even a fragility of self (M3 hypothesis) might have been triggering the problem sequence as well as constraining the implementation of an adaptive solution sequence.

With the complexity of numerous hypothesizing metaframeworks at play, the therapist and the clients had to develop an initial, coherent plan for the therapy. At first glance, this was not easy, because there was a cogent argument for focusing on one or any combination of the hypothesizing metaframeworks, but the IST essence diagram guides the therapist to work directly to establish a solution sequence. Further, the therapy's starting point is influenced by the cost-effectiveness and temporal guidelines. The cost-effectiveness guideline asserts that the therapist and key clients should use interventions that are more direct, less expensive (in terms of time or duration and money), and less complex before moving, in the face of failure, to less direct, more expensive, and more complex interventions. Stated simply, take the shortest and most direct route before taking a longer, less direct, and more complex route. The temporal guideline asserts that therapy should begin by focusing on the here-and-now and should move to the past only as necessary in the face of the failure of the here-and-now–focused strategies to transform the problem sequence.

With that in mind, the therapist decided to draw from the top three planning metaframeworks—(a) action, (b) meaning/emotion, and (c) biobehavioral—in implementing a solution sequence. Starting with the action metaframework, the therapist believed that part of the problem was that the couple did not know how to stop the escalating sequence. Thus, he planned to start by identifying, labeling, and interrupting the problem sequence. This is akin to the notion of "see it, name it, change it." That is, the therapist planned to help the couple see and understand the sequence. The therapist would then do some psychoeducation about how to interrupt it by teaching them how to implement a successful "time-out." He intended to practice with them in session as well as assign it as an "experiment" for them to try between sessions. In addition, the therapist would do some behavioral exposure with them in session by helping them to talk about the hard topics they tended to avoid.

The meaning/emotion metaframework is connected to the action metaframework in that conducting a successful time-out means being able to regulate one's emotions. Thus, the therapist planned to do some psychoeducation about maladaptive emotions and teach the couple important tactics such as scaling to implement a successful time-out. The therapist would also help them identify maladaptive narratives that constrain the implementation of the solution sequence. With the establishment of the time-out procedure, the therapist would focus on helping them have a healthy and direct expression of authentic emotion by helping the clients move from secondary emotions, such as defensive anger, to softer primary emotions, such as vulnerability and shame. A fair bit of work would also be focused on helping them to accept each other given their sensitivity to being judged and their predilection to judge each other.

Last, the therapist planned to recommend that Jane see a cognitive behavior therapist for her anxiety. This was based on the understanding that Jane's anxiety, which was painful for her and triggering for Adam, constrained implementation of the solution sequence (productive discussion of difficult, but important, topics). The message would be given that both of them had to understand and accept the anxiety they bring to the relationship, take responsibility for managing it, and get help, if needed, to not let it constrain their ability to connect. After conceptualizing and planning, the therapist met with them conjointly to share feedback and propose a plan for how to proceed with the therapy. The therapist realized that the planning would require buy-in from the couple and, further, that over the course of therapy, the road to solutions may wind in ways not accounted for by the initial conceptualization.

The Feedback Session

Therapist: How are both of you doing?

Adam: I am excited and anxious to hear your feedback.

Jane: Ditto.

Therapist: I will definitely give you my feedback, but before I do, I have a couple of questions for you. First, upon reflecting on the individual sessions, is there anything you forgot to mention or would like to expand upon? [With this question, the therapist continues to promote a collaborative alliance by letting them know that they can always bring up something from a previous session.]

Jane: I can't think of anything.

Adam: Me either.

Therapist: OK. My second question is can the two of you provide me with a little update about how things have been going since I've last seen you? [The therapist is mindful that a lot can change over the course of three sessions. Thus, he requests a temperature reading to make sure the feedback was presented in a manner that recognized the current state of the relationship.]

Jane: We have been on our best behavior since starting couples therapy. So, things have actually gotten better in that we have not been fighting.

Adam: I agree, but I also don't completely trust it. I feel that we are fairly vulnerable to slipping back into our old patterns.

Therapist: I am very pleased to hear that things have improved! I also understand you don't completely trust the progress. In fact, let me expand on that. It is important for both of you to know that change in therapy is not a straight line. Although the goal is to end up at a better place than you started, it will not be a direct path. Some weeks you will come in and make a lot of progress, and other weeks you may come in and feel like you are back at square one. Although it may feel like that at times, in reality, you are not at square one, and it will be easier to get back to the higher place by building on past progress. Does that make sense?

Adam: Yes. I think that makes sense.

Jane: I agree. You may need to remind us of this, though.

Therapist: Will do. As we move on to my feedback, I want you to know that couples typically have one of three reactions to it. The first reaction is that you feel I completely nailed it! That I understood you and your relationship problems. The second reaction is that you feel I completely missed the boat! That you wonder if I was even listening to you during the session. The third reaction is something like "Huh, that's interesting. I haven't thought about that before. I will have to take some time to let that digest." All three of those reactions are completely normal. [Adam and Jane both nod in a manner to indicate that they understand. In reality, the second reaction is rare. However, the importance of including it is to model for the couple that it is OK to disagree with or to question the therapist. Normalizing a couple's reaction conveys a therapist's openness to feedback.] OK, for starters, I want to mention a few of the many good signs that I see. First, and arguably most importantly, the two of you have very similar versions of the problem. Many partners come in with different stories about the problem, and we can't start implementing solutions if we are not all on the same page with what the problem actually is. In fact, on the questionnaire you filled out, you both were in agreement as to which problems were causing significant distress and which areas of your relationship are positive. Second, it is quite positive that the two of you are coming in before getting married. Many couples see therapy as a last resort before divorce; however, in those situations, it is not uncommon for couples to come in too late because of the years of anger and resentment that have built up. Third, you both indicated a very high level of commitment. Change in therapy involves flexibility and a willingness to do things differently. Having a high level of commitment is critical in regard to your willingness to inconvenience yourselves for the betterment of your partner and your relationship. So from where I sit, there are some very positive aspects to your relationship that strongly suggest you can benefit from therapy. [Starting out with the positive is particularly important in IST because the model operates from a strength perspective that encourages therapists to identify and capitalize on clients' strengths to remove constraints and solve or improve their problems.]

Adam: It's reassuring to hear that. Our fighting has caused me a lot of distress and even doubt about our relationship.

Jane: I agree because I know that my mind tends to drift towards focusing on the negative. I have to remember the positive as well.

Therapist: It is also important that there are two primary pathways to relationship distress. [The therapist draws on the research of Karney and Bradbury (2000).] The first is a pile-up of external stressors, such as loss of a job, death in the family, moving. The second involves characteristics of the couple relationship, such as poor communication or poor conflict resolution. In terms of external stressors, Adam, your parents recently filed for divorce, your sister is pregnant and getting married, and the two of you have become engaged. It can be challenging to hold onto hope when you are also seeing the end of your parents' long-term marriage. That can be confusing and distressing.

Adam: That is exactly right. I have been questioning marriage in a way that I never did before because my parents are getting a divorce.

Therapist: I understand. I also think it is important to acknowledge the developmental stage of your relationship because every stage in a relationship has different stressors and different goals that need to be met in order to move on to the next phase. The two of you are engaged, so this is a time of hope and excitement. But the hope and excitement can be challenged by the alarming reality of your parents' divorce. And, unlike couples who have been married for a long time who have faced significant challenges and developed some confidence that they can overcome problems, premarital couples do not have that history and therefore can lack the confidence that they can overcome their problems. [With this feedback, the therapist opens the development metaframework to help normalize and contextualize their fears. This metaframework may also be useful in helping the couple identify developmental milestones that have to be met.]

Jane: I haven't thought much about the stage of our relationship. It makes sense. [The couple then provides further background information and discusses how the developmental frame for their relationship seemed to fit. The discussion is lively and demonstrates their ability to use the concept to improve their understanding of their relationship.]

Therapist: Let's talk about the conflicts that brought you into therapy. You have described the escalation process [problem sequence]. As I understand it, it primarily boils down to the two of you getting triggered with anxiety and insecurities when discussing hard topics that highlight differences in your relationship, which in turn can be threatening to your future together. This can come about when talking about money or sexual fantasies or what commitment looks like in the context of being bisexual. Other topics, like money and unemployment, can also bring conflict. These triggers turn into anxieties or fears, which quickly turn into anger. In fact, I believe the ultimatums and threats you throw at each other reflect the anxiety that results from not being able to control the situation or influence your partner's perspective. How is this sitting with each of you?

Adam: That makes a lot of sense to me.

Jane: [With tears in her eyes] I struggle so much with anxiety that it is overwhelming, and I have tried to cope with that anxiety by getting more controlling, which only fuels my anger. This is a heavy bag that I want to let go of.

Therapist: I very much appreciate your candor, and the good news is that I think I can help. I am wondering if you would be interested in seeing someone for your anxiety. Specifically, I want to recommend cognitive behavior therapy, as it is the most effective treatment for anxiety. [Referring one member of a couple can be tricky because couples therapy is always a balancing act, especially with the alliance. Thus, as a general rule, IST therapists try to minimize splitting up the system. That being said, an exception can be made when referring one member of the couple for specialized treatment like CBT for anxiety. Individual therapy as an adjunct to couples therapy works best when the individual therapy is not focused on the relationship but rather on a specific symptom. This keeps the relational issues in the couples therapy context.]

Jane: Yes, I would appreciate that referral. Adam went through CBT, and it really helped him. [Adam then shares how his therapy was helpful for him and expresses his hope that Jane will have the same benefit. Jane is appreciative and asks a couple of questions about the approach. Adam responds to her questions then defers to the therapist, who provides some explanatory information. Jane expresses concern about the cost, and Adam assures her they can afford it. The therapist agrees to look for someone in their insurance network, which is reassuring to Jane.]

Therapist: Great, I will work on that and have a referral for you next week. My first suggestion for our work here is to teach you some skills for managing conflict. I'd like to go over a step-by-step approach for preventing the escalation. Once you have the skills down, then I want to help the two of you increase your tolerance for hard conversations. Look, the central task of any romantic relationship is the management of differences. Quite simply, couples who manage their differences better tend to have a higher relationship satisfaction. Those who don't, tend to have lower relationship satisfaction. Thus, I want to help the two of you to be less reactive to your differences and be able to focus on staying connected especially when discussing hard topics. How does this sound to you?

Adam: This is exactly what I was looking for. I know that the way we communicate now isn't working, but I don't know of a different way. The idea that we will learn some skills is encouraging.

Jane: Yes, a plan to manage our differences gives me hope.

Therapist: I'm glad to hear that. In fact, Jane, you raise another important aspect to the therapy. I know it can be hard to have these arguments so early in your relationship, but I am hoping that this therapy can help the two of you develop a sense of confidence, a sense of security that you can face whatever life throws at you.

Jane: I am feeling much better about our relationship. I think you have a really good understanding of our problems and goals.

Adam: I agree, and I'm excited to get started.

Therapist: Good. So at our next session let's start digging into learning the tools for managing conflict, and Jane, I will work on getting you a referral.

One of the potential benefits of the four-session introductory format is the strengthening of the alliance that can occur. For example, as stated earlier, both members of the couple were a little apprehensive about starting couples therapy, especially Adam. The alliance scale of the questionnaire the therapist used assesses how clients feel about the therapist and the therapy on a scale of 1 to 7, with higher being better. After the first session, Adam gave a rating of 4, and Jane gave a 5. After the fourth session, Adam's rating improved to 6.5, and Jane's rating improved to 7. The alliance is central to IST, and given the research demonstrating that therapists are not good judges of the alliance, having an objective measure of it is helpful.

Early to Middle Phases of Therapy

Enacting solution sequences and working with here-and-now constraints are important focuses in the early phase of therapy. Depending on progress, the middle phase may be more about maintenance of progress, moving on to other therapy goals, or investigating constraints of a more historical nature.

> *Therapist:* I'm wondering what thoughts or conversations, if any, you have about the feedback session?
>
> *Adam:* We both left your office feeling hopeful and excited to get started. [Jane nods in agreement.]
>
> *Therapist:* Good. Before we get started, Jane, I spoke to one of my colleagues who is a well-respected cognitive behavior therapist. She usually has a waiting list, but she said if you can give her a call that she will fit you in.
>
> *Jane:* Thanks. I will contact the cognitive therapist later today. I want to try the CBT first. If that does not help, I can consider medication.
>
> *Therapist:* Great. Part of how I work is that I'd like to be able to coordinate with your other providers to ensure we are all on the same page and are able to give you the best care possible. In order for that to happen, I would need for you to sign a release so that I can speak with her. I will always let you know if I have spoken with one of your care providers, and if something comes up in our therapy session that leads me to think it would be good to contact either of them, I will also let you know. How does that sound? [As part of being an IST therapist, working collaboratively with other providers is essential to maintain a systemic perspective. A good alliance between providers mitigates possible iatrogenic effects that can arise with multiple therapists working on a client system.]

Jane: Of course. I would prefer for all of you to communicate whenever possible, so whatever I need to sign to make that happen I will.

Therapist: Good.

Adam: Question for you. Will you share information about me with the CBT therapist?

Therapist: Good question. I will not share any specific information about you with the therapist. I will be discussing Jane in response to you, but I will not go into any detail about your current life or history.

Adam: OK. And it is fine if you do share information about me; I was just curious.

Therapist: No problem. It's a good question. So let's get started. One of the primary problems is your difficulty having hard conversations without having them escalate. So what I'm going to go over is a strategy for how to prevent the escalation. Please keep in mind that this is not how to resolve the conflict but rather how to stop and prevent the conversation from spiraling out of control. [Both Adam and Jane nod their heads.] In essence, I am going to teach the two of you how to do a time-out. There are several steps to doing a proper time-out, and each step comes with the risk of not doing it correctly. What I want each of you to pay attention to is what step is going to be the hardest one for you. [They both continue to nod their heads affirmatively.]

The therapist carefully and painstakingly explained the time-out procedure, discussing in detail the step-by-step process of taking a time-out: (a) recognizing the physiological cues for when to take a time-out (louder voice, faster speech, increased heart rate), (b) finding a respectful way to call a time-out (stating the importance of the topic, indicating one's need to calm self, and committing to come back to talk more about it), (c) accepting a partner's need for a time-out, (d) executing an effective time-out period (engaging in a calming activity, then engaging in self-reflection about one's part in the escalation and how to more productively approach the next conversation), and (e) calling "time-in" (initiated by the person who called the time-out—"I am ready to talk when you are"). In reviewing the steps, the therapist gave humorous examples about how not to take a time-out that illustrated how it could go wrong. This brought shared laughter that seemed to strengthen the therapeutic relationship.

Jane: I really like the steps. It seems this will help us slow down. We have done parts of this but never the whole procedure.

In fact, the times it didn't work we didn't do one or more of the steps, so I think this will really be helpful. I know I will have trouble engaging in activity during the time-out. I tend to ruminate, which, like you said, just makes me more upset.

Adam: I think this will work. I know that I will struggle the most with taking the time-out. I tend to want to keep going, so if she calls a time-out, I am going to have to work on letting that happen, and I will have to work on calling the time-out myself as I probably stay in the conversation too long when I'm already upset.

Therapist: I'm glad to you both articulated what you will struggle with the most. One of the general principles of successful couples therapy is the ability to turn the mirror on ourselves rather than on our partner. That is, it is always better to call yourself out than to point out the flaws in your partner. It's hard enough to change ourselves, so to think we are going to change our partners is near impossible. [They both nod in agreement.] Let me provide an important guideline. If you think your partner is upset, it is not going to go too well if you tell your partner, "I think you need to take a time-out!" [They both burst out laughing.] Sometimes it is true that our partners realize we are upset before we do. However, the way to handle it is by observing the sequence between the two of you. If you see that the conversation is going in a bad direction, then take a time-out by saying, "Our conversation is going in a bad direction, and I am concerned that my number [rating of frustration or anger] is going up." This allows for being authentic without throwing gasoline on the fire. [They both indicate agreement.] OK, because you are both excellent students, I have an experiment for you. [They both smile.] I want you to review the steps repeatedly, as the only way to implement this successfully is to overlearn it. And I don't want either of you to expect perfection. If you have to take a time-out, it will likely not go perfectly. So, I am not interested in perfection but rather in your attempt to implement it. When you mess up on a step, I want you to try and figure out what went wrong and what you can do better the next time.

This segment of the first session after the initial evaluation sessions operationalized the IST education guideline in that the therapist educated the couple on why and how to take a time-out. The assumption was that the couple would continue to engage in the problem sequence of conflict escalation because they lacked the knowledge of a viable alternative. The hope was that the time-out would be a solution sequence for the escalation and a building block for better overall communication.

Next Session: Initial Follow-Up on the Experiment

    Therapist: So, how was the week?

    Adam: Well, it wasn't great. We got into a series of arguments. We tried to implement the time-out, but as you predicted, we had limited success.

    Jane: I agree. We tried, and it helped some, but we kept arguing.

    Therapist: Although I'm sorry to hear that you had arguments and struggled with the procedure, I am glad that you report trying to use it as a technique that takes practice. So why don't you tell me any patterns you observed and take me through one of the failed attempts. [The therapist understands the importance of the details when trying to implement a behavioral intervention and thus hopes to identify the constraints to help the couple lift them and implement the solution sequence.]

    Adam: The part that was so upsetting was that we started arguing about stupid stuff. It is one thing if we had an argument about a real problem, but this was about dumb stuff. I had a really difficult day at work as I was up against a deadline and couldn't fix a problem at work. When I got home, I just wanted to vent about my day, have a nice meal, and spend some time with Jane. When I got home, I saw that Jane hadn't cooked dinner. I mean she is at home all day—how hard is it to cook dinner? She then laid into me about all of my shortcomings, and I lost it! I stormed out of the room, and she said don't walk away, and I then reminded her that she has to let me take a time-out. We argued some more but agreed to take a time-out for the next hour.

    Therapist: Jane, do you agree with Adam's account of the fight?

    Jane: Yes. It was very demoralizing! And it seems like we get into a lot of fights after work.

    Therapist: So how did it get resolved? [In IST it is important to understand the entire sequence, so the therapist wants to be sure to understand how it ended.]

    Jane: Well, Adam went out for a walk like he sometimes does, and although I always get anxious when he walks by himself at night, I let him have some time to cool off, and then when he came home he apologized, and I accepted.

Therapist:	Well, it actually sounds like you had some success.
Adam:	I shouldn't have yelled at her about something silly like dinner.
Jane:	And I could've been less defensive and owned up to not honoring our agreement, which is that I would do the cooking since I'm not working.
Therapist:	I'm glad that you are both able to see your contribution to the problem sequence. Adam, you came home pretty tense from work. It seems like you entered the home at about a 4 or 5 [on a 10-point scale of stress or frustration].
Adam:	Yeah, that sounds right.
Therapist:	The key to a time-out is to recognize your number and to be able to call the time-out before you get to a bad place. I also want the two of you to pay particular attention to points of transition during the day. For instance, leaving for work and coming home are often frequent times when couples have fights. So I have another experiment for the two of you. When you come home, I would like for the two of you to start your transition to home by not only checking in about your days but also giving a rating for how you are feeling on a scale of 1 to 10. So let's say your level of frustration is a 7, then tell your partner what happened. The partner's goal is not to see if the 7 is an accurate rating but rather to understand what factors contribute to your partner having a good or bad day. In essence, your job is to be a good student of your partner, which can only happen by being curious rather than judgmental. The other benefit to this is that if you do it as soon as you get home, and your partner tells you they are not in the best place, then you can give your partner some slack. How does this sound to the two of you? [They both state that they agree and feel that it would help.]

Subsequent Sessions: Establishing and Maintaining a Solution Sequence

The therapist read the feedback that the time-out was not entirely successful, worked to identify the constraints, and proposed a more nuanced solution sequence aimed at lifting the constraint. In subsequent sessions the therapist reviewed the steps to conducting a time-out and identified and addressed additional constraints to the procedure through the iterative process of hypothesizing, planning, conversing, and reading the feedback. Over time the couple was more successful at taking time-outs and being considerate of the other partner's stress level. The sessions also involved enactments in which the couple discussed hard topics with the support of the therapist, the practice of emotion regulation techniques, and even taking a time-out in session as needed. After a few months, they mastered the time-out and were much better at regulating their emotions. This was confirmed by improvement on their questionnaire.

The therapist also had conversations with Jane's CBT therapist. The two therapists and the couple all agreed that Jane's anxiety had decreased. In fact, her anxiety symptoms went into the normal range on the questionnaire. Although progress was undeniable, it was also clear that the couple was still unable to have conversations at home about difficult topics, including their families of origin, marriage, sex, money, and children. They were able to implement the time-out, but whenever these topics came up, they still would have visceral reactions that interfered with communication. Thus, consistent with IST's failure-driven principle, after 3 months of significant progress with de-escalation, but insufficient progress with communication, the therapist decided that the upper matrix interventions involving communication skills and conflict resolution were not sufficient to address Jane and Adam's hot topic triggering issues. The therapist planned to explore constraints that were based on their family-of-origin experiences.

Middle to Late Phases of Therapy: Addressing Historical Constraints

In the next session, the therapist initiated a conversation about progress in therapy. After a collaborative discussion of progress, he decided to propose a plan for exploring factors in the couple's past that may have been constraining communication.

> *Therapist:* The two of you have made some really nice progress, as you are better able to stop the escalation, and you are better able to prevent some of the fights about nothing, such as division of labor. However, every time the two of you discuss certain topics like your families or sexual identity or sex, it triggers visceral fights. Although you can take a time-out and recover from them quicker, the same sequence plays out almost every time. So what I would like to do is spend the next couple of sessions talking about your families of origin and early childhood experiences to see if it may help us learn about what keeps you from changing this pattern. As I do this, I will spend most of the session focused on one of you, and I would like the other to listen and seek to simply understand. Then in the next session I will focus on the other's family background. How does that sound? [In this statement, the interpersonal guideline was used in that the therapist believed it was beneficial and perhaps essential

that each partner witness the family-of-origin session of the other to help contextualize the behavior that the partner did not understand. In fact, this can help humanize a partner and facilitate an understanding of the etiology of a partner's vulnerabilities, which will hopefully translate into better understanding and greater intentionality for responding to those vulnerabilities in a different manner. That is, conjoint sessions focused on family-of-origin experiences, especially those that contain traumatic histories, have potential for healing.]

Adam: I am all for it as we need to be able to have these harder conversations.

Jane: This is scary, but probably what is needed. I'm tired of feeling so drained from these topics.

Therapist: OK. Adam, I would like to start with you next week. Would you both be comfortable with that?

Adam: Sure.

Jane: Absolutely.

Adam's Family-of-Origin Session

Therapist: Today is Adam's day. [Adam and Jane chuckle.] Ready to explore some of the relationship issues in the context of Adam's background? [Both nod and indicate they are ready.] Jane, I ask you to just listen and remain curious. [The therapist then describes the relational sequence involving Jane's anxiety and Adam's reaction to it and provides a recent example of the sequence to elicit thoughts and feelings related to it. After some discussion of this, the therapist begins to explore the origin of Adam's strong reaction to Jane's anxiety.] Adam, I hear that you get very activated when Jane is anxious about something. In fact, it almost seems intolerable, and you have a sense of urgency that she needs to be able to take care of herself.

Adam: Yes, that is very true. It really upsets me when she gets stressed out by something like her family. Whenever her family calls her, she almost has a panic attack, and I can't take it! I begin to fear that she will always be anxious and that this is something that we will always struggle with.

Therapist: Just to play devil's advocate for a minute, let's say that is the case. What's so bad about that? All couples have things they have to accept about their partner and have to manage. So if

	this is one of the things you will have to manage throughout your life, why is that so bad?
Adam:	[He takes a long sigh and is silent for a while.] I don't know why.
Therapist:	Well, I remember from our individual session that you shared that your mom was dependent on your dad and that no matter how hard your dad tried, he could not console your mom.
Adam:	Yes.
Therapist:	And not only did your dad fail at it but then you had to take care of your mom, especially when she was drunk or sick, and it wasn't easy for you either.
Adam:	[Gets quiet and a little teary eyed.] Yes, I tried hard to please my mom, and when I was able to take care of her adequately, it felt great because that was the time she said she loved me. But I also resented the fact that I had to be her caretaker as I couldn't just be myself. [As the session progresses, the therapist continues to interview Adam about his relationship with his mother. Adam shares specific events that occurred, as well as his overall sense of his role in the family and what he feels it had cost him. The therapist is empathic and does not hesitate to point out both how Adam was resourceful enough to find ways to cope with a difficult situation and how those ways of coping may not always fit well within the context of the relationship with Jane.]
Therapist:	It's like your identity became fused with being your mom's caretaker.
Adam:	I never had a life.
Therapist:	I wonder if when Jane seems helpless because of her anxiety that it brings you right back to what it was like when you had to take care of your mom. It also seems that it is difficult for you when you make efforts to soothe Jane and she doesn't seem consolable. It may even on an unconscious level bring you back to feelings about caring for your mom and how difficult that was. I wonder if not being able to take care of Jane when she is upset triggers fears about whether or not she loves you because you learned from your childhood that being loved means successfully making a distressed loved one feel better. [Adam now has more tears in his eyes, as does Jane.] Adam, what are you feeling?

Adam:	I can't believe I have treated Jane like my mom! [He bursts out crying, and Jane, also crying, moves over to him and puts her arms around him.] Jane, I love you so much, and I don't mean to come at you with anger and turn you into my mom.
Therapist:	And worse than being your caretaker is trying to be your caretaker and failing at it.
Adam:	Jane, I am so sorry!
Jane:	Me too.
Therapist:	I'm so glad that the two of you are having this conversation. This is the beginning of a journey, of healing.

In this session, the therapist opened up the family-of-origin and mind metaframeworks (specifically an M2 object relations hypothesis). The rest of the session elaborated on the hypothesis that connected his early experience to current day interactions with Jane and raised the issue of his current struggle with differentiation from his parents. In IST, the purpose of going historical is to remove constraints to the solution sequence, so the therapist is using object relations to link past family-of-origin experiences to current feelings and thoughts that constrain solutions.

Jane's Family-of-Origin Session

Therapist:	Today I want to talk with you, Jane, about your background. And Adam, as a reminder, I would like for you to listen and remain curious. Your goal is to look for ways to connect and to remain compassionate.
Adam:	OK.
Therapist:	Jane, I notice that one of the triggers for you is when Adam tries to share thoughts about his bisexual identity. As I understand it, you react like you don't want to hear about it. I know your reaction is not because you have any stigmatizing thoughts, but you seem to automatically assume that he wants to have an open relationship, which I know is a deal breaker for you. However, Adam has mentioned many times that he does not want an open relationship; he just wants to be able to talk about his coming out process.
Jane:	I know, I know . . . I mean I know he says that, but I have a hard time believing him.
Therapist:	Is there anything in your past that might help explain this? [The therapist looks for opportunities to link the past to the present.]

Jane: Well, my parents, especially my dad, never wanted me.

Therapist: What do you mean?

Jane: My dad would say that he wished I was a boy and that I am ugly and that no one would ever love me! [She begins to cry.] So why would Adam or anyone love me? The only time someone loves me is for sex, so I'm basically a sex object for men! That is why my dad molested me because that is all I was good for!

Adam: That is not true! I love you! [Adam reaches out to her.]

Therapist: Jane, I wonder if because of the messages you received in your childhood if you sometimes wonder, even now, if you are lovable?

Jane: [Whispering, barely audible due to crying.] Yes. [Jane is shaking, and Adam is holding her. The therapist decides not to say anything for several minutes because silence can sometimes be a powerful intervention.]

Therapist: This is clearly an important and healing moment. Both of you seem to be in a similar boat, albeit for different reasons. You both struggle with believing that you are lovable, and thus your interactions are driven by fear due to unhealed trauma and unresolved family-of-origin experiences, which is why your reactions to each other are so powerful. You both unintentionally trigger the other. The good news is that we can work on changing these sequences. In fact, I believe your relationship can be a context for healing. How does that sound to the two of you? [While holding each other, they both say it sounds hopeful.]

The session continued to explore Jane's experiences in her family of origin as well as the way her fears of not being lovable seemed to interact with Adam's feeling powerless to help her and consequently feeling unworthy of her love. The therapist led a discussion about how their awareness of this deeper pattern might help them begin to modify their communication about hard topics.

Consolidating, Tapering, and Terminating

Working with interventions from the bottom of the matrix involves patience and repetition. For the next year, the therapy focused on helping the couple to have a different experience of each other. Moreover, the work involved helping them to see that their thoughts and feelings about each other were reflections of internalizations of themselves and each other that were formed from early family relationships and childhood experiences. M2 strategies and interventions were drawn from object relations and internal family systems approaches, providing insights with constant linkage of the past to the present problem sequences.

Another major thrust of the therapy was working on their sexual relationship. This included managing their different sexual expectations because Adam's libido was higher than Jane's. A particular challenge was that Adam's homosexual desires had never been acted on, yet he was signing up for a monogamous relationship. Thus, several sessions were spent helping him grieve and accept that his desires would remain fantasies. The therapist also helped the couple understand the emotional aspect of sex above and beyond a biological urge. Thus, because they were able to manage their triggers better and become more emotionally connected, their sexual connection also improved. The progress was gradual and led to the two of them setting a date for the wedding and then finally getting married.

Not surprisingly, getting married served as a major trigger for some regression. The regression involved activation of their dependency issues and exacerbation of key problem sequences, but they worked successfully to understand their reactions, dampen their reactivity, and settle into their developing patterns of interdependence. The therapy became less didactic and behavioral and moved to being more experiential. The healing was an iterative process with attachment injuries serving as opportunities to have corrective emotional experiences. The therapist provided reminders of how the couple resolved past difficulties to remind them that their relationship was safe and that they were fortunate to have found each other. The couple started to respond to each other in more healing ways, and the questionnaire showed that all the scales were in the normal range.

Termination involved a tapering of sessions from weekly, to every other week, to monthly, and finally to every other month. There was always the explicit message that they could call the therapist at any time if a situation arose. After almost two years of therapy, the couple and therapist decided to take a break. The therapist led a discussion of their significant progress, the strengths they had as individuals and as a couple, and the challenges they may face going forward. He presented the idea of couples therapy being analogous to family medicine. That is, couples therapy and family therapy are available throughout the life span as needed. Different developmental stages and transitions can engender new challenges, and so the therapist advised them to never hesitate to call. The therapist gave the strong recommendation to resume therapy if and when they got pregnant because that is a difficult life transition for any couple. The therapist wanted to give the message that they could do well on their own (promoting independence) but also that returning to therapy is normative (minimizing shame and abandonment issues). In the last session, both members of the couple were teary eyed and extremely grateful for the work.

11

THE INTEGRATIVE SYSTEMIC THERAPY APPROACH TO WORKING WITH INDIVIDUALS

Though the integrative systemic therapy (IST) approach to individual therapy, or what we more accurately call *individual context work*, incorporates concepts and strategies from existing models of therapy, it differs from most forms of individual therapy. Four critical aspects of IST distinguish its approach to individual work. The first part of our clinical case example illustrates the distinguishing characteristics of IST individual work.

HOW IS INTEGRATIVE SYSTEMIC THERAPY WORK WITH INDIVIDUALS DISTINCT?

Client: Hi. My name is Guillermo Gonzalez. I was given your name by a friend who thought that you might be able to help me.

Therapist: Guillermo, what kind of help are you looking for?

http://dx.doi.org/10.1037/0000055-011
Integrative Systemic Therapy: Metaframeworks for Problem Solving With Individuals, Couples, and Families,
by W. M. Pinsof, D. C. Breunlin, W. P. Russell, J. L. Lebow, C. Rampage, and A. L. Chambers

Client:	I am not sure. I have a lot of anxiety and fears and would like to feel better.
Therapist:	How long has this been going on?
Client:	Most of my life, but it seems to be getting worse.
Therapist:	Any idea why it might be getting worse now?
Client:	Well, I got married about 6 months ago, and my wife, Lucy, is also concerned that I get so uptight so often.
Therapist:	Is she forcing you to get therapy, or are you choosing to do it now yourself?
Client:	She doesn't even know I'm calling you. I am choosing to do something about my problems now.
Therapist:	Would you consider telling her that you've called me to set up an appointment?
Client:	Not now. I am not ready to tell her that.
Therapist:	Why?
Client:	I need to talk to you about some private things, and I know she will be full of questions that I don't want to answer at this point.
Therapist:	OK, let's see if we can find a time to meet. How about 10:00 Friday morning?
Client:	That would be great. Where is your office?

Individuals Are Always Part of Larger Systems

As this vignette illustrates, the first critical difference between IST and other forms of individual therapy is the concept of the client system (see Chapter 2, this volume). The IST therapist viewed Guillermo as ineluctably part of a larger biopsychosocial system. Although Guillermo was presenting as an individual client, the therapist was curious about the network of relationships that made up his intimate life and seized on the interpersonal component of Guillermo's explanation of why his anxiety had gotten worse. In asking whether Guillermo was seeking therapy because his wife was pressuring him, the therapist opened the door of that relationship. In clarifying that he had chosen to pursue therapy, Guillermo began to define his relationship with his wife by informing the therapist that she was not even aware that he was seeking therapy. This led the therapist to begin hypothesizing about Guillermo's relationship with his wife and his issues about autonomy and intimacy.

Others Can Help Inform the Individual Client's Therapy Experience

The second aspect of IST that distinguishes its approach to individual work is the interpersonal guideline, which asserts that, when possible and appropriate, it is better to do an intervention, regardless of its nature, within an interpersonal (family or couple) as opposed to an individual context. Typically, when individuals present for individual therapy, the IST therapist explores the possibility, as early as possible, of involving other relevant members in the direct client system. The purpose of this involvement is not necessarily to change the modality from individual to couples or family therapy, but rather to engage other members of the client system in helping to define and understand the presenting problems. IST therapists involve relevant others in an individual's therapy to develop a more comprehensive picture of the problems than the individual client can typically provide. It also helps to build the alliance with the relevant others in the client's life. In terms of the direct–indirect client system boundary, other client system members are invited to cross the boundary and join the direct system temporarily as guests of the presenting client. They may or may not remain in the direct system and become "clients" as opposed to "guests," depending on the information that emerges in the conjoint episodes.

In asking Guillermo whether he would consider telling his wife that he had decided to go into therapy, the therapist was testing a variety of hypotheses. First, he was trying to understand further what might be behind Guillermo's statement "She doesn't even know I'm calling." Was it fear, and if so, fear of what? The therapist was also somewhat indirectly suggesting an intervention—"Would you consider telling her" about the therapy. Guillermo's response was clear and emphatic—"Not now." But his response held out hope that perhaps he would consider telling her sometime in the future that he was in therapy.

If Guillermo had answered the therapist's "Would you . . ." query by saying that he would consider telling his wife, the therapist might have gone further in planning with Guillermo over the phone how he might do that. If Guillermo had responded to the therapist's query with "That's a good idea; I will tell her," the therapist might even have explored the possibility that Guillermo's wife might join them for the first appointment. In other words, even if the therapy ended up focusing primarily on Guillermo's anxiety and fears, his wife's presence, at least episodically, might have facilitated the therapy and broadened the systemic alliance.

As With Couple and Family Contexts, the Alliance Predominates

The third aspect of IST that defines individual work is the concept of the integrative therapy alliance. As specified previously, this alliance addresses the alliance with Guillermo and the therapist, the alliance with the other key members of the client system (e.g., his wife), and the alliance between Guillermo and his wife in regard to his engagement and work in the therapy. In the vignette, the therapist decided not to challenge Guillermo's refusal to tell his wife because his alliance with Guillermo was just beginning and was, therefore, relatively weak. To insist that he tell his wife at this point could well discourage Guillermo from participating in the therapy and getting the help he clearly needed. This moment illustrates the "alliance predominance" concept, in which developing and preserving the alliance takes priority over the interpersonal guideline.

Also, Guillermo's statement about "private things" and questions he did not want to answer at that point raised the possibility that what he wanted to tell the therapist may have realistically jeopardized his relationship with his wife, and until the therapist had a better understanding of what Guillermo wanted to talk about, it was prudent to grant him the privacy and confidentiality he desired. For instance, if Guillermo were struggling with being gay or if he were engaged in an affair that had led him to question his desire to continue in the marriage, it would probably have been less destructive and more effective to initially help Guillermo address these aspects of his life individually and then find a way to integrate this information into his marriage.

Assessment and Intervention Start With the Initial Phone Call and Continue Throughout

The last aspect that defines individual work in IST is the inseparability of assessment (reading feedback and hypothesizing) and intervention (planning and conversing) as co-occurring processes that span the entire course of therapy. More specifically, this vignette illustrates how the therapist was beginning to develop and test hypotheses about the presenting problem and the web of constraints ("How long has this been going on?"), simultaneously suggesting that Guillermo might change his behavior with his wife ("Would you consider . . ."). In other words, the conversation over the phone was not just about taking factual information and setting up the first session; it was an active intervention in which the therapist was deciding who would be involved in the first session and who would know about who would be involved in the first session.

The first phone call is a chance to "test the waters" and see how the caller responds. This is particularly the case when the caller, unlike Guillermo, presents their unhappiness with their spouse or partner as a major problem. In this case, couples therapy may make sense; moreover, starting off by seeing one of the partners alone may well skew the therapy and constrain the development of the alliance with the nonparticipating spouse or partner. Similarly, if a parent is calling for individual therapy for a child, it makes sense for the parents (and possibly siblings) to attend the first session. In other words, the first phone call is a critical therapeutic interaction that lays the groundwork for the entire therapy and provides invaluable information about the client system.

ADDRESSING GUILLERMO'S WORKPLACE ANXIETY

In the first and second sessions, the therapist thoroughly explored Guillermo's current social context and his concerns about anxiety and fear (his initial presenting problem). Guillermo shared that he was a second-generation Mexican American. His parents emigrated from Mexico when they were teenagers. His mother had received an American citizenship, but his father had not. Spanish was spoken in the home, and Guillermo reported that his parents raised the family with Mexican values. Guillermo acculturated as a child, and in high school, he had many battles with his parents as he pressed to have the autonomy of American teenagers. Guillermo met Lucy in high school. They lost touch when Lucy went to college, but they started dating again when they met at an immigration rally. They were married 3 years later despite Lucy's father's opposition to the wedding.

The therapist began to build an alliance by being respectful, listening carefully, and demonstrating concern about the things being presented in therapy. Guillermo shared that his anxiety was highest in situations that might involve conflict. He recently had become a manager at his job at an agency in the federal government. His anxiety had increased as he faced the challenges of holding employees accountable and dealing with their requests, concerns, and complaints. Guillermo indicated that the job was important to him and that he wanted to find a way of handling the anxiety. Problem sequences were mapped out, and in the third session, they agreed that self-calming and facing (vs. avoiding) interpersonal challenges would be important solution sequences. The interventions provided by the therapist included relaxation exercises, role-playing work scenarios, and a plan to face a hierarchy of difficult circumstances in vivo. During Sessions 3 to 6, Guillermo worked steadily in therapy and began to make significant progress in reducing his anxiety.

UNCOVERING ANOTHER PROBLEM AND SEQUENTIALIZING IT

In Session 7, Guillermo began to open up to the therapist about another problem.

Therapist: How was your week, Guillermo?

Guillermo: I feel like I am making progress. This week, I told one of my staff members that I wanted his reports done on time—

	pretty much how we practiced it. It wasn't easy, and I think he may not have liked it, but I did it.
Therapist:	Great. I agree that you are making significant progress. How has the anxiety been for you?
Guillermo:	It is improving overall, but I have been anxious about telling you—well, not telling you—something. I have been too embarrassed to tell you this, but I want to tell you today.
Therapist:	I'm glad you feel safe enough to share this with me today. What is it?
Guillermo:	I was in therapy before, and I thought things got better, but after I stopped, things got worse again.
Therapist:	When was this?
Guillermo:	About a year ago.
Therapist:	Tell me more about that therapy.
Guillermo:	I really liked the therapist. I felt he understood me and helped me talk about painful stuff that happened in my childhood that I never told anybody about. I began to understand where my fear and shame come from and began to not feel so alone or like such a freak.
Therapist:	Why do you think the changes did not last?
Guillermo:	I don't know. He moved away, and we had to stop therapy. Maybe I wasn't done.
Therapist:	Did you feel ready to stop when he moved away?
Guillermo:	Not really. I wanted to be able to make it on my own, but maybe I wasn't ready.
Therapist:	How did you feel about his moving away and you having to stop when you weren't ready?
Guillermo:	I felt it had to be, and there was nothing I could do about it.
Therapist:	What does it feel like to you when something you don't want has to be, and you can't do anything about it?
Guillermo:	I am not sure what you are getting at.
Therapist:	You know, sometimes when people kind of feel abandoned by someone they have grown to trust and care about, they feel alone, sad, and maybe even mad.
Guillermo:	I think I felt sad but knew there was nothing I could do about it.

Therapist:	I wonder if you also felt helpless and alone again?
Guillermo:	Yeah, there was nothing I could do, and there was no one I could talk to.
Therapist:	I imagine that you did not want your wife to know about that therapy either and that you could not talk to her about your sad and lonely feelings.
Guillermo:	That's right. We weren't married yet, but it is true that she did not know.
Therapist:	Guillermo, when you look back on your life, when was the first time that you can remember feeling that combination of sadness, helplessness, and aloneness?
Guillermo:	I don't want to talk about that. I am not ready.
Therapist:	Do you mean that you don't know me well enough yet, or trust me enough yet, to tell me about what happened to you?
Guillermo:	Well, it is not that I don't trust you. You seem to know your stuff. It's just that I'm not ready. This stuff is hard to talk about.
Therapist:	Would it be safe for me to say that it is hard for you to trust and confide in other people and that you have felt alone and sad much of your life?
Guillermo:	I guess so. When people get to know me, I am not sure they are going to like or accept me. I have to be very careful. I pull back a lot.
Therapist:	What about with your wife? She obviously likes and loves you.
Guillermo:	But she doesn't really know me.
Therapist:	Does she know about the painful stuff that happened in your childhood that you talked about with your previous therapist?
Guillermo:	No, and I don't want her to ever know about that stuff.
Therapist:	Because you feel ashamed about what happened and she might react in a way that makes you feel even more ashamed?
Guillermo:	I don't know if I can ever tell anyone again.
Therapist:	Does any part of you feel that your therapist discontinued your therapy because of what you told him?
Guillermo:	I don't know. I just felt like I poured my heart out with him, and it was on the floor, and he left me with it like that.

Therapist:	That sounds very painful and sad. He left you opened up and vulnerable. You weren't finished or closed up or healed, and he was gone.
Guillermo:	Yeah. [With tears in his eyes] But it wasn't his fault.
Therapist:	I know that you feel you are to blame for whatever happens to you, and it is hard for you to ever blame or feel angry at someone else. Do you think that he bears some responsibility for how he left you and that it is OK for you to have feelings about it? [Guillermo nods.] I do too. Do you worry that I will leave you like that if you ever feel safe enough to pour your heart out to me and let me know what happened?
Guillermo:	Yeah, I do worry about that.
Therapist:	I know you worry about that because it is so hard to talk about those things. It is like unloading dynamite.
Guillermo:	Yes, it's very tricky and dangerous for me.
Therapist:	Well, you know they say that men plan and God laughs. But setting that aside, I have no plans to leave my practice or you, and I hope that we can unpack this dynamite together when you are ready. I appreciate your courage to speak to this today.

In this vignette, the therapist worked with Guillermo on multiple things simultaneously. First, they identified an additional presenting problem—Guillermo's fear of being shamed and abandoned. They also began to sequentialize that problem. Guillermo thought about what happened to him, felt shame and a host of other feelings, assumed that others would feel the same way, and kept it all inside, ending up isolated and with tremendous feelings of loneliness, sadness, and pain. This vignette reflects an evolution in Guillermo's problem presentation. He started moving away from focusing on his concerns about anxiety and fear, to talking about social isolation, intense shame and self-blame, and distrust of others. The therapist understood that these feelings might constrain Guillermo from feeling more comfortable and less anxious. Guillermo also put on the table a clearly identified trauma, a trauma that was opaque to the therapist in that it had not yet been described. The clear trauma was the loss of his previous therapist and his subsequent feelings of anger, guilt, and humiliation. The opaque trauma was whatever happened in his childhood that the therapist had begun to hypothesize might be at the core of Guillermo's web of constraints. The two traumas began to link up in this vignette, but the therapist, heeding the feedback that Guillermo was not ready to discuss the historical trauma, chose to leave it alone.

The interpersonal process of this vignette is also relevant. Guillermo articulated his embarrassment about exposing himself to his previous therapist, getting better, then being abandoned and subsequently deteriorating. The therapist supported and validated Guillermo's acknowledgment of his embarrassment and shame and carefully explored that traumatic episode of Guillermo's life. The therapist also noted that Guillermo did not tell his wife that he had been in therapy previously or about the painful and traumatic aspects of that experience. Nor had he told his wife about the early, opaque trauma. Although noted, the therapist left the lack of transparency and communication with his wife, as well as Guillermo's early trauma, alone. The goal at this moment was to build the alliance with Guillermo, particularly what has been called the *bond component* of the alliance (Bordin, 1979; Horvath & Greenberg, 1989; Pinsof & Catherall, 1986). The therapist hypothesized that the growth of the bond, as a result of the empathic explorations of the clear, more recent trauma, would lay the relational groundwork for both the exploration of the early trauma and, ultimately, the sharing with his wife of that trauma and Guillermo's experiences in therapy.

The therapist also brought Guillermo's concern about disclosing and being abandoned directly into the therapy by asking Guillermo whether he feared he would open up and then be abandoned by the therapist. In other words, the therapist used his relationship and Guillermo's ambivalence about trusting him as a real-life example of Guillermo's problem. He implicitly said, "I know you are not sure you can trust me, and I want to directly address that issue with you." In other words, he was trying to give Guillermo a courageous and metacommunicative language in which they could talk about their relationship with each other. He also told Guillermo that he would do everything in his power to not abandon him if and when Guillermo opened up about his early trauma and terrible sense of shame.

Moving From Action Strategies to Meaning/Emotion Metaframework Strategies

In terms of the planning matrix, the therapist moved from using strategies from the action planning metaframework to address anxiety to using strategies from the meaning/emotion planning metaframework to explore what Guillermo experienced in his last therapy and what that meant to him. The trauma work in this vignette is reasonably proximal, focusing on what happened at the end of the prior therapy. The proximal work lays the emotional and relational infrastructure for the more distal trauma work that would occur later and draw on strategies from lower in the matrix.

In the eighth, ninth, and 10th sessions, the therapy had a dual focus, supporting Guillermo's gains in the workplace and building the therapeutic alliance through attunement and openness to his thoughts and feelings. Guillermo shared that he always felt he was different from other people because of what had happened to him and he had felt sad, ashamed, and lonely much of his life. The therapist hypothesized that this was a function of a traumatic history and that sharing that history within the context of a safe relationship would be a step toward reducing Guillermo's pain and isolation. The plan for this phase of therapy was to establish safety, provide a space for the material to emerge, and allow Guillermo to control the pace. The therapist continued with this plan in the next session.

Putting Guillermo in Charge of Telling His Trauma Story

Therapist: How are things going?

Guillermo: I am functioning OK at work, but I am realizing how isolated I feel. At this point, no one outside of this office understands or knows me.

Therapist: And how does that feel to you?

Guillermo: Lonely. Bad.

Therapist: I know. You've felt that loneliness most of your life, but now you are becoming more aware of it—more in touch with yourself.

Guillermo: And it does not feel good.

Therapist: I know it does not feel good, but I am glad that you can share the feelings with me. At least you're beginning to feel that you can open up to and trust me somewhat.

Guillermo: But not all the way yet.

Therapist: Yeah, not yet trusting or safe enough with me to tell me what happened when you were younger?

Guillermo: I have been thinking a lot about that. I want to tell you, but feel afraid you will think I'm disgusting or awful.

Therapist: Guillermo, although we are still getting to know each other, based on what you have seen and felt in this office, how likely is it that I will think you are disgusting or awful?

Guillermo: I guess it's not very likely.

Therapist: But you are afraid nevertheless because you trusted your previous therapist and were left opened up on the emotional surgery table.

Guillermo: Yeah, but if I can't trust you, who can I trust?

Therapist:	Yeah, I guess I am the best of the whole untrustworthy lot at this point in your life.
Guillermo:	You're better than that.
Therapist:	But not by that much. [They both laugh.] However, I think there are some things that we can do to minimize your sense of opening up and being left high and dry.
Guillermo:	Like what?
Therapist:	I think that we should plan our sessions exploring your early trauma so that they unfold in three segments. The first is touching base and catching up. The second is you telling me about the trauma and as much as you remember about your thoughts and feelings at the time. The last part of our session will be talking about what we talked about, what it means, and how it may impact your life. That part also involves some planning for our next session. How does that sound?
Guillermo:	That sounds like a good idea. So we close up after each day's surgery?
Therapist:	Exactly, and we only go as far each session as you are comfortable. You set the pace, and I follow.
Guillermo:	That sounds OK with me. When do we start?
Therapist:	We can start as soon as you are ready.
Guillermo:	Do you think I should start now?
Therapist:	Yeah. If you feel ready. You can say no if it is too soon. We can do it next session.
Guillermo:	No, we might as well get started.
Therapist:	OK, lead the way.
Guillermo:	I know you probably suspected this, but I was sexually abused by my oldest brother, Paco.
Therapist:	I would like to know more about you and Paco and what happened. Can you tell me how old was he and how old were you at the time?
Guillermo:	It began when I was 7 and ended when I was around 10. He must have been about 15 when it started and 18 when it ended. That's when he moved out to California.
Therapist:	Tell me about your brother. What was he like?
Guillermo:	Paco was an angry kid. He had a terrible relationship with our father. My father beat him a lot, and my brother was like a broken person. But I looked up to him. He was my

older brother, almost like a little father. As you know, my father was never around—worked all the time, traveled back and forth to Mexico, and would be gone for a month or more. He left Paco in charge when he was gone. That's when it started.

Therapist: How do you mean?

Guillermo: Sometimes, when I was scared I would get into Paco's bed and sleep with him. We slept in the same room. My other brother, Ronaldo, who was 11, had his own room because he talked and screamed in his sleep and would wake anyone near him up.

Therapist: Was your mom around? Why wouldn't you have gotten into bed with her when you were scared?

Guillermo: She was exhausted, and my twin sisters were her major focus—I was 5 when they were born. They were always in and out of her bed. There was no room for me.

Therapist: So you would get into Paco's bed when you were scared?

Guillermo: Yeah. In my last therapy, I was able to remember and describe some things that happened. I have a memory—I'm just going to say it—of him taking my hand and putting it on his penis. He told me to—you know—give him a hand job. I think I was shocked at the time and then disgusted. It is disgusting to me now when I think of how he made me clean it up. I had to go get toilet paper. He just rolled over and went to sleep, without a word. I think that happened a lot.

Therapist: How did you feel?

Guillermo: I felt confused. I did not know what semen was, and I didn't know that men came. I guess I still thought babies came from God or the stork. I had a sense that what we were doing was bad, but I knew it made my brother feel good. I wanted to please him, and I wanted him to like me.

Therapist: What happened after that?

Guillermo: Paco would tell me to get into bed with him most nights. He made me give him oral sex. Then sometimes he would touch me, but most of the time he would make me touch him or give him oral sex.

Therapist: What was that like for you?

Guillermo: It was awful—I hated it, especially oral. He would hold my head down, and it was hard to breathe. I felt like choking.

I remember throwing up one time. I can't remember all the things that happened.

Therapist: You must have dreaded going to bed.

Guillermo: I would try to go to bed and be asleep by the time Paco came in. But he would wake me up. I even asked my mom if I could sleep in Ronaldo's room, but it was like a closet— no room.

Therapist: Did you tell your mom why you wanted to sleep in Ronaldo's room?

Guillermo: No, I was afraid to. Paco told me that this was our secret, and if I told anyone else, he would tell them I was crazy and telling lies. He said he would tell them I was a *maricón*.

Therapist: What is a *maricón*?

Guillermo: It means homosexual or gay. It is like "fag" or "homo."

Therapist: So you felt trapped. You could not get away, you could not tell anyone, and Paco was forcing you to have sex with him.

Guillermo: He even tried anal sex, but I screamed because it hurt so much, and he stopped.

Therapist: So awful for you, but it sounds like you were not totally powerless. Vomiting and screaming put some limits on what you would let him do with you.

Guillermo: I guess that's right. But I began to feel like a robot when I would get into his bed. It was like I was almost not there.

Therapist: You dissociated from the experience. It was a way to protect yourself, like the vomiting and screaming.

Guillermo: Yeah, that's what my previous therapist called it. But I never thought of it as a way to protect myself.

Therapist: Guillermo, you have been phenomenally open with me about what happened. I would like to switch now and talk about how you are feeling about having been so open and explicit with me today.

Guillermo: I feel OK. I didn't feel too much emotion while telling you about it. Maybe some disgust. I am glad I was able to say what happened, though. And it feels different to tell you about it. I feel a little out of it, but I heard from you that maybe I wasn't just a victim or totally helpless. I realize that I did kind of fight back in my own way. I don't feel so ashamed.

This vignette reflects enormous progress in the therapy. The therapist began by querying Guillermo's readiness to trust him and tell him about what happened in response to Guillermo's expression of feeling so lonely and isolated. The therapist even brought some humor into the conversation ("I guess I am the best of the whole untrustworthy lot"). When the prospect of Guillermo telling the therapist about what happened became a reality, the therapist, in the service of building the alliance and creating a structure for addressing Guillermo's remote trauma, proposed a structure for the disclosure sessions. This was a way to let Guillermo know that the structure of therapy would be sufficient, in every sense, to contain his disclosure. In launching the process, the therapist explicitly placed Guillermo "in charge" by saying "lead the way."

Pinpointing Constraints and Strengths

As Guillermo told his story, the therapist asked questions that elaborated the familial context in which the abuse occurred. Because of the cultural constraint that some Mexican families stigmatize homosexuality, Guillermo could not see how he could have gone to his parents. So he suffered in silence. Moreover, having internalized and generalized a belief that you cannot talk about difficult things, Guillermo spent his life ashamed and unsupported.

A critical piece, coming out of the IST strength guideline, which encourages the therapist to see and build on the strengths of the clients, is the therapist's identification of Guillermo's agentic or assertive behaviors in the process of victimization. He commented on how Guillermo's vomiting and screaming effectively stopped certain types of abusive behavior, and he defined Guillermo's feeling like a robot as a way of dissociating from the abuse and protecting himself. In other words, the therapist implicitly told Guillermo that although he was horribly victimized by his brother, he was not totally a helpless victim. He used the power available to him to minimize the abuse and the damage to himself. In elaborating this narrative thread, the therapist also laid the groundwork for Guillermo to increasingly experience himself as someone who had power, who could act, and who was, and was not then, helpless even in the face of unavoidable abuse.

At the end of Guillermo's self-disclosure, the therapist asked him for feedback on the experience. Guillermo clearly picked up on the therapist's agentic emphasis and commented that it diminished his sense of shame about what happened. As the session drew to a close, the therapist talked more with Guillermo about his sense of shame and how he felt "broken" by his brother's abuse of him. He commented that he felt as if he was "stained" by what happened and could never be normal, particularly in regard to his sexuality. He also felt he could never tell anybody about what had happened and that it had marked him as being different and alone.

The next week Guillermo called to cancel, but confirmed for the following week. During the next session (the 12th) the therapist asked him about the cancellation, noting that it was the first cancellation and that it followed Guillermo's talking about the abuse. Guillermo did not immediately see a connection, but subsequent to the discussion, he agreed that on some level he may have been taking a break from the therapy. Further work in this session led to Guillermo crying hard and grieving for what had been lost to him in childhood. In the 13th session, the work continued to focus on the abuse, Guillermo's response at the time (which did show strength), how he had been affected by it, and how he had managed to thrive in many ways despite it.

In Session 14, recounted next, the therapist worked with Guillermo using the internal representation planning metaframework.

Modifying an Internalized Problem Sequence

Therapist: Guillermo, we have been talking about what happened with Paco, how it cut you off from your family and the world. You could never tell anybody about it, yet it had marked or changed you. Since then you told your previous therapist, and now you've told me. I'd like to talk with you about how you would feel about telling, Lucy, your wife, that you are in therapy and about Paco's abuse.

Guillermo: I knew we were going to get to this sooner or later. How do I feel about telling her? I feel scared. I am afraid that she will see me as defective—not good enough—that she might think I am a *maricón* and want to divorce me.

Therapist: So you think she will see you as that critical and judgmental part of you sees you—you know, that part of you that bought the humiliation story that Paco threatened you with—that you are stained, that there is something irreparably wrong with you, and that you are gay. And therefore she cannot be married to you.

Guillermo: Yeah, that's about it. All the negative shit that Paco piled up to silence me so that I would be too ashamed to tell anyone about what he was doing to me.

Therapist: So how realistic do you think those fears are in regard to Lucy? Is she a very critical and judgmental person? Does she think victims of sexual abuse are defective and forever blemished? Does she dislike and reject gay people?

Guillermo: No. We have become good friends with a lesbian couple who have adopted a child, and Lucy is completely supportive of their relationship and the idea that gays and lesbians should be able to marry just like anybody else. She is a very compassionate person and very accepting.

Therapist: The more you talk about her, the more I am convinced that you married the right person. I would really like to meet her. So, given what you know about her, how probable is it that she will react negatively to your telling her about our therapy and the fact that you were abused?

Guillermo: Not very likely. I too am convinced I married the right person. But I am still scared.

Therapist: I know. I think we have to talk more about that part of you that judges you as stained, as less than, as permanently marked with an A for abuse.

Guillermo: I know it's crazy, but that is how I sometimes feel and think.

Therapist: [Stands up, goes over to the wall, picks up an empty chair, and brings it into a triangle with his chair and Guillermo.] Guillermo, I want you to imagine that that judgmental and critical part of you is in that chair. When you get an image of it, tell me.

Guillermo: [Fidgeting and looking at the empty chair.] I see it. It is a person that looks like a cross between my brother and my father—older than me.

Therapist: How old does he look?

Guillermo: About early 40s.

Therapist: What is the look on his face when he looks at you?

Guillermo: He will not even look at me. He is looking away.

Therapist: Does he have a name or can you give him one?

Guillermo: His name is Francisco. Paco is the nickname for Francisco. It was my father and my brother's formal name.

Therapist: They had the same name?

Guillermo: Yes.

Therapist: Guillermo, I want to try something. When you feel ready, I want you to go and sit in that chair and imagine that you are that man—that you are Francisco.

Guillermo:	[After sitting and looking at the empty chair for about 30 seconds, stands up and sits in the empty chair.] OK.
Therapist:	Now I want to look away at that wall, and I want you to tell Guillermo that you are too disgusted with him to even look at him. You can add anything you want after that.
Guillermo:	[Looking at his vacant chair.] You disgust me. I cannot even look at you. What you did was your fault, and you make me sick.
Therapist:	Tell him what you think about people who participate in those kind of acts.
Guillermo:	[To the empty chair] You are a fag, a *maricón*. You are a sissy, and I should put a dress on you. You cannot even defend yourself.
Therapist:	Guillermo, when you are ready I want you to come back to your chair and look at Francisco.
Guillermo:	[Gets up slowly and moves back to his chair.]
Therapist:	Is Francisco looking at you?
Guillermo:	No.
Therapist:	Tell him to look at you.
Guillermo:	Look at me. [Raising his voice.] Look at me. [Almost shouting.] Look at me, *pendejo* [prick].
Therapist:	Tell him how you feel about the things he said to you. Tell him your truth.
Guillermo:	You are wrong. There is something wrong with you. You are sick and afraid. You pick on people who are weaker and cannot defend themselves. You are a bully. I hate you. [He is shouting and starting to cry.]
Therapist:	Talk to him through your tears.
Guillermo:	You did not protect me. You took advantage of me. You broke the law, but you didn't break me.
Therapist:	Tell him how he didn't break you, how you are still whole.
Guillermo:	I am still whole. I have a wife. We will have a family. I will be a better man and father than you. You have taught me how not to be. I will never be like either of you. I can love.
Therapist:	Say that again.

Guillermo: I can love. I can protect my wife, and I will protect and love my children. They will not grow up afraid and sad. [They both sit quietly. Guillermo wipes his eyes but keeps looking at the empty chair. He slowly turns and faces the therapist.] Wow.

Therapist: Wow is right.

At the beginning of this vignette, the therapist raised the issue of Lucy, Guillermo's wife, being told that he was in therapy and that he was abused. Working primarily in the action and meaning/emotion planning metaframeworks, the therapist challenged Guillermo's catastrophic expectations about his wife's response, and Guillermo acknowledged the low probability that she would respond negatively. As the therapist tested the reality of Guillermo's catastrophic fears, he also affirmed Lucy's role and value in Guillermo's life, as well as Guillermo's wisdom in marrying her. The therapist also defined Guillermo's catastrophic expectations as being associated with a part of him that was linked to Paco and the fears and threats that Paco used to silence him. In doing so, the therapist differentiated the threatening part from the rest of Guillermo's personality, implicitly stating that "these thoughts and feelings about yourself are not your totality, they are just one of many parts of you." The therapist shifted down the matrix to address this M2 hypothesis.

The therapist drew an intervention from the internal representation planning metaframework by bringing in the "empty chair" (L. S. Greenberg, 1979; Perls, 1968; R. Schwartz, 2013) and asking Guillermo to imagine the part they had just defined sitting in the chair. As a further internal differentiation strategy, the therapist asked Guillermo to name that part of himself, to which he responded with the name Francisco, the formal name of both his father and the brother that abused him. The therapist then conducted a two-chair interaction in which Guillermo identified with and played out his Francisco part and then came back to his Guillermo part and challenged the negative attributions about him that the Francisco part embodied. The therapist invited Guillermo to take control of the two-chair interaction by telling him to tell Francisco to look directly at him—to see him. He heightened Guillermo's anger at Paco and the Francisco part, and then the rocket of Guillermo's rage ignited. In essence, the therapist differentiated key parts of Guillermo and then used here-and-now strategies (stimulating direct interaction and eliciting/heightening emotion) to begin to transform the internal representations from his childhood. All this work was in the service of helping Guillermo to be less anxious, fearful, passive, and withdrawn. The therapist helped Guillermo change the internal cognitive and emotional sequences that played out in his mind in the here-and-now with the two-chair tactic.

This session was followed by several sessions elaborating the way in which the Francisco part of Guillermo dominated his thinking and his action. He reported feeling more confident and less frightened in his interactions with people. He also felt better about himself. This led the therapist to move back up the matrix to reexplore the action plan for Guillermo's telling his wife his truth. The therapist hypothesized that one of the reasons Guillermo's gains did not last after his last therapy was that the only person who knew his truth—his therapist—had left him. Guillermo had not told anyone else. The therapist hypothesized that if Guillermo could tell his wife, he would actually build his new emerging reality more permanently into his life. He would not be so alone anymore with his painful reality. The question in the therapist's mind was whether it would be better for Guillermo's disclosure to occur in or outside of therapy. This was explored in the next (18th) session.

HELPING GUILLERMO ENACT SOLUTION SEQUENCES WITH HIS FAMILY

Guillermo: I am feeling a lot better these days. I almost feel like I don't need therapy anymore.

Therapist: That's great. I'm glad that you're feeling better. You have been doing great work in therapy, and it feels to me like you are coming out of your shell and your fog.

Guillermo: Except I feel so angry at Paco for what he did to me and at my father for what he did to Paco and at both my parents for not protecting me. The fog protected me from these feelings. The fog and my robot were friends.

Therapist: That's right. Now you are seeing with greater clarity and honesty. And you are also feeling—no more robot.

Guillermo: I guess that's better than not feeling mad or sad and just being a crazy, anxious robot.

Therapist: Yeah. But I want to go back to your feeling that maybe you don't need therapy anymore. I have a theory and a potential plan that I want to discuss with you and see what you think.

Guillermo: Shoot.

Therapist: I think that one of the reasons your progress from your previous therapy did not last, besides the fact that you were unable to continue your therapy because he moved away, was that you never shared your truth with a real person in your life. This is not to say that we therapists are not real people, but there is a way in which, too often, what happens in therapy, particularly individual therapy, stays in therapy. I think that you need to tell Lucy.

Guillermo: You are probably right. I also feel ready to do that. I think she will hear me and not pick up the phone to call a lawyer.

Therapist: I believe you're right. The next question for me is where and how should this happen. Specifically, do you want to do it here with me or on your own at home? Obviously, the first option would require you to tell her you are seeing me and would like her to come in for a couple of sessions as your guest.

Guillermo: What do you think I should do?

Therapist: Well, my selfish desire is that you invite her in here because I would like to meet her. However, as your therapist, I would also recommend that option because I think I could help you and Lucy process the emergence of all this new information between you in a way that would help both of you going forward.

Guillermo: I like the option of inviting her in. I have a little fear that if we did it at home, it could get out of control. I think you could help Lucy understand me and the abuse and a lot of the connections that I might be too overwhelmed to remember.

Therapist: If we go with inviting her in, I would want to rehearse with you what you want to say when she comes in. I would prefer to do as little talking to her for you as possible. It is really important that you tell her your truth—that she hears your voice. I'll be there to help, but you will be the star.

Guillermo: OK, when do we do this?

Therapist: I think we will need another session to plan and think through the sessions with Lucy. First off, we're talking about at least two guest sessions. Second, I think you should invite her in right after our next session. Too much time between the invitation and the session could lead to a lot of anxiety on both of your parts.

Guillermo: What do I tell her?

Therapist: What do you think you should tell her?

Guillermo: Well, first I need to tell her that I'm in therapy and a little about you. Then I need to invite her to come in for the next session. Why should I say I want her to come in?

Therapist:	What do you think you should say about why you want her to come in?
Guillermo:	Because my therapist wants to check you out and see if you're a whack job?
Therapist:	[Laughing.] I would not recommend that.
Guillermo:	I think I should her tell that I have some things that I would like to talk about, and you and I think it would be best to talk about those things in therapy rather than outside. But then she is going to get scared that I am going to tell her I want a divorce or something.
Therapist:	I think you need to tell her enough that she is not scared that you are going to tell her you want out of the marriage or anything like that, but don't get into the content of the abuse with her. If you open that door, it will be very hard to close it. You also don't want to lie to her so she feels betrayed or set up.
Guillermo:	Maybe I should tell her that I am learning stuff about myself that I want to share with her, but I don't want to get into it until we are in therapy. I can also tell her that you and I believe my telling her will make me and our marriage stronger. That will reassure her.
Therapist:	Great plan.

This session began with Guillermo acknowledging his progress and emerging feelings of power and autonomy. The therapist validated these feelings, but then presented his thinking to Guillermo about why his changes did not last from his previous therapy and why they should try something different. The therapist, consistent with the strength guideline, treated Guillermo as a coinvestigator and codecision-maker in their therapy. He invited him into his theorizing and elicited Guillermo's response. He also did not want to discourage or depotentiate Guillermo and his new feelings of power and autonomy, but he also believed that stopping without doing this piece of conjoint work would be a mistake. Guillermo agreed with him, and then they got into planning the invitation.

At the outset of the planning process, the therapist set the stage for this episode (or series of sessions) of work. Lucy was coming in (joining the direct therapy system) as Guillermo's guest, not an invitee of the therapist. The episode would be for at least two sessions, which would give all three of them enough time to address the impact and meaning of the disclosure. Most important, the therapist made it clear to Guillermo that he would be the "star" of the conjoint episode. He would be talking to Lucy about himself, rather than the therapist telling Lucy about Guillermo. In making this clear at the outset, the therapist implicitly began the process of empowering Guillermo. He was going to do the work and experience the gain. The therapist would be there to help, but it was going to be Guillermo's show. The therapist kept putting Guillermo's questions about the invitation back on Guillermo to answer. He was following the IST policy of getting the client to do as much of the work as possible and just being a "good enough therapist" (Pinsof, 1995; Winnicott, 1962). Not surprisingly, Guillermo was able to think through out loud and with thoughtfulness and sensitivity some of the challenges and issues he would have to address with Lucy. The therapist validated his thinking and plan.

The First Session With Lucy

Guillermo: Lucy, this is _____, my therapist.

Therapist: Lucy, it's a pleasure to meet you. Come on in and sit down. [They all sit.] Lucy, I'd like to begin by asking you how you feel about being here today, with me and Guillermo?

Lucy: A little nervous, but I guess that's normal.

Therapist: It sure is. Is this the first time that you have ever met with a therapist?

Lucy: No. I was in individual therapy for a while before I met Guillermo.

Therapist: Was that a good experience?

Lucy: It was. It helped me overcome my fears about commitment and paved the way for Guillermo and me to find each other and get married.

Therapist: I'd be interested in your expectations about what is going to happen today.

Lucy: Well, I know that Guillermo wants to tell me something about his past.

Therapist: That's right. I'd just like to clarify that I see my role today as doing whatever I can to help the two of you talk to each other, rather than talking to me or me leading the conversation. Does that make sense? [Lucy nods.] Also, in addition to meeting today, I would like us to have at least one more meeting of the three of us next week. Is that OK? [Lucy nods.] But before we jump in, is there anything that you would like to ask me? Anything is fair game.

Lucy: Guillermo told me about you this week, and I don't really have any questions at this point. I am glad that he found you and that you are helping him.

Therapist:	Good. Guillermo, want to take it from here?
Guillermo:	Lucy, thank you for coming in today. I have been thinking about this session for a long time, and I am glad that it is finally here. I need to tell you about something that happened to me when I was a kid. Between the ages of 7 and 10 I was sexually and emotionally abused by Paco. You know I slept in the same room as him, and when I was little, I would get in bed with him if I was scared. When I was 7, he started to force me to do things with him.
Lucy:	Oh, no. Like what kind of things?
Guillermo:	Like masturbate him and give him blow jobs.
Lucy:	Oh, Guillermo. I feel so bad for you. How long did this go on?
Guillermo:	About 3 years, until he moved out to California.
Lucy:	It makes me feel like throwing up. I could kill him.
Guillermo:	I know. I have felt that way myself, particularly since I started talking about it. I hate him.
Lucy:	Did you tell anyone—your parents?
Guillermo:	No, Paco told me that if I did, he would say I was crazy, that I made it up and that I was a little *maricón*.
Lucy:	He trapped you so he could abuse you, and you could not talk. What a monster he was. Have you ever talked to him about it, confronted him with what he did?
Guillermo:	No, I have never said a word to him about it since he went to California. Now when I see him at family events, I pretty much avoid him. The only people I have ever talked to about it before today was the previous therapist I told you about and _____. [Nodding toward the therapist.]
Lucy:	The next time I see him I don't know if I will be able to be civil. I would like to spit in his face and kick him you know where.
Guillermo:	We can talk about what we want to do with Paco. How are you feeling about me now that I have told you what happened?
Lucy:	I feel like I should have been able to protect you from him. I know that is crazy, I cannot go back in time, and you are not my child. But that's how I feel.
Guillermo:	Do you think I was bad for what happened? Do you see me as defective or blemished? [He has tears in his eyes.]

Lucy: No. You were a victim, and he was so much older and bigger. What could you do? You are not defective or blemished. You are a wonderful lover, and I love being with you.

Guillermo: [With more tears] Thank you. I am so lucky that you are in my life. [Lucy comes over to Guillermo and kneels at his chair and puts her arms around him. He cries. All three sit silently.] I feel relieved. Safe for the first time.

Therapist: Lucy, how are you feeling? [She rises, kisses Guillermo on the forehead, and goes back to her chair.]

Lucy: I am shocked, but not totally surprised. I suspected that something like this might have happened in his past. I never liked Paco, but now I feel rage at him. Also, I feel angry at his father, who I know physically abused Paco, and at his mother for not protecting him. They should have protected him.

Therapist: They should have. I know this news is fresh, but does it change how you see Guillermo and how you feel about him?

Guillermo: [To Lucy] He is asking these questions for me because he thinks I don't believe what you said before. But I guess I would like to hear your answers now again.

Lucy: It helps me understand the tremendous loneliness and uptightness in you. It also helps me understand better the distance that you keep from others. You have been afraid how they might see you if they knew the truth. But I am actually glad to know and very happy that you finally decided you could trust me enough to tell me. I think what I took as you being an introvert may not actually be the real you. Maybe there is an extrovert somewhere in there waiting to come out. It's like your brother put you into a shell that you are breaking out of. It is nice to watch and be part of your rebirth.

Guillermo: Thank you, Lucy. What you are saying means so much to me.

Therapist: Guillermo, I understand even more fully the wisdom behind your choice of a wife. Lucy, you are everything and even more than Guillermo has said. I am very moved and impressed by your reaction today. It is a real pleasure to see a couple like the two of you in my office.

Guillermo: Thanks.

The session ended shortly after this conversation with a plan to meet the following week for a follow-up. The work Guillermo did with the therapist in preparation for the session could be seen in the way Guillermo jumped in and took the lead. His skilled leadership was evident in his redirection of the conversation from Paco to Lucy's reaction to his disclosure. Also, his emerging leadership could be seen in his interjection to Lucy that the therapist was asking these questions so he could hear the answers he needed to disconfirm his catastrophic expectations about Lucy's reaction. In terms of sequences, this session marked the successful implementation of the solution sequence of Guillermo having the courage to tell Lucy difficult and shameful things and Lucy being able to hear them with love, empathy, and affirmation. Also, more generally, this session clearly reflected solution sequences in which Guillermo took charge of the interaction and showed his nascent leadership skills.

The therapist's and Guillermo's plan for the second session with Lucy (in the next section) was to address the issue, if appropriate, of what to do with Paco at that point in Guillermo's life. The plan was to focus the first conjoint session fully on the disclosure and discuss Paco in the following session, which was one of the reasons Guillermo deflected away from it in the first session with Lucy.

Supporting Guillermo's Plan to Break the Silence With His Brother

Therapist: I'd be interested in hearing how things have gone between the two of you this week after Guillermo's disclosure last session. Of course, I am also interested in how each of you are feeling individually about the whole thing.

Lucy: Well, Guillermo and I talked a lot about the whole thing. He went into more detail about what happened with Paco and how he resisted and prevailed. Guillermo was also talking about how he didn't just feel hatred for Paco, but that in certain ways, Paco was the only one who was there for him in his family. Also, that Guillermo had seen how his dad abused Paco.

Guillermo: As much as I feel so angry at Paco, I also know that he was a lost guy and used me to get something he felt he couldn't get from other boys or girls his own age. I can't help but think he was desperate for some comfort and affection and had no idea how to get it.

Therapist: Guillermo, I am so struck by the shift you are going through. You are clearly expressing empathy toward Paco and seeing the world as maybe he saw it—that you were someone who

	could give him some comfort or affection that he could not get from anyone else at that point in his life.
Guillermo:	That's right. But I still feel angry with him too and angry at how that abuse put a cloud over my life for so many years. I feel less shame but more sadness.
Therapist:	Because of the abuse, you have led a life constrained by shame and terrible feelings of being different and alone. You have missed a lot. You have not been fully engaged in your life—part of you always split off, alone and hidden. That is sad. [Guillermo gets tears in his eyes, and Lucy moves her chair closer to his and touches his arm.]
Guillermo:	But I am coming out and I feel much more present and engaged. As part of that, I am starting to think about what I want to do with Paco.
Therapist:	What are your thoughts?
Guillermo:	I am thinking that I would like to talk with him about what happened between us. We have never spoken about it for 23 years—since I was 10. It feels like talking with him would be the end of the secret and the end of my shame.
Therapist:	Lucy, where are you on this issue?
Lucy:	I am mixed up about it. On the one hand, I want to kill him for what he did to Guillermo. I also get it that he was abused and a really lost kid. I don't know if I could even be in the same room with him.
Guillermo:	You would not have to be with him. I would.
Therapist:	Guillermo, how are you thinking about doing this?
Guillermo:	I am not sure. Part of me wants to go out to Sacramento and do it face-to-face. I feel a little frightened about that getting out of hand. But he's a lot more stable than he was back then. He's married, and they have two little kids. He manages a car repair shop and makes a decent living.
Therapist:	What would be the alternative to going out there?
Guillermo:	You mean, I should invite him in here?
Therapist:	That's a possibility.
Guillermo:	I feel like I want to do it on my own. I want to think it through with you, but I don't think I need you to be there.
Therapist:	What about Lucy—would you want her there?

Guillermo: I am not sure. Lucy, you just said you cannot see yourself in the same room with him. It sounds to me like you don't want to be there.

Lucy: If you want me there, I will be there.

Therapist: I have a suggestion. I could envision a scenario in which you both go out to Sacramento. Guillermo, you meet first with Paco and tell him what you need to tell him. After you are finished or the next day, perhaps Lucy could join you. I think it is important for there to be some communication between Lucy and Paco, or you could end up miles ahead of her in the relationship with Paco. If you have a meaningful conversation with him and he owns up to what he did and apologizes, your feelings might shift because you went through that process with him. Lucy may still be over there with her feelings toward Paco unchanged. I'm afraid it could split the two of you, with Lucy still holding all the anger and you moving on in your feelings with Paco.

Lucy: I think that's a good point. I don't want you to become all warm and cozy with him and then I'm still back here with all of the anger. Maybe I should be there from the beginning.

Guillermo: If you were there from the beginning, you could be part of whatever happens. I don't know if he will be more uptight with you there, less likely to be honest, but if he knows that I have told you everything and that you need to be part of this, it might be OK.

Therapist: Guillermo, why don't you write him? Tell him that you have been in therapy and that you have been working on what happened between you and him in the years before he left for California. You decided in your therapy to invite Lucy in because you had never told her about what happened. Now that you both know the truth, you both would like to come out to Sacramento and meet with him and talk about what happened. You'd like to break the secret and address what happened. If you want to, you could offer him the option of coming out here and doing this with you and Lucy in therapy with me. He might feel safer with that option.

Guillermo: I think that's a good idea. I can see how he responds, and that will tell me where he's at with the whole thing. He may be in total denial that it even happened for all I know, although I doubt that.

Therapist: Lucy, what do you think?

Lucy: I think we've got a plan.

The therapist was impressed with Guillermo and Lucy's handling of his disclosure. The couple reported that Guillermo shared more about the abuse after they left the first conjoint session, and Lucy "got" how he had resisted and maintained some sense of his own agency during the abuse. She was surprised at the emergence of Guillermo's empathy toward his brother. The therapist validated and heightened Guillermo's movement from anger to sadness. Lucy comforted Guillermo, without distracting from his feelings. After some moments, Guillermo spontaneously began to address what to do with Paco. As part of his process of self-empowerment, Guillermo visualized an independent (outside of therapy) confrontation with Paco. This visualization reflected the fact that Guillermo felt strong enough in himself to face his brother on his own. His self-esteem and self-efficacy were on the rise.

As Lucy and Guillermo discussed whether she should go with him, the therapist presented his scenario of first Guillermo, then Lucy and Guillermo with Paco. The therapist's rationale rested on his hypothesis that if Guillermo did this alone, Lucy may have been left behind in the emotional triangle with Paco, which could result in an affective split or disequilibrium between them—Guillermo feeling closer, and Lucy still feeling alienated and angry. Lucy picked this up and spontaneously said, "Maybe I should go with him." The therapist then suggested that Guillermo write to Paco and lay out his thoughts about getting together. Guillermo liked that idea and further elaborated that reaching out in this way would let him "read the feedback" from Paco, which would help prepare him for whatever lay ahead. They all concurred.

It is interesting to note that as part of his empowerment, Guillermo was implicitly learning the IST blueprint. He was seeing his letter as a form of conversing coming out of a plan based on the hypothesis that he had to get some sense of where Paco was in regard to what happened between them. Guillermo's internalization of the IST way of thinking reflected the goal of helping clients internalize and integrate the therapist into their collective ego or mind. The client system learns to work in a new way that facilitates thoughtful trial and error learning—a core process in IST.

After the second conjoint session, Guillermo drafted a letter to Paco that he shared with Lucy and the therapist. All three of them wordsmithed the letter until it said what Guillermo wanted to say. He sent it, and Paco responded almost immediately. He said he was relieved to get the letter and had been expecting something like this for many years. He also said he and his wife had been in couples counseling, and his troubled childhood, including his relationship with Guillermo, had been a topic of conversation. He was glad for Guillermo and Lucy to come out, and he even proposed that his wife, Juana, join them in their conversation.

Guillermo and Lucy went in together for the next session and planned the meeting(s) with Paco and Juana. They rehearsed different scenarios. The therapist suggested they communicate with Paco and Juana the possibility that they would have more than one conversation while they were out there. The therapist thought this would ensure they had enough time and space to talk about what they needed to talk about. The therapist also coached them, suggesting that they have some discussion at the beginning of the first meeting, specifying that Juana and Lucy should primarily be witnesses to the conversation between their husbands and that they would have a chance to get into the action subsequently. The therapist cautioned that it might be too easy for the wives to jump in and talk for the men and that it was crucially important that the men do the work they had to do. In other words, the therapist was both prescribing and protecting the solution sequence between the brothers—that they deal directly with each other.

In the following session, the couple reported that Paco had sent an e-mail to cancel the meeting. He indicated that it was not a good time for him to meet and that he did not want to be pushed to do so. Guillermo and Lucy shared their disappointment with the therapist, but said they felt good about the progress in therapy and had hope for a meaningful discussion with Paco someday. They felt they would be ready for that day.

The therapist and Guillermo met for three more individual sessions to consolidate the gains of therapy and deal directly with what it meant to Guillermo to be discontinuing. Guillermo stated that he felt far more prepared for therapy to end than was the case in his first therapy. And he felt he could be open with Lucy about any anxiety or feeling of shame that he might feel. In the last session (the 26th), the therapist congratulated Guillermo on his courage and accomplishments in therapy and made it clear that Guillermo would be welcome to return for a session or sessions down the road. Guillermo expressed his gratitude and agreed to be in touch as needed.

About a year later, Guillermo called to schedule an appointment for Lucy and him. He reported that his father had had a nearly fatal heart attack and that he and Lucy, on a visit to Sacramento, had talked with Paco and Juana.

FOLLOW-UP AND CONSOLIDATION

Therapist: I'm happy to hear that your father is doing better. And it seems you have other news for me.

Guillermo: You're right. We talked with Paco and Juana, and it went as well as I could have imagined. In a way, I feel as if I got a brother back. We met at their house the first evening after the kids had gone to bed and talked for over two hours. Paco and I were definitely the main event. I began, and he listened. As he listened, tears came into his eyes, and Juana looked very distressed. Paco said that until he heard my story, he had blocked out a lot of what had happened, but that as I told him my memories, he denied nothing. He said that he was so lost at that time in his life, he did crazy and awful things like abuse me. He apologized and said that hearing my story was one of, if not the most, painful thing in his life. His apology felt real. I felt like crying but didn't. Juana said that she felt so sorry for me and what I went through. She said that if one of her kids, who are 5 and 7, went through something like that, it would break her. She said that she hated my father for what he did to Paco and how that led to his abuse of me.

Lucy: I felt that their response was very real. They both were so sad and upset by what Guillermo told them. Paco talked about how he did not even know how lonely and lost he felt at that time in his life. It drove him to do sick things. He then asked Guillermo if there was anything now that he could do to make it up to him. Guillermo said the only thing was what he and Juana were doing, which was to listen and take it in.

Guillermo: The next day we all got together again, and Paco said again that he was so sorry for what he had done to me and that he so appreciated how I handled reaching out to him and breaking the silence between us. He hoped that going forward he could be the brother he should have been to me in those days. I told him that was not necessary; he just needed to be my brother now. I said that how he had responded to me yesterday and today was like a real brother, and I truly appreciated that.

Therapist: How do you, Guillermo, feel after your trip out there?

Guillermo: I feel like a huge burden has lifted. Lucy knows my truth, and I have confronted and, in some sense, embraced my brother, and he, in turn, has apologized and embraced me. I feel so grateful to you for helping me face my truth and share it with the people I really needed to share it with— Lucy and my brother. *Muchisimas gracias y un abrazo para ti.* [Guillermo stands up and embraces the therapist. Both have tears in their eyes. Lucy then stands up and puts her arms around both men.]

In this session, Guillermo and Lucy consolidated their experience with Paco and Juana. Guillermo had confronted his abuser and, wonder of wonders, his abuser had accepted responsibility and apologized. Despite their abusive history, they could go forward as brothers. Lucy felt as close to Paco and Juana as Guillermo did. Being part of the conversation had allowed her to experience what Guillermo had experienced and to move ahead with him on the continuum of forgiveness.

This case illustrates how the IST therapist maintains an intensive and empathic focus on an individual client, while simultaneously maintaining awareness of and concern about the larger systems in which the client is embedded. Using this dual focus, the therapist was able to help Guillermo address his anxiety in the workplace and repair and heal himself in regard to his trauma and shame and, as part of that healing process, strengthen his relationship with his wife and build a new and impactful relationship with his brother.

12

LIFELONG LEARNING IN INTEGRATIVE SYSTEMIC THERAPY: BEGINNING, PRACTICING, SUPERVISING, AND CONTINUING TO GROW

The comprehensiveness of integrative systemic therapy (IST), which allows it to be applicable to most any problem and client system, requires that it be complex. It requires, and accordingly provides for, the incorporation and integration of many concepts, a variety of case-formulating factors, and a broad set of strategies for intervention. It is an open system in that each blueprint component accommodates extensive bodies of existing and emerging knowledge and practice. The resulting theoretical complexity establishes IST as an approach that is never completely mastered. There is always more to learn. In this sense, it invites ongoing study and reflection from the early phases of training, through the development of significant competence, to the assumption of mentoring and supervising functions, and ultimately, through the later career years.

In addition to inviting continuous development, IST provides a basis and structure for it. *Hypothesizing* uses a set of frameworks (hypothesizing

http://dx.doi.org/10.1037/0000055-012
Integrative Systemic Therapy: Metaframeworks for Problem Solving With Individuals, Couples, and Families,
by W. M. Pinsof, D. C. Breunlin, W. P. Russell, J. L. Lebow, C. Rampage, and A. L. Chambers

metaframeworks) that facilitate the description of the complex, multileveled functioning of the client system, especially with regard to strengths and constraints. *Planning* organizes strategies for enacting solution sequences and removing constraints into a set of frameworks (planning metaframeworks) that are applied according to the IST guidelines and in concert with evolving hypotheses. *Conversing* contains a body of knowledge about the linguistic choices and communication skills that are used to build alliances, learn about the client system, and execute interventions. Last, *feedback* contains a body of knowledge about types of information (client responses, therapist reactions, and empirical data) that inform the conduct of therapy. The four larger classes of information (hypothesizing, planning, conversing, and feedback) and their organization around the blueprint are illustrated in Figure 12.1, the "loaded" blueprint. The loaded blueprint, with its open-ended integrative schemata, provides a virtually limitless capacity to house and organize information about the conduct of therapy. For further discussion and examples of how the loaded blueprint can be used, download Bonus Chapter 1 from the APA website (http://pubs.apa.org/books/supp/pinsof/).

The value of an integrative structure in the facilitation of lifelong career development is supported by the research of Orlinsky and Rønnestad (2005) on psychotherapist development. In their international survey of over

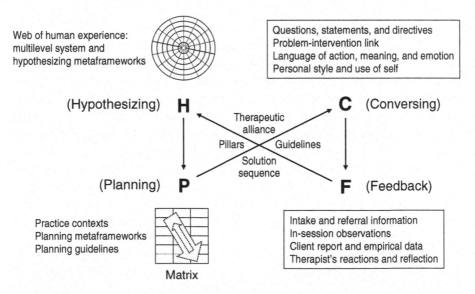

Figure 12.1. The loaded integrative systemic therapy blueprint. From "Integrative Problem-Centered Metaframeworks Therapy II: Planning, Conversing, and Reading Feedback," by W. M. Pinsof, D. C. Breunlin, W. P. Russell, and J. L. Lebow, 2011, *Family Process, 50*, p. 334. Copyright 2011 by John Wiley & Sons, Inc. Adapted with permission.

4,000 therapists, they found that "broad-spectrum integrative–eclectic practitioners were the 'most growing' therapists, being more likely than most others to experience progress" (p. 120), a pattern characterized by an experience of "much growth and little depletion" (p. 118). They suggested that this "may reflect a link between theoretical breadth and a tendency to experiment in practice" (p. 120). We maintain that IST's theoretical breadth, along with its blueprint for therapy and failure-driven guideline, does indeed invite systematic experimentation with new concepts, strategies, and techniques.

RECOGNIZING OPPORTUNITIES TO LEARN: CASE EXAMPLE

An example of recognizing opportunities to learn is an early-career therapist working with a family on the academic difficulties and video game preoccupation of a 15-year-old boy. The family consisted of a second-generation Mexican American heterosexual couple, Carlos and Mariana, and their son, Joaquin. Mariana had a bachelor's degree, worked as a lab tech, and had been a practicing Catholic all her life. Carlos's family of origin had been Catholic, but until recently, he had not engaged in religious practice. He had completed high school and for many years worked as a meter reader for the electric company, but his employment there was jeopardized because of his drinking during work hours. He had completed an intensive outpatient program for alcohol dependence 10 months before the family therapy and was, at that time, reinstated in his job. He became committed to sobriety, began attending church with Mariana and Joaquin, and at the time of therapy, attended several Alcoholics Anonymous (AA) meetings each week. Joaquin was in the final month of his first year in high school, where he had struggled academically.

In the first session, after welcoming the family and defining the concerns that had brought them to therapy, the therapist tracked the sequences for homework and video games and found that neither parent structured or monitored Joaquin's homework. Carlos had previously exercised a disciplinary role in relation to school performance, when necessary, but had stepped back from that role when he entered sobriety. Although Mariana placed high importance on Joaquin's education, her job, including a long commute, along with some medical issues, often left her feeling too tired at night to focus on Joaquin's work or work habits. The parents disagreed on what to do about the video games. Mariana wondered whether Joaquin should be prohibited from playing the games until he improved his performance in school. Carlos shared that before his treatment for alcoholism he had sometimes been demanding and overly hard on Joaquin. He felt that the video games were addicting and that Joaquin would have to come to terms with that when he was ready to do so. Mariana shared her worry that Joaquin's current pattern would continue and that he would not be successful in life.

The therapist's initial hypothesis was that Joaquin would benefit from more parental guidance and involvement with his schoolwork and video game access. This was proposed, with the explanation that the parents could help him develop productive habits by providing some further structure (homework time and limits on time allowed for video games). The father expressed his concerns about this, stating that his spirituality within the AA program suggested that he not try to control things over which he was powerless, such as the behavior of others. He stated that his sobriety was maintained by the peace he drew from accepting that he was powerless over such things. Such things he put in God's hands. He thought his son might have to "hit bottom" when it came to his schoolwork. Thus, he was not pressing Joaquin as he used to, though he confessed to "preaching from time to time." By opening the spirituality metaframework, the therapist realized and respected the profound change that AA's spirituality had wrought in Carlos's life, but she felt constrained and stymied by Carlos's application of that spirituality and the twelve-step beliefs to Joaquin's video game playing.

The therapist had knowledge of child and adolescent development and the family organizational patterns that tend to support achievement and felt that Joaquin would likely benefit from some structure to help him develop habits that would facilitate his taking responsibility for his time and schoolwork, but there did not seem to be a way forward to that type of solution sequence. The therapist stated that the husband's practice of acceptance was obviously important to him and that she would give some further thought to the types of solutions that would be feasible. The family agreed to give this some thought as well.

The therapist had a lot to think about. For one thing, the father's sobriety and emphasis on acceptance had begun just before Joaquin began high school. The development metaframework was relevant there. Also at issue was whether Carlos's strict adherence to acceptance served a function within the mind metaframework, such as managing emotion dysregulation. Most compellingly, IST's culture and spirituality metaframeworks called out to the therapist between sessions: "I need to understand more about the culture and spirituality of AA." She did not feel informed enough about these topics, but this was familiar turf in that, within IST, each case is expected to provide the opportunity and the necessity to incorporate new learning. The blueprint provides encouragement and structure for incorporating new information and experimenting with weaving it into the therapeutic conversation. To that end, some reading on AA and an extensive discussion with a friend who was in the AA program gave the therapist some information that would prove to be useful in therapy.

In the next session, the therapist summarized the dilemma defined in the first session and the family further discussed the AA spiritual issues. Mariana shared that she was happy that Carlos was sober and noted that he had become more spiritual and even-tempered since entering sobriety. She said she respected Carlos's spirituality. She stated that hers was also important but that she did not feel the "hitting bottom" approach fit for her when it came to Joaquin's schooling. Carlos discussed his spirituality further, and the therapist acknowledged the importance of faith in his life. Joaquin good-naturedly joked that his father had become "preachy." Carlos smiled, and the family and therapist shared a laugh.

The therapist then entered into a conversation with Carlos that was informed by what she had learned between sessions, namely, the distinction provided by the serenity prayer, essential within AA culture, which asks for "the serenity to accept the things I cannot change, courage to change the things I can, and wisdom to know the difference." The therapist and Carlos connected on this, and all agreed that Joaquin's achievement and his interest in video games were not things that were directly in Carlos and Mariana's control. The therapist shared the belief that Carlos and Mariana would certainly do whatever was in their power to help their son develop into a responsible and effective adult. They agreed. She asked whether, if they thought that providing more structure for Joaquin was good for his development, they would do it, as long as they did not try to take responsibility for the outcome, which was ultimately beyond their control. The conversation continued and reached a point at which all agreed that fostering conditions for Joaquin's growth, including providing structure for his day, was something they could do without the spiritual risk of trying to control something they could not change. The therapist wondered whether Carlos would want to talk with his sponsor about this from an AA and sobriety perspective. Carlos agreed to do so. In the next session, he reported that his sponsor saw no problem with the plan, as long as Carlos did not become excessively controlling or reactive. Then the parents, in concert with Joaquin, established a structured daily homework time with limited video game time as a reward for a job well done. Mariana felt relieved. Joaquin agreed to it.

Valuing the continual process of learning and appreciating the theoretical breadth provided by the metaframeworks, this therapist learned about spirituality in AA, explored this with the family, and experimented in a conversation that integrated three hypothesizing metaframeworks (spirituality, development, and organization) such that there was a shared rationale for a change in how the family interacted regarding the presenting concerns of achievement and video game usage. The therapist understood that there might be other twists and turns in the case, other constraints to identify, and other alliance issues to manage, but it felt good to have established a working relationship with the family and to have agreed on what seemed to be a reasonable and hopefully effective solution sequence. Meanwhile, she had obtained new information that would likely apply to other cases. The process of gathering new information and learning new concepts and skills is an expected and ongoing process in IST. New learning is continually sought and then integrated onto the scaffolding provided by the components of the blueprint.

In addition to being an integrative therapy, IST is also a systemic therapy in that it conceptualizes cases within their multilevel context and, as appropriate, seeks to convene couples and families, as well as individuals. Even in the context of one case, the therapist may work in different therapy contexts (individual, couple, and family). This was true of the case of Carlos, Mariana, and Joaquin, in which the therapist met mostly with the whole family, but over the course of therapy had seen the parents without the son twice and the son alone twice. The result of this is that IST therapists accumulate experience in working in each of these various contexts (modalities). There is evidence that working in these modalities, a natural outgrowth of systemic, clinical decision making in IST, has positive effects on therapists' career development. Orlinsky and Rønnestad (2005) found that therapists who practiced a combination of individual, couples, and family therapy "most typically experience their work as an Effective Practice (58%) and only rarely as a Distressing Practice (7%)" and that "breadth and depth of case experience across multiple treatment modalities" (p. 95) were the strongest predictors of healing involvement in their work. These outcomes were significantly better than those for therapists who practice only individual therapy or only individual and group therapy, although the outcomes for the latter group may be influenced also by the context of practice (group therapy being practiced more often in institutionalized settings).

In sum, IST's breadth of focus, its complexity, its systemic and integrative nature, and the organization of its components provide support for lifelong learning and professional development. The motivation for learning and development, however, comes from the individual practitioner. A major finding of Rønnestad and Skovholt (2003) was that "an intense commitment to learn propels the developmental process" (p. 30). Thus, each therapist is responsible for their own development that is, in large part, a function of the commitment they make and sustain over time. Whether, for a particular therapist, the commitment to learn and develop is best housed in IST is an essential question to ask.

THERAPIST FIT WITH INTEGRATIVE SYSTEMIC THERAPY

Although we hold that virtually any problem can be treated with the IST approach and that IST provides an effective platform for lifelong learning for its practitioners, we clearly do not suggest that IST should be the model of choice for all therapists. Rather, we subscribe to the idea that the core assumptions and operative requirements of a model of therapy have to fit with the therapist's worldview. Simon (2003) advanced the argument that therapy benefits from being an expression of the therapist's view of the human condition. When the therapy model is syntonic with the therapist's belief system, a more authentic encounter between therapist and client(s) is the result. Simon (2006) proposed to reconcile the common factors and model-specific approaches to family therapy through an emphasis on the self-of-the-therapist. He hypothesized that "a therapist becomes maximally effective when he or she uses a model of proven efficacy whose underlying worldview closely matches his or her own" (p. 343). Although this hypothesis has not, to our knowledge, been tested, it makes good sense that both a set of common factors and the specific operations of a therapeutic approach are potentiated by a therapist's fit with the approach, as well as comfort with and commitment to it. Furthermore, fit is a requirement for both long-term adherence to a model of therapy and career satisfaction.

This raises the question "For whom is IST a good fit?" IST's pillars (see Chapter 2, this volume) and therapy guidelines (Chapter 6; summarized in the Appendix) provide philosophical and practical direction and shed light on the question of fit. We encourage readers to review them in a systematic way and consider how well they line up with their worldviews. In addition, we highlight here a few of what seem to be the most prominent issues of fit. Any of these factors can contribute to fit, and having several of them present may suggest a very good fit.

First and foremost, IST is designed for therapists who are committed to a systemic approach. Family therapists, social workers, psychologists, and counselors who view human problems in the context of a multilevel biopsychosocial system fit well with IST, particularly if they have interest in involving family members, as appropriate, in the treatment of individuals who present for therapy. Further, a strong interest in the patterns (sequences) within client systems is an indicator of fit because IST prioritizes a focus on sequences of action, meaning, and emotion.

Second, IST tends to fit well for therapists who have a strong belief in the inherent strengths and resources that exist in individuals and their families. IST is problem centered and systematically acknowledges factors in the system that constrain solutions (including, in some cases, profoundly impactful constraints), but never loses sight of the abilities and good intentions of clients. This awareness is, in a sense, an article of faith. The therapist's faith in human nature provides a basis for a collaborative approach to therapy.

Third, therapists preferring a focused and planful therapy may find that IST is a good fit for them. This is particularly true if they are comfortable beginning therapy with a straightforward problem-solving focus but are open to considering more complex formulations of cases as needed.

Fourth, there is fit for therapists who value autonomous decision making and their own improvisation. IST emphasizes the unique nature of each therapy system (unique client system and unique therapist). Within IST's procedures and decision-making structure, the therapist and clients determine how to build their relationship and engage in problem solving. The approach is planned and focused, but in a manner that allows therapists to exercise their judgment and use their creativity (in concert with client feedback) in the way they integrate bodies of knowledge, concepts, and techniques. This is in contrast to approaches that prescribe particular interventions (often manualized) for particular problems. Although IST incorporates elements of empirically supported, manualized therapies and, at times, may work faithfully within such an approach for a series of sessions, it remains committed to selecting strategies and designing interventions to specifically address the unique problem sequences and constraints of a particular client system (vs. simply matching the therapy to a problem type). IST therapists are not mired in required procedures, nor are they adrift. Rather, they enjoy the freedom to improvise within the structure of the IST essence and use the blueprint and guidelines to guide their decision making along the way.

A fifth fit issue has to do with the breadth of practice. IST is certainly useful for therapists who have a specialized practice (e.g., sexual problems in couples), but it is especially advantageous for therapists who work with a variety of presenting problems and/or particular problems that call for using several modalities (i.e., contexts of therapy: family, couple, and individual).

SOURCES OF LEARNING AND DEVELOPMENT

IST provides a vehicle for professional development over the course of one's career by providing a structure to organize and house new information, concepts, strategies, interventions, insights, and skills. These additions come from three sources: (a) the various activities that are part of the practice of psychotherapy; (b) the many sources of knowledge generated within a society; and (c) the experience of living a full, examined life.

Therapists learn and grow through professional activities that include clinical practice, clinical supervision, case consultation, collaboration with colleagues, workshops, classes, and professional reading. The knowledge accrued through these activities is loaded onto the scaffolding of the IST blueprint. For therapy to be a source of learning, therapists must let their clients teach them about their life dilemmas. Each case is a journey in which therapist and clients learn together. Challenges encountered in clinical work present opportunities for therapists to learn from the process of therapy and identify the need to expand knowledge and skills.

Another source of learning in clinical practice occurs through making referrals and coordinating care. Contacts with teachers, doctors, attorneys, community agencies, and other therapists help therapists better understand a client system's ecology by providing different perspectives grounded in other professional training and experience. For example, a therapist working with a married, heterosexual couple suspected that the husband might have adult attention-deficit/hyperactivity disorder (ADHD). The therapist referred the man to a psychiatrist for evaluation and began to work collaboratively to coordinate care. The diagnosis of ADHD was made, and the psychiatrist, who had a specialization in adult ADHD, commented on common relational patterns in couples with one member who has this diagnosis. As a result of the discussion, the therapist better understood the burden the wife carried, the shame the husband felt, and the interactional sequence that carried these emotions. The therapist was inspired to do some further research on the topic. Within a few weeks, the therapist was substantively more knowledgeable about ADHD and its impacts on couples and substantially better prepared to help this couple (and other couples) find solutions to their challenges.

Societal sources shed light on many aspects of the human experience that are related to therapy. Therapists learn and grow as they experience the world around them. Observing a couple arguing in a park or a mother pleading with a child in the grocery store reveals problem sequences that elaborate on what we hear from clients. Articulation, analysis, and interpretation of society through news reports, current events, films, television, the Internet, novels, biographies, art, music, science, and sports expand our ability to hear our clients and understand the human condition. Hearing a piece of music that evokes sadness or seeing a film that depicts grieving in a family may establish a basis for empathizing more deeply with a client's sense of loss. A relational pattern depicted in a novel may help the therapist understand what is transpiring within a family. Reading about a scientific study on patterns of weight loss and gain may give a therapist a better understanding of a client's struggle with weight.

An important source of learning and growth is living an examined life that includes personal reflection on ourselves and all the relational systems in which we participate. Personal challenges, joyous events, relational patterns, health practices, life cycle transitions, traumatic experiences, and losses all contribute to the development of the self-of-the-therapist. Included in this category is the therapist's own use of therapy.

Living life presents countless opportunities to learn and grow. For example, as therapists become parents, they deepen their understanding of the joys, concerns, and fears young parents face. Further, life is a great leveler: Both clients and therapists have to live it and experience the themes and challenges of being human. Therapists and clients have complementary roles that invite a sense of difference, but life reminds therapists of the commonality of human experience.

For therapists to use lifelong learning in these ways, they must cultivate a spirit of curiosity and a habit of reflection both in their daily lives and in their practice. Along with personal and professional support systems, these factors protect against career stagnation and dissatisfaction and maximize learning across the various phases of development.

PHASES AND DIMENSIONS OF DEVELOPMENT IN INTEGRATIVE SYSTEMIC THERAPY

IST can function as an effective vehicle for lifelong learning, but how therapists use it varies with the phase of their development. In particular, use of IST is influenced by developmental issues such as level of comfort with professional role and responsibilities, levels of competence and autonomy, and congruence of professional and personal selves.

On the basis of a cross-sectional and longitudinal qualitative study of 100 therapists, Rønnestad and Skovholt (2003) proposed a model that included six phases of professional development: (a) lay helper, (b) novice student, (c) advanced student, (d) novice professional, (e) experienced professional, and (f) senior professional. In discussing the development of IST therapists, we draw on this research, but we collapse the analysis to four phases most closely related to IST: beginning, practicing, supervising, and continuing to grow.

Beginning

Because of its comprehensiveness and complexity, learning IST requires a commitment to careful study and supervised clinical practice. This commitment, in turn, requires an attraction to a systemic, integrative approach and a good fit with IST, as discussed earlier. Anyone learning a new approach to therapy faces the challenge of finding room for new concepts and frameworks within or alongside existing cognitive schemata. How this challenge plays out varies with, among other variables, the level of experience of the therapist. The earlier in one's career IST is studied and the more intensively one studies it, the more readily it is adopted and used as a framework for professional development. The further along one is in their career, the more challenging it is to adopt a new set of organizing principles for practice.

Essentially, therapists study IST in one of two circumstances: as graduate students in a program providing IST training or later in their career after they have studied other perspectives and had to accommodate them to what IST has to offer. In either case, learning IST is challenging but is accompanied by significant rewards.

Learning Integrative Systemic Therapy in Graduate School

Much of our experience in training IST therapists has occurred in the context of a master's degree program in marriage and family therapy. Before entering the program, students may have been exposed to psychotherapy through undergraduate study and/or their own therapy. They may also have acted as "lay helpers" (Rønnestad & Skovholt, 2003, p. 10) with friends and family members. They have views on the process of helping others, but these views are typically not strongly established. They choose to enter the program with the understanding that IST will be the cornerstone of their training. Their openness to new learning is further supported by factors associated with their developmental phase (Rønnestad & Skovholt, 2003, 2013) in which they are highly motivated to be taught how to practice therapy and rely heavily on factors external to them, including their professors, supervisors, and relevant readings. With few exceptions, these students learn and internalize IST quickly and by graduation have achieved a basic level of competence in its practice.

Early in their training, graduate students typically (and understandably) are anxious about assuming the roles and responsibilities of therapist. Not only must they sit and work with real clients for the first time, but they must also learn a complex way of thinking about therapy (IST). Several strategies facilitate this initial period of training: first, providing practical, basic training in how to conduct sessions while concurrently teaching the over-arching IST perspective; second, helping students to "keep it simple" in session (defining problems, forming alliances, tracking sequences, providing support and encouragement to clients) while using supervision meetings to discuss solution sequences, constraints, and plans; and third, teaching students specific strategies of intervention they can begin to use in session to help clients solve their problems. At this early stage, we encourage students to be patient with the process of internalizing and using IST and to depend on their supervisors for guidance in conceptualizing their cases.

As training progresses, students begin to internalize IST's essence diagram and blueprint. They progressively demonstrate their ability to read feedback, think on their feet, and identify solution sequences and constraints.

They feel less anxious and less cautious and begin to experience a greater relatedness and effectiveness with their clients. They are moving to the advanced student phase. We find that students at this point in their training benefit from reminders that what they seek to learn is neither finite nor entirely attainable. We encourage them to embrace the excitement and challenge of continual learning and accept that they are, and will continue to be, "works in progress."

Rønnestad and Skovholt (2013) described five developmental tasks required of advanced students. All programs that train therapists provide instruction and supervised clinical experience to address the first two tasks: (a) learning conceptual knowledge and (b) acquiring procedural competence. Our IST-based program, as rated by graduating students, is a strong vehicle for both these tasks. The other three tasks assist students in grasping and managing the enormous complexity of psychotherapy. For these tasks, IST training is especially qualified because its integrative frameworks (essence, guidelines, and blueprint) help students to both appreciate and manage that complexity. The third task is (c) remaining open "to information and theory at a meta level" (Rønnestad & Skovholt, 2013, p. 71) while selecting specific theories and techniques. The extensive array of information provided by the hypothesizing and planning metaframeworks along with the decision-making process of the blueprint are tools for accomplishing this task. The fourth task is (d) modifying "unrealistic and perfectionistic images of psychotherapy" (p. 71) and of the therapist role. The failure-driven and alliance priority guidelines help students achieve perspective on this. The fifth task is (e) managing the confusion associated with discovering just how complex psychotherapy is. IST was created, in part, to address this task. As students learn to use it, they learn to tolerate and reduce the confusion associated with doing therapy.

We encourage our students to see these developmental tasks as continuing opportunities for growth that will be with them over the course of their careers. To continue their development and stay current in the field, therapists have to integrate new learning and manage the complexity of their work. We encourage them to use IST as a tool for deutero-learning (Bateson, 1972; Breunlin, 2016)—that is, learning to learn. Graduates of the program recognize that they are just at the beginning of an exciting career that will be enriched by each new case they treat and by the opportunity to incorporate into IST advances in the field as they occur.

Because of the centrality of the therapeutic alliance in IST, the program also emphasizes the development of the self-of-the-therapist (Aponte & Kissil, 2016; Baldwin, 2013). Through course work, clinical work, supervision, and often their own therapy, students grow in their understanding of themselves and become more attuned human instruments in the therapeutic process. Greater self-awareness enables them to manage their emotional responses to clients, access their strengths as therapists, and recognize and repair alliance ruptures. With a solid foundation in the practice of IST and significant development of the self-of-the-therapist, students complete the program prepared to engage in continuous reflection on their work. This reflection is essential to professional development throughout the life cycle of therapists (Rønnestad & Skovholt, 2003, 2013).

Adopting Integrative Systemic Therapy as an Experienced Therapist

Experienced therapists come to IST from different therapeutic perspectives. A first group comprises those who enjoy drawing concepts and interventions from multiple perspectives. They have been practicing an eclectic therapy but without clear organizing principles. This group of therapists is likely to show interest in IST because they appreciate that the integrative schemata of IST are more thorough and precise than those they had developed intuitively. IST brings greater clarity to their decisions about what to do when in therapy. A second group is therapists who have practiced primarily within a particular theoretical model. They have found that their approach is only effective with some clients or certain presenting problems, and they wish to expand their view of therapy to be more effective with a greater cross section of clients. Essentially, they have recognized the need for a more integrative practice (Breunlin, Rampage, & Eovaldi, 1995). A third group is composed of specialists who are committed to practicing empirically supported treatments designed for a specific problem or population. For these therapists, IST can constitute the big picture into which a specialist practice fits. Although not fully practicing IST, they can use it as a tool to recognize when they have to add another therapeutic resource to their treatment plan. For example, a cognitive behavior therapist treating a child for an anxiety disorder might use IST to hypothesize that the anxiety is exacerbated by the parents' marital distress and refer the parents for marital therapy.

Experienced therapists seeking to fully adopt IST may be challenged by the need to rethink some of their assumptions and practices. With a strong interest, a sense of good fit, and IST supervision or consultation they can readily learn IST and integrate within it their preexisting knowledge, skills, and personal style. Once on board, they will continue the trajectory of practicing, supervising, and continuing to grow, but because of previous clinical training and experience will likely be accelerated in their development in terms of clinical expertise with IST and readiness to supervise within it.

Because IST has many discrete concepts (e.g., sequence, constraint, multilevel system, therapy context) and components (e.g., the essence diagram, blueprint, web of human experience, matrix), it can be appealing to therapists who choose to adopt parts of it that fit well with their existing practice. These adaptations are more readily accomplished than the full-scale adoption of IST and do not require extensive study and supervision. In such cases, the IST concept or component is incorporated into their preexisting schema for therapy.

Practicing

This section discusses IST therapist development from the first job through the acquisition of significant professional experience and competence. Experienced therapists who study IST might benefit from the linguistic suggestions provided in the discussion of novice IST therapists but, otherwise, will find themselves in the subsection on experienced IST therapists.

Developmental Issues for Novice Integrative Systemic Therapy Therapists

Starting that first job ushers therapists into the novice professional phase, which is said to last 2 to 5 years (Rønnestad & Skovholt, 2003, 2013). This phase typically involves factors such as adjustment to practicing more autonomously, a struggle to reconcile graduate school training with the reality of the job, a search for a mentor, improved boundaries regarding the work, and increased reliance on inner resources as a focus of their development. Although this is a challenging time, many therapists begin to feel more relaxed in their professional role and see, increasingly, how they can express their unique personality in their work.

IST provides a framework broad enough to be used in most any work context, but novice IST therapists are generalists who have not learned all they need to know about working with the specific populations, problems, and circumstances they encounter on the job. Given this, they are highly motivated to learn new concepts, interventions, and skills. The task is to incorporate new learning, including the strategies used by supervisors and coworkers, into IST. Being open to new learning and organizing their learning within the IST frameworks both increases competence and further deepens their operative understanding of IST. Continued IST supervision supports ideal development and assures maintenance of a strong footing in IST.

The more IST-supportive the work context (or at least supportive of integrative, systemic therapies), the more likely the footing in IST will strengthen. In contexts that are less supportive of integrative, systemic approaches (emphasizing individual therapy or a particular model of therapy), novice therapists may be challenged in their commitment to IST. A common challenge is working with coworkers from different professions or theoretical orientations. Although in some cases this can lead to some erosion in commitment to IST, for others, IST commitment remains strong, and they find they can significantly influence other professionals in the work context.

The complexity of IST presents a challenge for newly minted therapists to briefly and adequately describe their perspective. Two recommendations to aid in describing how they work are essentially linguistic in nature. The first recommendation is to prepare a brief description of IST that can be used to explain it to coworkers. It need not be more than 100 to 150 words. For example:

> I was trained in integrative systemic therapy (IST). It is a systemic approach in that it views the presenting problems of families, couples, and individuals within a relational and biopsychosocial context. It looks to solve problems by changing the patterns of how people act and interact. IST is integrative in that it organizes a broad range of theories about what can prevent problem solving and selects interventions from various therapy models to address the specific factors relevant to a particular case. In IST it is better to begin with direct, action-oriented, problem-solving strategies when possible, but it can address a wide variety of constraining factors by using strategies of intervention derived from models as diverse as experiential, cognitive, narrative, neurobiological, and psychodynamic. IST takes a collaborative approach to therapy, recognizing client strengths and paying special attention to the problem-solving alliance with clients.

There is no one, correct "elevator pitch" for IST, but practitioners are encouraged to develop and memorize one for themselves. It can be tailored for different audiences, and it will likely evolve and become more colloquial over time. It will invite questions, which are further opportunities to explain the approach.

Because some IST terms are not used by non-IST therapists, a second recommendation is to avoid using terms such as *metaframework* and *blueprint* until or unless the other party has become familiar with them. The concepts of problem sequence, solution sequence, and constraint are relatively easy to explain, but in the absence of such explanation, they can be referred to, respectively, as patterns of interaction, solutions, and factors that keep the clients from solving the problem. Terms such as *strengths*, *therapeutic alliance*, and the names of the hypothesizing metaframeworks (e.g., *developmental factors*, *spiritual issues*, *family organization*, *gender issues*) will be familiar to other therapists. The actual interventions selected from the matrix are also common parlance.

Novice IST therapists are encouraged to think about relationships with colleagues in terms of alliance theory and to bring systemic case formulations to their discussions with them. A recently graduated family therapist with a strong commitment to IST took her first job in a psychiatric hospital inpatient unit. Her colleagues came from a variety of backgrounds, including social work, counseling, and clinical psychology. Her duties included working with families as they transitioned their loved ones back home, working with clients individually on trauma and emotion regulation, and running process groups, as well as cognitive behavioral and dialectical behavioral skills groups. The program favored behavioral approaches, and most of the therapists specialized in cognitive behavior therapy. This context, therefore, was foreign soil for an IST therapist. Her colleagues did not think systemically, tended to match the therapy to the problem (vs. problem sequence), and did not share her core assumptions (IST pillars and guidelines). The therapist shared with a mentor that, despite these challenges, she felt her colleagues appreciated her case-conceptualizing skills. She used her elevator speech to explain her approach but did not try to sell it. She established a collaborative alliance with her colleagues and shared her thinking on specific cases. She noted that although colleagues tended to ascribe pathology to patients and family members, they responded well when she commented on client and family strengths. She found there was room for her integrative, systemic approach to the work and that her point of view did significantly influence her colleagues.

Developmental Issues for Experienced Integrative Systemic Therapy Therapists

Over time, therapists develop greater competence and confidence and move into what Rønnestad and Skovholt (2003, 2013) called the *experienced professional phase*. Developmental tasks during this phase include maintaining professional growth while avoiding stagnation and/or burnout, integrating one's personal and professional self, and finding or creating a work role and context highly congruent with one's professional self. Professional growth in this phase is driven by reflection on personal and professional experience. Experienced therapists have a more internal and less external focus for learning, though new information from outside sources continues to enhance their knowledge base.

For IST therapists at this phase of development, clinical work becomes more intuitive as the use of the essence tasks, guidelines, and blueprint flows naturally—a function of simply doing what they do. For example, they search for solution sequences without thinking, "My next step in this therapy is to search for a solution sequence." They hypothesize without necessarily thinking, "OK, what is my hypothesis?" One highly experienced IST therapist described this intuitive process as a function of having internalized IST concepts and procedures and integrated them with an evolving self-of-the-therapist. This therapist went on to say the following:

> Sessions are very much in flow, and I am immersed in the present moment. My work feels anchored to me, and I think perhaps this is based on unconscious reasoning or intuition that comes from extensive experience with IST. It feels like a wisdom that grows out of continual practice. I think beginning therapists often don't feel that anchor, and that creates

anxiety for them. Conscious reasoning often happens in between sessions when I've had a chance to reflect on the work, when I've been able to metabolize and synthesize all of the feedback from the in-session work. I then carry this awareness into the next session. (S. Goldstein, personal communication, March 14, 2016)

At this stage of development, the challenge is to balance intuition with conscious reflection, careful hypothesizing, and the pursuit of new learning. Another experienced IST therapist who finds her work to be intuitive reported being more conscious with her IST thinking when she feels stuck or uncertain:

If I have to make careful steps, I have to consciously think about why I'm moving to the next action and how I am going to do it. I could see this happening in the moment in session or outside the session (either in consult or alone on reflection). That's when the IST training comes in a more conscious way for me. For example, I will ask myself, "Who should I invite in from the indirect system?" "What is constraining this person?" "How should I tackle this constraint?" Another time when I am especially conscious in my reasoning is when I'm trying to explain what I'm thinking to my client(s). When I am explaining this, I have to put into words the assumptions and beliefs I have about change and about the dynamics going on within the system that are constraining them. (J. Kinsman, personal communication, March 14, 2016)

Another therapist and author of this book put it this way:

I do think there is something to the idea that the use of IST becomes more intuitive. Not that the work is increasingly based on uninformed gut or instinct, but that the gut plays a role and that the gut itself becomes informed by IST. For example, I will automatically notice strengths because, at a deep level that is essentially intuitive now, that is what I have learned to do. This occurs without conscious reasoning telling me to look for strengths. Without consciously thinking about the IST guidelines, I just start with the problem and problem sequences, seek an action intervention when feasible, and maintain attention to the alliance. At other times in session, I am more consciously hypothesizing or planning. Particular feedback may lead to my being very careful in my thinking. I appreciate this more thoughtful mode and know that I need to use it to ensure quality care and identify areas for my own learning and growth. (W. P. Russell, personal communication, April 16, 2016)

In this phase, IST therapists use familiar concepts and interventions in a flexible and highly personalized manner. They have evolved their own style of working. Although faithful to IST, they are less mechanical and more fluid in the use of its frameworks. It might be said that they more inhabit than use IST. They are skilled in the art of therapeutic conversation, masterful in reading client feedback, and adept at making course corrections. These therapeutic conversations can be compared to jazz. Jazz is structured (melodies and rhythms) and yet improvisational. Jazz musicians improvise around the structure and create the music as they play. Further, the musicians continually react and respond to each other with the aspiration that their sound as a whole will be greater than the sum of its parts. The music produced on any particular occasion is idiosyncratic and unique. Whatever magic happens will never happen quite the same way again. Each set (of music), like each session of therapy, provides an opportunity to cocreate something new and worthwhile.

Experienced therapists continue to integrate new concepts and interventions into IST. For example, having attended a workshop on cognitive behavior therapy, they would abstract ideas and interventions from the workshop that can be incorporated into their work. Although such learning from external sources continues, experienced therapists increasingly look inward for their primary source of expertise (Rønnestad & Skovholt, 2003, 2013). They rely on their experience and an established pattern of reflection on their work both in terms of the process of intervention (hypothesizing, planning, conversing, reading feedback) and the use of self. We do recommend, however, that practitioners, regardless of their level of experience, have regular consultation or supervision to test their clinical perspectives and to receive support from other professionals. The combination of personal reflection and clinical consultation can prevent or mitigate what Trotter-Mathison, Koch, Sanger, and Skovholt (2011) called *meaning burnout* (p. 152), caused by reduced feeling of challenge in the work, not feeling helpful to clients, or losing touch with the reasons a career as a therapist was chosen, and *caring burnout* (p. 154), caused by the repeated process of attaching, working, and ending with clients, as well as the risks of compassion fatigue (Figley, 1995, 2002) and vicarious traumatization (McCann & Pearlman, 1990).

Supervising

After a number of years of practice, therapists often become clinical supervisors. Although this developmental step is fairly typical, it is not universal. For therapists who do become supervisors, there are multiple benefits. Supervision is generative because it contributes to the profession and represents a way to give back. It also stimulates professional growth by heightening and broadening the supervisor's ability to reflect on the process of therapy. Finally, the lens of supervision develops the self-of-the-supervisor or therapist. The brief discussion of supervision that follows addresses issues associated with becoming an IST supervisor.

Advantages of Systemic, Integrative Supervision

Rigazio-DiGilio (2014) argued that integrative approaches to supervision "offer a more robust understanding of supervisee and client development and adaptation" (p. 252). Integrative supervisors have access to multiple perspectives and a means to decide when to draw on these perspectives, leading to a supervision that is tailored to specific needs, culture, and context of participants. In IST, the metaframeworks provide the multiple perspectives the supervisor uses to understand and intervene in the process of supervision.

The arguments we presented Chapter 2 for an integrative, systemic approach to therapy apply equally to an integrative, systemic approach to supervision. Specifically, IST's concepts of a multilevel system (ontology pillar) and recursion in systems (causality pillar) are useful in understanding the process of supervision. The supervisory system is conceptualized as a multilevel system that includes the clients, therapist, and supervisor (and sometimes the supervisor's mentor), as well as the relationships among all these levels. This means that the supervisor is charged with considering the needs of clients, the learning goals of the therapist, and his or her own functioning and development as a supervisor. IST supervision requires attention to the relationship between therapist and supervisor as well as the relationship between the therapist and client system.

When to Become a Supervisor

As is the case with all approaches to therapy, becoming an IST supervisor involves taking responsibility for both the clinical work and the development of supervisees. Therapists planning to supervise will have to understand the roles and responsibilities of being a supervisor, acquire a range of supervisory methods, understand the relational aspects of supervision, and comprehend the ethical aspects of it. Further, because a supervisor is responsible for ensuring the therapy provided meets professional standards, an intermediate level of competence, confidence, and autonomy as a therapist is a prerequisite. Given a strong commitment to a process of reflection on their IST practice and an interest in becoming a supervisor, IST therapists may be ready to begin training as supervisors as soon as their third year of postdegree clinical practice. The emphasis here is on "begin training." In the tradition of the field of marriage and family therapy, IST is committed to the practice of training supervisors to supervise.

Readiness to supervise is also a function of the experience level of the supervisee. Both supervisor and supervisee have to feel that the supervisor has a level of knowledge and experience sufficient to benefit the supervisee. Our experiences in a graduate program in marriage and family therapy have supported the training and use of early-career IST supervisors. Exit interviews with graduating students have shown that year after year, students are extra-ordinarily pleased with supervision, ranking it as one of the most highly valued assets of the program. Who are these supervisors who get such glowing reviews? For the most part, they are graduates of the program with at least 2 years of postdegree clinical experience (this timing corresponds to the eligibility to become licensed). A comparison of feedback given for the most experienced compared with the least experienced supervisors has revealed that, although experience is valued, similar learning outcomes are achieved so long as the supervisor is competent and garners the respect of the students.

The experience with supervision reported here is contextualized by the accreditation of our program by the Commission on Accreditation for Marriage and Family Therapy Education that stipulates that accredited programs must use American Association for Marriage and Family Therapy (AAMFT)–approved supervisors or approved supervisor candidates (supervisors-in-training) who have been meticulously trained in the practice of supervision. A systemic model for the learning objectives and supervisory competencies for supervision is provided by AAMFT (2014). Parallel to the process of learning to be a therapist, learning to be a supervisor includes participation in lecture, discussion, supervision practicum, and supervision mentoring (supervision of supervision). This process typically takes 2 to 3 years.

Application of Integrative Systemic Therapy Concepts to Supervision

IST supervision involves more than guiding supervisees in the practice IST. It also involves using IST to understand the process of supervision and to support the therapist in the acquisition of core competencies. Rather than give an exhaustive description of IST supervision, we present a few IST concepts that supervisors must learn to apply to the process of supervision.

Alliance

Breunlin (2016) established how alliance theory, including the dimensions of tasks, goals, and bonds (Bordin, 1979; Pinsof & Catherall, 1986), unifies seemingly disparate training goals and can serve as a "centerpiece for training" (p. 524). The goals and tasks dimensions of the alliance provide a directive aspect to supervision whereby the supervisee learns to implement the planning metaframeworks. Supervision addresses bonds, including emotional reactions to clients and associated coping mechanisms, through work on the self-of-the-therapist.

In addition to the alliance among clients and supervisee, the supervisor also focuses on the alliance between supervisor and supervisee. Does the supervisee feel respected, emotionally safe, and sufficiently challenged? Are supervisor and supervisee in agreement on the tasks and goals of supervision?

For example, if the supervisor hesitates to give concrete suggestions to a supervisee early in training, the supervisee may become more anxious and frustrated with supervision. Or if the supervisee repeatedly fails to bring video recordings of sessions, the supervisee and supervisor may not be aligned regarding the task of learning through watching videotapes of sessions. Such misalignments must be addressed to develop the alliance and accomplish the training goals.

Essence of Integrative Systemic Therapy

The essence diagram provides an effective supervision tool. It can be used to encourage the supervisee to be aware of which essence task they are working on in therapy. This brings clarity of purpose to particular moments or sessions in therapy. The supervisor can also use the essence diagram as a problem-solving guide to address any problems that develop during the therapy or the supervision. From a training perspective, the competencies instilled in supervisees through supervision are essentially solution sequences for becoming a better therapist. If the supervisee struggles to implement a solution sequence (master a competency), the supervisor and supervisee search for constraints and look for ways to lift them. For example, if a supervisee hesitates to intervene in conflictual sequences between members of a family, a specific plan (solution sequence) to address this can be developed, practiced in role-playing, implemented in session, and reviewed in live or video supervision. If the solution sequence is not implemented, the supervisor asks what kept the therapist from doing it. This question facilitates the identification of constraints within one or more of the hypothesizing metaframeworks.

Blueprint

The decision-making process of the blueprint is applied to the processes of supervision. The supervisor collaboratively tests hypotheses related to how the supervision system is functioning, what factors may be constraining it, and what strengths can be mobilized to address constraints and implement solution sequences (including supervisor competencies). The hypothesizing metaframeworks of IST (organization, development, culture, mind, gender, biology, and spirituality) represent the classes of constraints that can exist in the supervisory system. In the example of the supervisee who struggled with intervening with conflict, the supervisor asks, "What keeps you from intervening?" or "How do you feel when you think about intervening?" If the supervisee identifies fear as a constraint, the supervisor and supervisee can develop a plan to manage or reduce fear so the supervisee can work effectively with the case and acquire competency in handling conflict. If the supervisee also reports that open conflict and the expression of anger is discouraged in his or her culture and family of origin, this issue will also have to be addressed.

Integrative Systemic Therapy Guidelines

IST supervisors apply the IST guidelines to the process of supervision. They assume strengths at all levels of the system and guide both the therapy and the development of the supervisee with direct, here-and-now, straightforward solutions before considering more complex, indirect solutions. Further, shifts in plans for the client system or supervisee are pursued as a result of the failure-driven principle and with consideration of the alliances within the system.

The supervisor, mindful of the application of IST guidelines to the development of the supervisees, respects their strengths and believes that clinical competencies can be implemented with direct coaching (strength guideline) unless supervisees demonstrate an inability to do so. Further, action strategies for supervisory intervention are favored both as the initial means of incorporating competence (cost-effective and temporal guidelines) and as a step toward identifying the constraints to that competence. In the case of the supervisee who hesitates to intervene in the conflict of clients, the supervisor would likely begin with encouraging the direct implementation of the clinical competency (sequence replacement and cost-effectiveness guidelines)—"Go ahead and stop the interaction and redirect the process." If this action-oriented, "just-do-it" approach does not begin to establish the clinical competency, then exploration of constraints would lead to a plan to remove them or manage them differently to allow the competency to develop.

Although IST supervisors strongly encourage all new therapists to enter therapy (to have the experience of being in the client's shoes, to manage the stress of becoming a therapist, and to develop greater awareness of self), recommending therapy for a practice-related constraint is considered a less direct and more complex way of addressing the constraint; thus, the supervisor does not recommend therapy for a specific constraint (cost-effectiveness and temporal guideline) until it is established that direct efforts to implement the competencies and work with constraining emotions and beliefs do not lead to the acquisition of the competence (failure-driven guideline). This practice builds, when necessary, a more cogent, practical argument for entering therapy for supervisees who have not entered it on the basis of the general recommendation to do so.

Impact of Supervising on Development

Becoming a supervisor suggests that one has attained a significant level of experience and expertise. Although supervising carries this status, we find that therapists supervise primarily because they simply love doing it. Fostering the development of therapists brings meaning and satisfaction, contributes to the profession, and promotes the supervisor's own personal and professional growth.

By "giving back," supervisors also reflect on their professional beliefs, practices, and use of self. Supervision facilitates looking at one's practice and career from several new angles. First, to be helpful to supervisees, supervisors must clarify how they think about their work. This provides an opportunity to reexamine practices that may have become habitual or solely intuitive. Second, supervisors see the work and the world through the eyes of their supervisees, thus broadening the supervisor's worldviews. Third, the multi-level focus of IST supervision strengthens the supervisor's ability to conceptualize and formulate complex systems. Fourth, supervision cultivates the habit of reflection, which has been shown to facilitate professional development at all levels of experience (Rønnestad & Skovholt, 2003, 2013).

Continuing to Grow

A skeleton can serve as a fitting metaphor for IST, which provides the skeletal structure for both the conduct of therapy and for a career as a therapist. A skeleton supports the body and provides a framework for movement. It bears weight, defines and allows many different movements, carries the organ systems, and houses and protects the heart and brain.

As therapists become more experienced (and IST is in their bones), they concentrate less on how and where to move the joints and instead move them spontaneously. They move in a manner consistent with what the IST skeleton allows, but also according to their personal preferences and style of movement. Further, "the heartbeat and the blood flow of the therapy, though not prescribed by the model, come to inhabit the model (the skeleton) and flow from the self-of-the-therapist" (S. Goldstein, personal communication, March 14, 2016). IST organizes bodies of knowledge and strategies of intervention relevant to the practice of therapy and provides structure and guidelines for how to use them. The heart of the work, including empathy, emotional intelligence, relational competence, and use of self, is a function of the self-of-the-therapist. Each practitioner brings "heart" and integrates it within the constructs of IST.

The development as an IST therapist has three foci: (a) maintaining IST's integrative, systemic, and empirically informed basis for practice; (b) continuing to acquire and integrate new knowledge and skill; and (c) continuing to develop the self-of-the-therapist. With experience, these foci become increasingly integrated and congruent. Learning and professional development, though, is lifelong, and IST is never fully mastered. There are always new concepts, knowledge, and skills to integrate and new developments within the self-of-the-therapist. Even as therapists move into the later years of their careers, there is a progressive, continuous, and never-completed process of mastering IST.

Rønnestad and Skovholt's (2003, 2013) last phase of development is the senior professional phase. They found that the modal length of time in practice to reach this phase was 20 to 25 years. Senior clinicians are typically well established, competent, and satisfied with their work. Because of growing life expectancy, senior clinicians may operate in this phase for 20 or more years. Rønnestad and Skovholt identified developmental risks for these clinicians that included intellectual apathy, cynicism about "new" approaches to therapy, and boredom with routine tasks. IST's theoretical breadth, comprehensiveness, and openness to new ideas and interventions provide some protection from these risks. We believe, however, that continued, long-term protection from stagnation, cynicism, and apathy for any senior clinician is more likely achieved by clinicians who engage in regular peer clinical consultation, supervise, provide clinical consultation, or teach courses or workshops because these activities support reflection on clinical work and provide connection with other therapists.

At this phase of development, senior therapists are likely to have experienced significant losses and other highly impactful life experiences. They have traversed most of the life cycle stages and faced the adversity associated with them. They also live with anticipatory loss. These experiences, and the knowledge accrued from them, will likely deepen their understanding of life's challenges and increase their capacity to do meaningful therapy. IST welcomes and readily accommodates these developments, though the level of wisdom achieved is less a function of IST or any model of therapy and more a function of personal adaptation to life experience and continued reflection and introspection about it.

THE UNFOLDING FUTURE OF INTEGRATIVE SYSTEMIC THERAPY

Given its organization, breadth of focus, integrative nature, and room for individual style and preferences, IST is an ideal framework for continuous professional growth and lifelong learning. A final consideration relates to the unfolding life cycle of IST. As the practice of psychotherapy and related scientific fields continues to evolve, so also will IST. IST will accommodate new findings into the web of human experience and new interventions into the matrix. New research on communication, relationships, and the therapeutic alliance will be incorporated into the components of conversing and feedback. Further, the structure of IST will likely be modified, as it has been in recent years, to increase its capacity to accommodate emerging knowledge and practices. For example, the original conceptualization of the web of constraints (Breunlin, Schwartz, & Mac Kune-Karrer, 1992, 1997) conceptualized biology as a level of the system (which, of course, it still is), but advances in neurobiology and its utility in understanding the mind–body connection (D. Siegel, 2007) and interpersonal relationships (Fishbane, 2007; D. Siegel, 1999), the study of illness and families (Rolland, 1994a, 1994b, 2003), and a biopsychosocial model of genetics (Rolland & Williams, 2005) have led us to view biology as a metaframework. This facilitates hypothesizing about biological constraints. IST is built to last—not as a final authority on the practice of therapy but as a perspective that will evolve with the field, as well as support the evolution and professional growth of its practitioners.

APPENDIX

Integrative Systemic Therapy Guidelines

1. The problem centered guideline	All interventions should be linked, in some way, to the client system's presenting problems or concerns.
2. The strength guideline	Until proven otherwise, it is assumed that the client system can use its strengths and resources to lift constraints and implement adaptive solutions with minimal and direct input from the therapist.
3. The assessment and intervention "inseparability" guideline	Assessment and intervention are two inseparable and co-occurring processes that span the course of therapy and lead to increasingly refined hypotheses and therapeutic plans that facilitate problem resolution.
4. The sequence replacement guideline	The primary task of the therapist is facilitating the replacement of the key problem sequences with alternative, adaptive sequences that eliminate or reduce the problem.
5. The empirically informed guideline	The practice of psychotherapy must be continually informed with empirical and scientific data in order to be maximally effective and efficient.
6. The educational guideline	Therapy is an educational process in which therapists give away their skills, knowledge, and expertise as quickly as clients can integrate them.
7. The cost-effectiveness guideline	Therapy begins with less expensive, more direct, and less complex interventions and moves to more expensive, indirect, and complex interventions as needed.
8. The interpersonal guideline	When possible and appropriate, it is always better to do an intervention, regardless of its nature, within an interpersonal as opposed to an individual context.
9. The temporal guideline	Therapy generally begins with a focus on the here-and-now and progresses to a focus on the past as more complex and remote constraints emerge within the therapy.
10. The failure-driven guideline	Therapeutic shifts occur when the current interventions fail to modify the constraints sufficiently to permit implementation of an adaptive solution to the presenting problem.
11. The alliance-priority guideline	Growing, maintaining, and repairing the therapeutic alliance takes priority over the principle of application (planning matrix arrow) unless doing so fundamentally compromises the efficacy and/or integrity of the therapy.

Note. From "Integrative Problem-Centered Metaframeworks Therapy I: Core Concepts and Hypothesizing," by D. C. Breunlin, W. Pinsof, W. P. Russell, and J. Lebow, 2011, *Family Process, 50*, p. 301. Copyright 2011 by Wiley. Reprinted with permission.

REFERENCES

Adams, J., & Boscolo, L. (2003). Milan systemic therapy. In L. L. Hecker & J. L. Wetchler (Eds.), *An introduction to marriage and family therapy* (pp. 123–148). New York, NY: Haworth Press.

American Association for Marriage and Family Therapy. (2014). *Approved supervision designation: Standards handbook.* Retrieved from http://dx5br1z4f6n0k.cloudfront.net/imis15/Documents/Supervision/2016%20Supervision%20Forms/Jan_2014_AS_Handbook_ver_Oct_%202016.pdf

American Cancer Society. (2009). *Cancer facts and figures 2009.* Retrieved from https://www.cancer.org/content/dam/cancer-org/research/cancer-facts-and-statistics/annual-cancer-facts-and-figures/2009/cancer-facts-and-figures-2009.pdf

Anderson, C. M., Hogarty, G., Bayer, T., & Needleman, R. (1984). Expressed emotion and social networks of parents of schizophrenic patients. *The British Journal of Psychiatry, 144,* 247–255. http://dx.doi.org/10.1192/bjp.144.3.247

Aponte, H. J. (2009). The stress of poverty and the comfort of spirituality. In F. Walsh (Ed.), *Spiritual resources in family therapy* (2nd ed., pp. 125–140). New York, NY: Guilford Press.

Aponte, H. J., & Kissil, K. (Eds.). (2016). *The person of the therapist training model: Mastering the use of self.* New York, NY: Routledge.

Baer, R. A. (2003). Mindfulness training as a clinical intervention: A conceptual and empirical review. *Clinical Psychology: Science and Practice, 10,* 125–143. http://dx.doi.org/10.1093/clipsy.bpg015

Baker, K. A. (1999). The importance of cultural sensitivity and therapist self-awareness when working with mandatory clients. *Family Process, 38,* 55–67. http://dx.doi.org/10.1111/j.1545-5300.1999.00055.x

Baldwin, M. (Ed.). (2013). *The use of self in therapy* (3rd ed.). New York, NY: Routledge.

Bandura, A. (1969). *Principles of behavior modification.* New York, NY: Holt, Rinehart and Winston.

Bandura, A. (1989). Human agency in social cognitive theory. *American Psychologist, 44,* 1175–1184. http://dx.doi.org/10.1037/0003-066X.44.9.1175

Bandura, A. (1991). Social cognitive theory of self-regulation. *Organizational Behavior and Human Decision Processes, 50,* 248–287. http://dx.doi.org/10.1016/0749-5978(91)90022-L

Barlow, D. H. (2008). *Clinical handbook of psychological disorders: A step-by-step treatment manual* (4th ed.). New York, NY: Guilford Press.

Barlow, D. H., Craske, M. G., Cerny, J. A., & Klosko, J. S. (1989). Behavioral treatment of panic disorder. *Behavior Therapy, 20,* 261–282. http://dx.doi.org/10.1016/S0005-7894(89)80073-5

Barlow, D. H., Raffa, S. D., & Cohen, E. M. (2002). Psychosocial treatments for panic disorders, phobias, and generalized anxiety disorder. In P. E. Nathan & J. M. Gorman (Eds.), *A guide to treatments that work* (2nd ed., pp. 301–335). London, England: Oxford University Press.

Barsky, A. E. (2010). Assumed privilege: A double-edged sword. In S. K. Anderson & V. A. Middleton (Eds.), *Explorations in diversity: Examining privilege and oppression in a multicultural society* (pp. 139–148). Boston, MA: Cengage Learning.

Bateson, G. (1972). *Steps to an ecology of mind: Collected essays in anthropology, psychiatry, evolution, and epistemology*. Northvale, NJ: Jason Aronson.

Baucom, D. H., Epstein, N. B., LaTaillade, J. J., & Kirby, J. S. (2002). Cognitive–behavioral couple therapy. In A. S. Gurman & N. S. Jacobson (Eds.), *Clinical handbook of couple therapy* (3rd ed., pp. 31–72). New York, NY: Guilford Press.

Baucom, D. H., Epstein, N., & Norman, B. (1990). *Cognitive–behavioral marital therapy*. Levittown, PA: Brunner/Mazel.

Beck, J. S. (2011). *Cognitive behavior therapy: Basics and beyond* (2nd ed.). New York, NY: Guilford Press.

Berg, I. K. (1994). *Family-based services: A solution-focused approach*. New York, NY: Norton.

Beutler, L. E., Consoli, A. J., & Lane, G. (2005). Systematic treatment selection and prescriptive psychotherapy. In J. C. Norcross & M. R. Goldfried (Eds.), *Handbook of psychotherapy integration* (pp. 121–143). London, England: Oxford University Press.

Birdwhistell, R. (1962). An approach to communication. *Family Process, 1,* 194–201. http://dx.doi.org/10.1111/j.1545-5300.1962.00194.x

Blume, L. B., & Blume, T. W. (2003). Toward a dialectical model of family gender discourse: Body, identity, and sexuality. *Journal of Marriage and Family, 65,* 785–794. http://dx.doi.org/10.1111/j.1741-3737.2003.00785.x

Blumenthal, J. A., Babyak, M. A., Doraiswamy, P. M., Watkins, L., Hoffman, B. M., Barbour, K. A., . . . Sherwood, A. (2007). Exercise and pharmacotherapy in the treatment of major depressive disorder. *Psychosomatic Medicine, 69,* 587–596. http://dx.doi.org/10.1097/PSY.0b013e318148c19a

Bordin, E. S. (1979). The generalizability of the psychoanalytic concept of the working alliance. *Psychotherapy: Theory, Research & Practice, 16,* 252–260. http://dx.doi.org/10.1037/h0085885

Boszormenyi-Nagy, I., & Krasner, B. (1986). *Between give and take*. New York, NY: Brunner.

Boszormenyi-Nagy, I., & Spark, G. M. (1973). *Invisible loyalties: Reciprocity in intergenerational family therapy*. New York, NY: Harper & Row.

Bowen, M. (1974). Toward the differentiation of self in one's family of origin. In F. Andres & J. Lorio (Eds.), *Georgetown family symposium* (Vol. 1, pp. 222–242). Washington, DC: Georgetown University Medical Center.

Bowen, M. (1978). *Family therapy in clinical practice*. Northvale, NJ: Jason Aronson.

Bowen, M. (2004). Family reaction to death. In F. Walsh & M. McGoldrick (Eds.), *Living beyond loss: Death in the family* (2nd ed., pp. 85–98). New York, NY: Norton.

Boyd-Franklin, N. (2012). *Reaching out in family therapy: Home-based, school, and community interventions*. New York, NY: Guilford Press.

Breunlin, D. C. (1979). Non-verbal communication in family therapy. In S. Walrond-Skinner (Ed.), *Family and marital psychotherapy: A critical approach* (pp. 106–131). London, England: Routledge and Kegan Paul.

Breunlin, D. C. (1988). Oscillation theory and family development. In C. J. Falicov (Ed.), *Family transitions: Continuity and change over the life cycle* (pp. 133–158). New York, NY: Guilford Press.

Breunlin, D. C. (1989). Clinical implications of oscillation theory: Family development and the process of change. In C. Ramsey (Ed.), *The science of family medicine* (pp. 135–149). New York, NY: Guilford Press.

Breunlin, D. C. (1999). Toward a theory of constraints. *Journal of Marital and Family Therapy, 25*, 365–382. http://dx.doi.org/10.1111/j.1752-0606.1999.tb00254.x

Breunlin, D. C. (2016). Advancing training and supervision of family therapy. In T. L. Sexton & J. L. Lebow (Eds.), *Handbook of family therapy* (pp. 517–529). New York, NY: Routledge.

Breunlin, D. C., & Jacobsen, E. (2014). Putting the "family" back into family therapy. *Family Process, 53*, 462–475. http://dx.doi.org/10.1111/famp.12083

Breunlin, D. C., Pinsof, W., Russell, W. P., & Lebow, J. (2011). Integrative problem-centered metaframeworks therapy I: Core concepts and hypothesizing. *Family Process, 50*, 293–313. http://dx.doi.org/10.1111/j.1545-5300.2011.01362.x

Breunlin, D. C., Rampage, C., & Eovaldi, M. L. (1995). Family therapy supervision: Toward an integrative perspective. In R. H. Mikesell, D.-D. Lusterman, & S. H. McDaniel (Eds.), *Integrating family therapy: Handbook of family psychology and systems theory* (pp. 547–560). Washington, DC: American Psychological Association.

Breunlin, D. C., & Schwartz, R. C. (1986). Sequences: Toward a common denominator of family therapy. *Family Process, 25*, 67–87. http://dx.doi.org/10.1111/j.1545-5300.1986.00067.x

Breunlin, D. C., Schwartz, R. C., & Mac Kune-Karrer, B. (1992). *Metaframeworks: Transcending the models of family therapy*. San Francisco, CA: Jossey-Bass.

Breunlin, D. C., Schwartz, R. C., & Mac Kune-Karrer, B. (1997). *Metaframeworks: Transcending the models of family therapy* (Rev. ed.). San Francisco, CA: Jossey-Bass.

Brody, S. (2010). The relative health benefits of different sexual activities. *Journal of Sexual Medicine, 7*, 1336–1361. http://dx.doi.org/10.1111/j.1743-6109.2009.01677.x

Bronfenbrenner, U. (2005). *Making human beings human: Bioecological perspectives on human development.* Thousand Oaks, CA: Sage.

Chambers, A. L. (2012). A systemically infused, integrative model for conceptualizing couples' problems: The four session evaluation. *Couple and Family Psychology: Research and Practice, 1,* 31–47. http://dx.doi.org/10.1037/a0027505

Chambers, A. L., & Kravitz, A. M. (2011). Understanding the disproportionately low marriage rate among African Americans: An amalgam of sociological and psychological constraints. *Family Relations, 60,* 648–660. http://dx.doi.org/10.1111/j.1741-3729.2011.00673.x

Chambers, A. L., & Lebow, J. (2008). Common and unique factors in assessing African American couples. In L. L. Abate (Ed.), *Toward a science of clinical psychology: Laboratory evaluations and interventions* (pp. 263–281). New York, NY: Nova Science.

Christensen, A., Doss, B. D., & Jacobson, N. S. (2014). *Reconcilable differences: Rebuild your relationship by rediscovering the partner you love—without losing yourself* (2nd ed.). New York, NY: Guilford Press.

Christensen, A., Jacobson, N. S., & Babcock, J. C. (1995). *Integrative behavioral couple therapy.* New York, NY: Guilford Press.

Claiborn, C. D., & Goodyear, R. K. (2005). Feedback in psychotherapy. *Journal of Clinical Psychology, 61,* 209–217. http://dx.doi.org/10.1002/jclp.20112

Claiborn, C. D., Goodyear, R. K., & Horner, P. A. (2001). Feedback. *Psychotherapy: Theory, Research, & Practice, 38,* 401–405. http://dx.doi.org/10.1037/0033-3204.38.4.401

Clarkin, J. F., Hurt, S. W., & Mattis, S. (1994). Psychological and neuropsychological assessment. In R. E. Hales, S. C. Yudofsky, & J. A. Talbott (Eds.), *The American psychiatric press textbook of psychiatry* (2nd ed., pp. 247–276). Washington, DC: American Psychiatric Association.

Cole, E. R. (2009). Intersectionality and research in psychology. *American Psychologist, 64,* 170–180. http://dx.doi.org/10.1037/a0014564

Coontz, S. (2005). *Marriage, a history: How love conquered marriage.* New York, NY: Penguin Books.

Craske, M. G. (1999). *Anxiety disorders: Psychological approaches to theory and treatment.* New York, NY: Basic Books.

Curlin, F. A., Lawrence, R. E., Odell, S., Chin, M. H., Lantos, J. D., Koenig, H. G., & Meador, K. G. (2007). Religion, spirituality, and medicine: Psychiatrists' and other physicians' differing observations, interpretations, and clinical approaches. *The American Journal of Psychiatry, 164,* 1825–1831. http://dx.doi.org/10.1176/appi.ajp.2007.06122088

Decuyper, M., De Bolle, M., & De Fruyt, F. (2012). Personality similarity, perceptual accuracy, and relationship satisfaction in dating and married couples. *Personal Relationships, 19,* 128–145. http://dx.doi.org/10.1111/j.1475-6811.2010.01344.x

De Jong, P., & Berg, I. K. (2001). Co-constructing cooperation with mandated clients. *Social Work, 46,* 361–374. http://dx.doi.org/10.1093/sw/46.4.361

Dell, P. F. (1984). The first international conference on epistemology, psychotherapy and psychopathology: Charge to the conference. *Journal of Strategic & Systemic Therapies, 3,* 43–49. http://dx.doi.org/10.1521/jsst.1984.3.1.43

Dell, P. F. (1986). In defense of "lineal causality." *Family Process, 25,* 513–521. http://dx.doi.org/10.1111/j.1545-5300.1986.00513.x

de Shazer, S. (1985). *Keys to solutions in brief therapy.* New York, NY: Norton.

de Shazer, S., Berg, I. K., Lipchik, E., Nunnally, E., Molnar, A., Gingerich, W., & Weiner-Davis, M. (1986). Brief therapy: Focused solution development. *Family Process, 25,* 207–221. http://dx.doi.org/10.1111/j.1545-5300.1986.00207.x

Doherty, W. J. (2009). Morality and spirituality in therapy. In F. Walsh (Ed.), *Spiritual resources in family therapy* (2nd ed., pp. 215–228). New York, NY: Guilford Press.

Drum, D. J., Brownson, C., Burton Denmark, A., & Smith, S. E. (2009). New data on the nature of suicidal crises in college students: Shifting the paradigm. *Professional Psychology: Research and Practice, 40,* 213–222. http://dx.doi.org/10.1037/a0014465

Edwards, T. M., & Patterson, J. E. (2006). Supervising family therapy trainees in primary care medical settings: Context matters. *Journal of Marital and Family Therapy, 32,* 33–43. http://dx.doi.org/10.1111/j.1752-0606.2006.tb01586.x

Ekman, P. (2003). *Emotions revealed.* New York, NY: Henry Holt.

Faiver, C. M., Ingersoll, R. E., O'Brien, E., & McNally, C. (2001). *Explorations in counseling and spirituality: Philosophical, practical, and personal reflections.* Pacific Grove, CA: Brooks Cole.

Fiese, B. H. (2006). *Family routines and rituals.* New Haven, CT: Yale University Press.

Fiese, B. H., Foley, K. P., & Spagnola, M. (2006). Routine and ritual elements in family mealtimes: Contexts for child well-being and family identity. *New Directions for Child and Adolescent Development, 2006*(111), 67–89. http://dx.doi.org/10.1002/cd.156

Fiese, B. H., Tomcho, T. J., Douglas, M., Josephs, K., Poltrack, S., & Baker, T. (2002). A review of 50 years of research on naturally occurring family routines and rituals: Cause for celebration? *Journal of Family Psychology, 16,* 381–390. http://dx.doi.org/10.1037/0893-3200.16.4.381

Figley, C. R. (1995). Compassion fatigue: Toward a new understanding of the costs of caring. In B. H. Stamm (Ed.), *Secondary traumatic stress: Self-care issues for clinicians, researchers and educators* (pp. 3–28). Baltimore, MD: Sidran Press.

Figley, C. R. (2002). Compassion fatigue: Psychotherapists' chronic lack of self care. *Journal of Clinical Psychology, 58,* 1433–1441. http://dx.doi.org/10.1002/jclp.10090

Fishbane, M. D. (2007). Wired to connect: Neuroscience, relationships, and therapy. *Family Process, 46,* 395–412. http://dx.doi.org/10.1111/j.1545-5300.2007.00219.x

Fishbane, M. D. (2013). *Loving with the brain in mind: Neurobiology and couple therapy.* New York, NY: Norton.

Fraenkel, P. (2009). The therapeutic palette: A guide to choice points in integrative couple therapy. *Clinical Social Work Journal, 37*, 234–247. http://dx.doi.org/10.1007/s10615-009-0207-3

Framo, J. L. (1976). Family of origin as a therapeutic resource for adults in marital and family therapy: You can and should go home again. *Family Process, 15*, 193–210. http://dx.doi.org/10.1111/j.1545-5300.1976.00193.x

Framo, J. L. (1992). *Family-of-origin therapy: An intergenerational approach.* Hove, England: Psychology Press.

Freedman, J., & Combs, G. (1996). *Narrative therapy.* New York, NY: Norton.

Freud, S. (1920). *A general introduction to psychoanalysis.* http://dx.doi.org/10.1037/10667-021

Freud, S. (1994). The ego and the id: Part III. The ego and the super-ego (ego ideal). In R. V. Frankiel (Ed.), *Essential papers on object loss* (pp. 52–58). New York: New York University Press.

Freud, S. (2003). *Psychopathology of everyday life.* Mineola, NY: Dover.

Friedlander, M. L., Escudero, V., Heatherington, L., & Diamond, G. M. (2011). Alliance in couple and family therapy. *Psychotherapy, 48*, 25–33. http://dx.doi.org/10.1037/a0022060

Gallup. (2016). *Religion.* Retrieved from http://www.gallup.com/poll/1690/religion.aspx

Goldfried, M. R. (1982). *Converging themes in psychotherapy: Trends in psychodynamic, humanistic, and behavioral practice.* New York, NY: Springer.

Goldner, V. (1985). Feminism and family therapy. *Family Process, 24*, 31–47. http://dx.doi.org/10.1111/j.1545-5300.1985.00031.x

Goldner, V. (1988). Generation and gender: Normative and covert hierarchies. *Family Process, 27*, 17–31. http://dx.doi.org/10.1111/j.1545-5300.1988.00017.x

Goldner, V., Penn, P., Sheinberg, M., & Walker, G. (1990). Love and violence: Gender paradoxes in volatile attachments. *Family Process, 29*, 343–364. http://dx.doi.org/10.1111/j.1545-5300.1990.00343.x

Goldsmith, J. (2012). *Rupture–repair events in couple therapy: An exploration of the prevalence of sudden drops in couple therapy alliance, and their impact on therapy progress* (Doctoral dissertation). Retrieved from https://etd.ohiolink.edu/ap/10?0::NO:10:P10_ACCESSION_NUM:miami1334705054

Goodrich, T. J. (1991). *Women and power: Perspectives for family therapy.* New York, NY: Norton.

Goodrich, T. J., Rampage, C., Ellman, B., & Halstead, K. (1988). *Feminist family therapy: A casebook.* New York, NY: Norton.

Gopnik, A., & Seiver, E. (2009). Reading minds: How infants come to understand others. *Zero to Three, 30*, 28–32.

Gorske, T. T., & Smith, S. R. (2009). *Collaborative therapeutic neuropsychological assessment.* New York, NY: Springer.

Gottlieb, L. (2011, July/August). How to land your kid in therapy. *The Atlantic.* Retrieved from https://www.theatlantic.com/magazine/archive/2011/07/how-to-land-your-kid-in-therapy/308555/

Gottman, J. M. (1993). The roles of conflict engagement, escalation, and avoidance in marital interaction: A longitudinal view of five types of couples. *Journal of Consulting and Clinical Psychology, 61,* 6–15. http://dx.doi.org/10.1037/0022-006X.61.1.6

Gottman, J. M. (2001). Meta-emotion, children's emotional intelligence, and buffering children from marital conflict. In C. D. Ryff & B. H. Singer (Eds.), *Emotion, social relationships, and health series in affective science* (pp. 23–40). http://dx.doi.org/10.1093/acprof:oso/9780195145410.003.0002

Gottman, J. M., & Levenson, R. W. (2002). A two-factor model for predicting when a couple will divorce: Exploratory analyses using 14-year longitudinal data. *Family Process, 41,* 83–96. http://dx.doi.org/10.1111/j.1545-5300.2002.40102000083.x

Gottman, J. M., & Notarius, C. I. (2000). Decade review: Observing marital interaction. *Journal of Marriage and the Family, 62,* 927–947. http://dx.doi.org/10.1111/j.1741-3737.2000.00927.x

Greenberg, J., & Mitchell, S. (1983). *Object relations in psychoanalytic theory.* Cambridge, MA: Harvard University Press.

Greenberg, L. S. (1979). Resolving splits: Use of the two-chair technique. *Psychotherapy: Theory, Research and Practice, 76,* 316–324. http://dx.doi.org/10.1037/h0085895

Greenberg, L. S. (2011). *Emotion-focused therapy.* Washington, DC: American Psychological Association.

Greenberg, L. S., & Iwakabe, S. (2011). Emotion-focused therapy and shame. In R. L. Dearing & J. P. Tangney (Eds.), *Shame in the therapy hour* (pp. 69–90). http://dx.doi.org/10.1037/12326-003

Griffith, M. E. (1995). Opening therapy to conversations with a personal God. In K. Weingarten (Ed.), *Cultural resistance: Challenging beliefs about men, women, and therapy* (pp. 123–139). http://dx.doi.org/10.1300/J086v07n01_12

Griffith, M. E. (1999). Opening therapy to conversations with a personal God. In F. Walsh (Ed.), *Spiritual resources in family therapy* (pp. 209–222). New York, NY: Guilford Press.

Gross, J. J., & Thompson, R. A. (2007). Emotion regulation: Conceptual foundations. In J. J. Gross (Ed.), *Handbook of emotion regulation* (pp. 3–24). New York, NY: Guilford Press.

Guntrip, A. S., & Rudnytsky, P. L. (2013). *The psychoanalytic vocation: Rank, Winnicott, and the legacy of Freud.* London, England: Routledge.

Guntrip, H. (1969). *Schizoid phenomena, object relations and the self.* New York, NY: Norton.

Gurman, A. S. (1983). Family therapy research and the "new epistemology." *Journal of Marital and Family Therapy, 9,* 227–234. http://dx.doi.org/10.1111/j.1752-0606.1983.tb01507.x

Gurman, A. S. (2008). Integrative couple therapy: A depth-behavioral approach. In A. S. Gurman (Ed.), *Clinical handbook of couple therapy* (4th ed., pp. 383–423). New York, NY: Guilford Press.

Haaga, D. A., McCrady, B., & Lebow, J. (2006). Integrative principles for treating substance use disorders. *Journal of Clinical Psychology, 62*, 675–684. http://dx.doi.org/10.1002/jclp.20257

Haley, J. (1976). *Problem-solving therapy*. San Francisco, CA: Jossey-Bass.

Haley, J. (1987). *Problem-solving therapy* (2nd ed.). San Francisco, CA: Jossey-Bass.

Haley, J., & Erickson, M. H. (1973). *Uncommon therapy*. New York, NY: Norton.

Hamill, S., & Goldberg, B. (1997). Between adolescents and aging grandparents: Midlife concerns of adults in the "sandwich generation." *Journal of Adult Development, 4*, 135–147. http://dx.doi.org/10.1007/BF02510593

Hayes, S. C., Strosahl, K., & Wilson, K. G. (1999). *Acceptance and commitment therapy: An experiential approach to behavior change*. New York, NY: Guilford Press.

Heru, A. M. (2014). Working with families in medical settings. *Journal of Child and Family Studies, 23*, 764–765.

Hodge, D. R. (2001). Spiritual assessment: A review of major qualitative methods and a new framework for assessing spirituality. *Social Work, 46*, 203–214. http://dx.doi.org/10.1093/sw/46.3.203

Holtzheimer, P. E., III, Snowden, M., & Roy-Byrne, P. P. (2010). Psychopharmacological treatments for patients with neuropsychiatric disorders. In S. C. Yudofsky & R. E. Hales (Eds.), *Essentials of neuropsychiatry and behavioral neurosciences* (2nd ed., pp. 495–530). Arlington, VA: American Psychiatric Publishing.

Hooley, J. M. (2007). Expressed emotion and relapse of psychopathology. *Annual Review of Clinical Psychology, 3*, 329–352. http://dx.doi.org/10.1146/annurev.clinpsy.2.022305.095236

Hopko, D. R., Robertson, S. M. C., & Lejuez, C. W. (2006). Behavioral activation for anxiety disorders. *The Behavior Analyst Today, 7*, 212–232. http://dx.doi.org/10.1037/h0100084

Horner, M. J., Ries, L. A., Krapcho, M., Neyman, N., Aminou, R., Howlader, N., . . . Edwards, B. K. (2009). *Surveillance, Epidemiology, and End Results Program: SEER cancer statistics review, 1975–2006*. Retrieved from http://seer.cancer.gov/csr/1975_2006/index.html

Horvath, A. O., & Bedi, R. P. (Eds.). (2002). The therapeutic alliance. In J. C. Norcross (Ed.), *Psychotherapy relationships that work: Therapist relational contributions to effective psychotherapy* (pp. 37–69). New York, NY: Oxford University Press.

Horvath, A. O., & Greenberg, L. (1989). Development and validation of the working alliance inventory. *Journal of Counseling Psychology, 36*, 223–233. http://dx.doi.org/10.1037/0022-0167.36.2.223

Imber-Black, E., Roberts, J., & Whiting, R. A. (Eds.). (1988). *Rituals in families and family therapy*. New York, NY: Norton.

Jacobson, N. S., & Margolin, G. (1979). *Marital therapy: Strategies based on social learning and behavior exchange principles*. Larchmont, NY: Brunner/Mazel.

Jacobson, N. S., Martell, C. R., & Dimidjian, S. (2001). Behavioral activation for depression: Returning to contextual roots. *Clinical Psychology: Science and Practice, 8*, 255–270. http://dx.doi.org/10.1093/clipsy.8.3.255

Jannini, E. A., Fisher, W. A., Bitzer, J., & McMahon, C. G. (2009). Is sex just fun? How sexual activity improves health. *Journal of Sexual Medicine, 6*, 2640–2648. http://dx.doi.org/10.1111/j.1743-6109.2009.01477.x

Johnson, S. M. (2002). *Emotionally focused couple therapy with trauma survivors: Strengthening attachment bonds*. New York, NY: Guilford Press.

Johnson, S. M. (2015). Emotionally focused couple therapy. In A. S. Gurman, J. L. Lebow, & D. K. Snyder (Eds.), *Clinical handbook of couple therapy* (5th ed., pp. 97–128). New York, NY: Guilford Press.

Kabat-Zinn, J. (2003). Mindfulness-based interventions in context: Past, present, and future. *Clinical Psychology: Science and Practice, 10*, 144–156. http://dx.doi.org/10.1093/clipsy.bpg016

Karney, B. R., & Bradbury, T. N. (2000). Attributions in marriage: State or trait? A growth curve analysis. *Journal of Personality and Social Psychology, 78*, 295–309. http://dx.doi.org/10.1037/0022-3514.78.2.295

Kazantzis, N., & L'Abate, L. (Eds.). (2007). *Handbook of homework assignments in psychotherapy: Research, practice, prevention*. http://dx.doi.org/10.1007/978-0-387-29681-4

Kazdin, A. E. (2011). Evidence-based treatment research: Advances, limitations, and next steps. *American Psychologist, 66*, 685–698. http://dx.doi.org/10.1037/a0024975

Keeney, B. P. (1982). What is an epistemology of family therapy? *Family Process, 21*, 153–168. http://dx.doi.org/10.1111/j.1545-5300.1982.00153.x

Kernberg, O. F. (1976). *Object relations theory and clinical psychoanalysis*. New York, NY: Jason Aronson.

Kerr, M. E., & Bowen, M. (1988). *Family evaluation: An approach based on Bowen theory*. New York, NY: Norton.

Kilpatrick, A. C., & Holland, T. P. (2005). *Working with families: An integrative model by level of need* (4th ed.). Boston, MA: Allyn & Bacon.

Knobloch-Fedders, L. M., Pinsof, W. M., & Mann, B. J. (2007). Therapeutic alliance and treatment progress in couple psychotherapy. *Journal of Marital and Family Therapy, 33*, 245–257. http://dx.doi.org/10.1111/j.1752-0606.2007.00019.x

Kohut, H. (1968). The psychoanalytic treatment of narcissistic personality disorders: Outline of a systematic approach. *The Psychoanalytic Study of the Child, 23*, 86–113.

Kohut, H. (1971). *The analysis of the self*. New York, NY: International Universities Press.

Kohut, H. (1977). *The restoration of the self*. New York, NY: International Universities Press.

Kohut, H. (1984). *How does analysis cure?* http://dx.doi.org/10.7208/chicago/9780226006147.001.0001

Kramer, C. H. (1980). *Becoming a family therapist: Developing and integrated approach to working with families.* New York, NY: Human Sciences Press.

Langer, E. J. (1992). Matters of mind: Mindfulness/mindlessness in perspective. *Consciousness and Cognition, 1,* 289–305. http://dx.doi.org/10.1016/1053-8100(92)90066-J

Lebow, J. L. (1995). Open-ended therapy: Termination in marital and family therapy. In R. H. Mikesell, D.-D. Lusterman, & S. H. McDaniel (Eds.), *Integrating family therapy: Handbook of family psychology and systems theory* (pp. 73–86). http://dx.doi.org/10.1037/10172-004

Lebow, J. L. (2014). *Couple and family therapy: An integrative map of the territory.* http://dx.doi.org/10.1037/14255-000

Lebow, J., & Newcomb Rekart, K. (2007). Integrative family therapy for high-conflict divorce with disputes over child custody and visitation. *Family Process, 46,* 79–91. http://dx.doi.org/10.1111/j.1545-5300.2006.00193.x

Lebow, J. L., & Sexton, T. L. (2015). The evolution of family and couple therapy. In T. L. Sexton & J. L. Lebow (Eds.), *Handbook of family therapy* (pp. 1–9). New York, NY: Routledge.

Levenson, H. (2010). *Brief dynamic therapy.* Washington, DC: American Psychological Association.

Lincourt, P., Kuettel, T. J., & Bombardier, C. H. (2002). Motivational interviewing in a group setting with mandated clients: A pilot study. *Addictive Behaviors, 27,* 381–391. http://dx.doi.org/10.1016/S0306-4603(01)00179-4

Linehan, M. M., Heard, H. L., & Armstrong, H. E. (1993). Naturalistic follow-up of a behavioral treatment for chronically parasuicidal borderline patients. *Archives of General Psychiatry, 50,* 971–974. http://dx.doi.org/10.1001/archpsyc.1993.01820240055007

Luborsky, L., & Barrett, M. S. (2006). The history and empirical status of key psychoanalytic concepts. *Annual Review of Clinical Psychology, 2,* 1–19. http://dx.doi.org/10.1146/annurev.clinpsy.2.022305.095328

Lucksted, A., McFarlane, W., Downing, D., & Dixon, L. (2012). Recent developments in family psychoeducation as an evidence-based practice. *Journal of Marital and Family Therapy, 38,* 101–121. http://dx.doi.org/10.1111/j.1752-0606.2011.00256.x

Madanes, C. (1981). *Strategic family therapy.* San Francisco, CA: Jossey-Bass.

Malpas, J. (2011). Between pink and blue: A multi-dimensional family approach to gender nonconforming children and their families. *Family Process, 50,* 453–470. http://dx.doi.org/10.1111/j.1545-5300.2011.01371.x

Mark, T. L., Levit, K. R., & Buck, J. A. (2009). Datapoints: Psychotropic drug prescriptions by medical specialty. *Psychiatric Services, 60,* 1167. http://dx.doi.org/10.1176/ps.2009.60.9.1167

Maturana, H. R., & Varela, F. J. (1980). *Autopoiesis and cognition: The realization of the living.* http://dx.doi.org/10.1007/978-94-009-8947-4

McAdams, D. P. (2001). *The person: An integrated introduction to personality psychology* (3rd ed.). Fort Worth, TX: Harcourt College.

McAdams, D. P. (2006). *The person: A new introduction to personality psychology* (4th ed.). Hoboken, NJ: Wiley.

McCann, I. L., & Pearlman, L. A. (1990). Vicarious traumatization: A framework for understanding the psychological effects of working with victims. *Journal of Traumatic Stress, 3,* 131–149. http://dx.doi.org/10.1007/BF00975140

McGrady, B. S., & Epstein, E. E. (2013). *Addictions: A comprehensive guidebook.* New York, NY: Oxford University Press.

McDaniel, S. H. (2005). The psychotherapy of genetics. *Family Process, 44,* 25–44. http://dx.doi.org/10.1111/j.1545-5300.2005.00040.x

McDaniel, S. H., Doherty, W. J., & Hepworth, J. (2013). *Medical family therapy and integrated care* (2nd ed.). Washington, DC: American Psychological Association.

McGoldrick, M., Gerson, R., & Petry, S. S. (2008). *Genograms: Assessment and intervention.* New York, NY: Norton.

Meichenbaum, D. (1977). Cognitive behaviour modification. *Cognitive Behaviour Therapy, 6,* 185–192.

Messer, S. B., & Warren, C. S. (1995). *Models of brief psychodynamic therapy: A comparative approach.* New York, NY: Guilford Press.

Miller, S. D., Hubble, M. A., & Duncan, B. L. (1996). *Handbook of solution-focused brief therapy.* San Francisco, CA: Jossey-Bass.

Miller, W. R., & Rollnick, S. (2012). *Motivational interviewing: Helping people change* (3rd ed.). New York, NY: Guilford Press.

Miller, W. R., & Rose, G. S. (2009). Toward a theory of motivational interviewing. *American Psychologist, 64,* 527–537. http://dx.doi.org/10.1037/a0016830

Minuchin, S. (1974). *Families and family therapy.* Cambridge, MA: Harvard University Press.

Minuchin, S. (1987). *Consultation interview.* Staten Island, NY: South Beach Psychiatric Center.

Minuchin, S., & Fishman, H. C. (1981). *Family therapy techniques.* Cambridge, MA: Harvard University Press.

Mojtabai, R., & Olfson, M. (2010). National trends in psychotropic medication polypharmacy in office-based psychiatry. *Archives of General Psychiatry, 67,* 26–36. http://dx.doi.org/10.1001/archgenpsychiatry.2009.175

Morgan, O. J., & Litzke, C. H. (2008). *Family intervention in substance abuse: Current best practices.* Philadelphia, PA: Haworth Press.

Morgan, O. J., & Litzke, C. H. (2013). *Family intervention in substance abuse: Current best practices* (Vol. 26). New York, NY: Routledge.

Nagoski, E. (2015). *Come as you are: The surprising new science that will transform your sex life*. New York, NY: Simon & Schuster.

Nathan, P. E., & Gorman, J. M. (2007). *A guide to treatments that work* (3rd ed.). http://dx.doi.org/10.1093/med:psych/9780195304145.001.0001

National Institute of Neurological Disorders and Stroke. (2014). *Brain basics: Understanding sleep*. Bethesda, MD: National Institute of Neurological Disorders and Stroke, National Institutes of Health.

Neff, L. A., & Karney, B. R. (2004). How does context affect intimate relationships? Linking external stress and cognitive processes within marriage. *Personality and Social Psychology Bulletin, 30*, 134–148. http://dx.doi.org/10.1177/0146167203255984

Neff, L. A., & Karney, B. R. (2009). Stress and reactivity to daily relationship experiences: How stress hinders adaptive processes in marriage. *Journal of Personality and Social Psychology, 97*, 435–450. http://dx.doi.org/10.1037/a0015663

Neugarten, B. L. (1968). *Middle age and aging: A reader in social psychology*. Chicago, IL: University of Chicago Press.

Nichols, M. P. (2009). *The lost art of listening: How learning to listen can improve relationships* (2nd ed.). New York, NY: Guilford Press.

Norcross, J. C. (Ed.). (2002). *Psychotherapy relationships that work: Therapist contributions and responsiveness to patients*. London, England: Oxford University Press.

Norcross, J. C. (2011). *Psychotherapy relationships that work: Evidence-based responsiveness* (2nd ed.). http://dx.doi.org/10.1093/acprof:oso/9780199737208.001.0001

Norcross, J. C., Hedges, M., & Castle, P. H. (2002). Psychologists conducting psychotherapy in 2001: A study of the Division 29 membership. *Psychotherapy: Theory, Research, Practice, Training, 39*, 97–102. http://dx.doi.org/10.1037/0033-3204.39.1.97

Norcross, J. C., Krebs, P. M., & Prochaska, J. O. (2011). Stages of change. In J. C. Norcross (Ed.), *Psychotherapy relationships that work: Evidence-based responsiveness* (2nd ed., pp. 279–300). New York, NY: Oxford University Press.

Norcross, J. C., & Lambert, M. J. (2011a). Evidence-based therapy relationships. In J. C. Norcross (Ed.), *Psychotherapy relationships that work: Evidence-based responsiveness* (2nd ed., pp. 3–22). http://dx.doi.org/10.1093/acprof:oso/9780199737208.003.0001

Norcross, J. C., & Lambert, M. J. (2011b). Psychotherapy relationships that work II. *Psychotherapy, 48*, 4–8. http://dx.doi.org/10.1037/a0022180

Norcross, J. C., & Wampold, B. E. (2011). Evidence-based therapy relationships: Research conclusions and clinical practices. *Psychotherapy, 48*, 98–102. http://dx.doi.org/10.1037/a0022161

O'Dell, M. (2003). Intersecting worldviews: Including vs. imposing spirituality in therapy. *Family Therapy Magazine, 2*(5), 26–30.

O'Donohue, W. T., Henderson, D. A., Hayes, S. C., Fisher, J. E., & Hayes, L. J. (Eds.). (2001). *A history of the behavioral therapies: Founders' personal histories.* Reno, NV: Context Press.

Oksenberg, J. R., & Hauser, S. L. (2010). Mapping the human genome with new-found precision. *Annals of Neurology, 67,* A8–A10. http://dx.doi.org/10.1002/ana.22061

Orlinsky, D. E., & Rønnestad, M. H. (2005). *How psychotherapists develop: A study of therapeutic work and professional growth.* http://dx.doi.org/10.1037/11157-000

Overholser, S. C. (1993). Elements of the Socratic Method. Systematic questioning *Psychotherapy: Theory, Research, Practice, Training, 30,* 67–74. http://dx.doi.org/10.1037/0033-3204.30.1.67

Padesky, C. A. (1993, September). *Socratic questioning: Changing minds or guiding discovery.* Paper presented at the meeting of the European Congress of Behavioural and Cognitive Therapies, London, England.

Patterson, G. R., Reid, J. B., & Dishion, T. J. (1992). *A social interactional approach: Vol. 4. Antisocial boys.* Eugene, OR: Castaglia.

Patterson, J. E., & Vakili, S. (2014). Relationships, environment, and the brain: How emerging research is changing what we know about the impact of families on human development. *Family Process, 53,* 22–32. http://dx.doi.org/10.1111/famp.12057

Paul, N. L., & Paul, B. B. (1986). *A marital puzzle: Transgenerational analysis in marriage counseling.* Hove, England: Psychology Press.

Perel, E. (2006). *Mating in captivity.* New York, NY: HarperCollins.

Perepletchikova, F., Hilt, L. M., Chereji, E., & Kazdin, A. E. (2009). Barriers to implementing treatment integrity procedures: Survey of treatment outcome researchers. *Journal of Consulting and Clinical Psychology, 77,* 212–218. http://dx.doi.org/10.1037/a0015232

Perls, F. S. (1968). *Gestalt therapy verbatim.* Boulder, CO: Real People Press.

Perls, F. S. (1969). *In and out the garbage pail.* Lafayette, CA: Real People Press.

Perls, F. S. (1971). *Gestalt therapy verbatim.* New York, NY: Bantam Books.

Piaget, J. (1952). *The origins of intelligence in children.* http://dx.doi.org/10.1037/11494-000

Pinsof, W. M. (1983). Integrative problem centered therapy: Toward the synthesis of family and individual psychotherapies. *Journal of Marital and Family Therapy, 9,* 19–35. http://dx.doi.org/10.1111/j.1752-0606.1983.tb01481.x

Pinsof, W. M. (1994a). An integrative systems perspective on the therapeutic alliance: Theoretical, clinical, and research implications. In A. O. Horvath

& L. S. Greenberg (Eds.), *The working alliance: Theory, research, and practice* (pp. 173–195). Oxford, England: Wiley.

Pinsof, W. M. (1994b). An overview of integrative problem centered therapy: A synthesis of family and individual psychotherapies. *Journal of Family Therapy, 16,* 103–120. http://dx.doi.org/10.1111/j.1467-6427.1994.00781.x

Pinsof, W. M. (1995). *Integrative problem-centered therapy: A synthesis of family, individual, and biological therapies.* New York, NY: Basic Books.

Pinsof, W. M. (2002). Integrative problem-centered therapy. In F. W. Kaslow (Ed.), *Comprehensive handbook of psychotherapy: Integrative/eclectic* (Vol. 4, pp. 341–366). Hoboken, NJ: Wiley.

Pinsof, W. M. (2017). The Systemic Therapy Inventory of Change—STIC: A multisystemic and multi-dimensional system to integrate science into psychotherapeutic practice. In T. Tilden & B. Wampold (Eds.), *Routine outcome monitoring in couple and family therapy* (pp. 85–101). New York, NY: Springer.

Pinsof, W. M., Breunlin, D. C., Chambers, A. L., Solomon, A. H., & Russell, W. P. (2015). Integrative problem-centered metaframeworks approach. In A. S. Gurman, J. L. Lebow, & D. K. Snyder (Eds.), *Clinical handbook of couple therapy* (5th ed., pp. 161–191). New York, NY: Guilford Press.

Pinsof, W. M., Breunlin, D. C., Russell, W. P., & Lebow, J. L. (2011). Integrative problem-centered metaframeworks therapy II: Planning, conversing, and reading feedback. *Family Process, 50,* 314–336. http://dx.doi.org/10.1111/j.1545-5300.2011.01361.x

Pinsof, W. M., & Catherall, D. R. (1986). The integrative psychotherapy alliance: Family, couple, and individual therapy scales. *Journal of Marital and Family Therapy, 12,* 137–151. http://dx.doi.org/10.1111/j.1752-0606.1986.tb01631.x

Pinsof, W. M., Goldsmith, J. Z., & Latta, A. T. (2012). Information technology and feedback research can bridge the scientist–practitioner gap: A couple therapy example. *Couple and Family Psychology: Research and Practice, 1,* 253–273. http://dx.doi.org/10.1037/a0031023

Pinsof, W. M., & Lebow, J. L. (2005). A scientific paradigm for family psychology. In W. M. Pinsof & J. L. Lebow (Eds.), *Family psychology: The art of the science* (pp. 3–19). New York, NY: Oxford University Press.

Pinsof, W. M., Tilden, T., & Goldsmith, J. (2016). Empirically informed couple and family therapy: Past, present, and future. In T. L. Sexton & J. L. Lebow (Eds.), *Handbook of family therapy* (pp. 500–516). New York, NY: Routledge.

Pinsof, W. M., Zinbarg, R., & Knobloch-Fedders, L. M. (2008). Factorial and construct validity of the revised short form integrative psychotherapy alliance scales for family, couple, and individual therapy. *Family Process, 47,* 281–301. http://dx.doi.org/10.1111/j.1545-5300.2008.00254.x

Pinsof, W. M., Zinbarg, R. E., Shimokawa, K., Latta, T. A., Goldsmith, J. Z., Knobloch-Fedders, L. M., . . . Lebow, J. L. (2015). Confirming, validating, and norming the factor structure of Systemic Therapy Inventory of Change Initial and Inter-session. *Family Process, 54,* 464–484. http://dx.doi.org/10.1111/famp.12159

Pisani, A. R., & McDaniel, S. H. (2005). An integrative approach to health and illness in family therapy. In J. L. Lebow (Ed.), *Handbook of clinical family therapy* (pp. 569–590). Hoboken, NJ: Wiley.

Poerksen, B., Koeck, A. R., & Koeck, W. K. (2004). *The certainty of uncertainty: Dialogues introducing constructivism.* Charlottesville, VA: Imprint Academic.

Pos, A. E., Greenberg, L. S., & Warwar, S. H. (2009). Testing a model of change in the experiential treatment of depression. *Journal of Consulting and Clinical Psychology, 77,* 1055–1066. http://dx.doi.org/10.1037/a0017059

Prochaska, J. O., & DiClemente, C. C. (1984). *The transtheoretical approach: Crossing traditional boundaries of therapy.* Homewood, IL: Dow/Jones Irwin.

Rampage, C. (2002a). Marriage in the 20th century: A feminist perspective. *Family Process, 41,* 261–268. http://dx.doi.org/10.1111/j.1545-5300.2002.41205.x

Rampage, C. (2002b). Working with gender in couple therapy. In A. S. Gurman & N. S. Jacobson (Eds.), *Clinical handbook of couple therapy* (3rd ed., pp. 533–545). New York, NY: Guilford Press.

Reid, W., & Epstein, L. (1972). *Task-centered casework.* New York, NY: Columbia University Press.

Rigazio-DiGilio, S. A. (2014). Common themes across systemic integrative supervision models. In T. Todd & C. Storm (Eds.), *The complete systemic supervisor: Content, philosophy, and pragmatics* (2nd ed., pp. 231–282). Chichester, England: Wiley.

Rogers, C. R. (1965). The therapeutic relationship: Recent theory and research. *Australian Journal of Psychology, 17,* 95–108. http://dx.doi.org/10.1080/000495 36508255531

Rolland, J. S. (1994a). *Families, illness, and disability: An integrative treatment model.* New York, NY: Basic Books.

Rolland, J. S. (1994b). In sickness and in health: The impact of illness on couples' relationships. *Journal of Marital and Family Therapy, 20,* 327–347. http://dx.doi.org/10.1111/j.1752-0606.1994.tb00125.x

Rolland, J. S. (2003). Mastering family challenges in illness and disability. In F. Walsh (Ed.), *Normal family processes: Growing diversity and complexity* (3rd ed., pp. 460–489). http://dx.doi.org/10.4324/9780203428436_chapter_17

Rolland, J. S., & Williams, J. K. (2005). Toward a biopsychosocial model for 21st-century genetics. *Family Process, 44,* 3–24. http://dx.doi.org/10.1111/j.1545-5300.2005.00039.x

Rønnestad, M. H., & Skovholt, T. M. (2003). The journey of the counselor and therapist: Research findings and perspective on professional development. *Journal of Career Development, 30,* 5–44. http://dx.doi.org/10.1177/089484530303000102

Rønnestad, M. H., & Skovholt, T. M. (2013). *The developing practitioner: Growth and stagnation of therapists and counselors.* New York, NY: Routledge.

Rooney, R. H. (2010). Task-centered interventions with involuntary clients. In R. H. Rooney (Ed.), *Strategies for work with involuntary clients* (2nd ed., pp. 167–217). New York, NY: Columbia University Press.

Ruddy, N., & McDaniel, S. H. (2016). Medical family therapy. In T. L. Sexton & J. L. Lebow (Eds.), *Handbook of family therapy* (pp. 471–483). New York, NY: Routledge.

Russell, W. P. (2005, February). *Action, meaning, and emotion in relational therapy.* Lecture presented at the Master of Science in Marriage and Family Therapy Program, Northwestern University, Evanston, IL.

Russell, W. P., Pinsof, W., Breunlin, D. C., & Lebow, J. (2016). Integrative problem centered metaframeworks (IPCM) therapy. In T. L. Sexton & J. Lebow (Eds.), *Handbook of family therapy* (pp. 530–544). New York, NY: Routledge.

Savege-Scharff, J., & Scharff, D. E. (2002). Object relations therapy. In J. Carlson & D. Kjos (Eds.), *Theories and strategies of family therapy* (pp. 251–274). Boston, MA: Allyn & Bacon.

Scharff, D. E., & de Varela, Y. (2005). Object relations couple therapy. In A. S. Gurman (Ed.), *Handbook of couples therapy* (pp. 141–156). Hoboken, NJ: Wiley.

Scharff, D. E., & Scharff, J. S. (2005). Psychodynamic couple therapy. In G. O. Gabbard, J. S. Beck, & J. Holmes (Eds.), *Oxford textbook of psychotherapy* (pp. 67–75). New York, NY: Oxford University Press.

Scharff, M. E. D. (Ed.). (1995). *Object relations theory and practice: An introduction.* New York, NY: Jason Aronson.

Scheflen, A. E. (1978). Susan smiled: On explanation in family therapy. *Family Process, 17,* 59–68. http://dx.doi.org/10.1111/j.1545-5300.1978.00059.x

Scheinkman, M., & DeKoven Fishbane, M. D. (2004). The vulnerability cycle: Working with impasses in couple therapy. *Family Process, 43,* 279–299. http://dx.doi.org/10.1111/j.1545-5300.2004.00023.x

Schwartz, P. (1995). *Love between equals: How peer marriage really works.* New York, NY: Touchstone.

Schwartz, R. (2013). *Evolution of the internal family systems model.* Oak Park, IL: Center for Self Leadership.

Selvini Palazzoli, M., Boscolo, L., Cecchin, G., & Prata, G. (1978). *Paradox and counterparadox: A new model in the therapy of the family in schizophrenic transaction* (E. V. Burt, Trans.). Lanham, MD: Jason Aronson.

Siegel, D. (1999). *The developing mind: Toward a neurobiology of interpersonal experience.* New York, NY: Guilford Press.

Siegel, D. (2007). *The mindful brain: Reflection and attunement in the cultivation of well being.* New York, NY: Norton.

Siegel, J. P. (2015). Object relations couple therapy. In A. S. Gurman, J. L. Lebow, & D. K. Snyder (Eds.), *Clinical handbook of couple therapy* (5th ed., pp. 224–245). New York, NY: Guilford Press.

Simon, G. M. (2003). *Beyond technique in family therapy: Finding your therapeutic voice.* Boston, MA: Allyn & Bacon.

Simon, G. M. (2006). The heart of the matter: A proposal for placing the self of the therapist at the center of family therapy research and training. *Family Process, 45,* 331–344. http://dx.doi.org/10.1111/j.1545-5300.2006.00174.x

Skenazy, L. (2009). *Free range kids: How to raise safe, resilient children.* San Francisco, CA: Jossey-Bass.

Skerrett, K. (2016). We-ness and the cultivation of wisdom in couple therapy. *Family Process, 55,* 48–61. http://dx.doi.org/10.1111/famp.12162

Solomon, A. H. (2001). *Stories of us: A qualitative analysis of sex differences in the relationship narratives of recently married women and men* (Unpublished doctoral dissertation). Northwestern University, Evanston, IL.

Sprenkle, D., Davis, S., & Lebow, J. L. (2009). *Common factors in couple and family therapy: The overlooked foundation for effective practice.* New York, NY: Guilford Press.

Stahl, S. M. (2013). *Stahl's essential psychopharmacology: Neuroscientific basis and practical applications.* Cambridge, England: Cambridge University Press.

Stanton, M., & Welsh, R. (2012). Systemic thinking in couple and family psychology research and practice. *Couple and Family Psychology: Research and Practice, 1,* 14–30. http://dx.doi.org/10.1037/a0027461

Stricker, G., & Trierweiler, S. J. (1995). The local clinical scientist. A bridge between science and practice. *American Psychologist, 50,* 995–1002. http://dx.doi.org/10.1037/0003-066X.50.12.995

Substance Abuse and Mental Health Services Administration. (2014). *Results from the 2013 National Survey on Drug Use and Health: Summary of national findings* (NSDUH Series H-48, HHS Publication No. SMA 14-4863). Rockville, MD: Author.

Sue, D. W., Capodilupo, C. M., Torino, G. C., Bucceri, J. M., Holder, A. M., Nadal, K. L., & Esquilin, M. (2007). Racial microaggressions in everyday life: Implications for clinical practice. *American Psychologist, 62,* 271–286. http://dx.doi.org/10.1037/0003-066X.62.4.271

Summers, F. (1994). *Object relations theories and psychopathology: A comprehensive text.* London, England: The Analytic Press.

Summers, F. (2013). *Transcending the self: An object relations model of psychoanalytic therapy.* New York, NY: Routledge.

Taffel, R. (2012). Are parents obsolete? The decline and fall of parental authority. *Psychotherapy Networker, 36*(1), 22.

Tarragona, M. (2008). Postmodern/poststructuralist therapies. In J. L. Lebow (Ed.), *Twenty-first century psychotherapies: Contemporary approaches to theory and practice* (pp. 167–205). Hoboken, NJ: Wiley.

Terkelson, K. (1980). Toward a theory of the family life cycle. In E. A. Carter & M. McGoldrick (Eds.), *The family life cycle: A framework for family therapy* (pp. 21–52). New York, NY: Gardner Press.

Thoma, N. C., & Cecero, J. J. (2009). Is integrative use of techniques in psychotherapy the exception or the rule? Results of a national survey of doctoral-level practitioners. *Psychotherapy: Theory, Research, Practice, Training, 46,* 405–417. http://dx.doi.org/doi:10.1037/a0017900

Tomm, K. (1987a). Interventive interviewing: Part I. Strategizing as a fourth guideline for the therapist. *Family Process, 26,* 3–13. http://dx.doi.org/10.1111/j.1545-5300.1987.00003.x

Tomm, K. (1987b). Interventive interviewing: Part II. Reflexive questioning as a means to enable self-healing. *Family Process, 26,* 167–183. http://dx.doi.org/10.1111/j.1545-5300.1987.00167.x

Tomm, K. (1988). Interventive interviewing: Part III. Intending to ask lineal, circular, strategic, or reflexive questions? *Family Process, 27,* 1–15. http://dx.doi.org/10.1111/j.1545-5300.1988.00001.x

Trotter-Mathison, M., Koch, J. M., Sanger, S., & Skovholt, T. M. (Eds.). (2011). *Voices from the field: Defining moments in counselor and therapist development.* New York, NY: Routledge.

Truax, C. B., & Carkhuff, R. R. (1967). *Toward effective counseling and psychotherapy.* Chicago, IL: Aldine.

Turkle, S. (2011). *Alone together: Why we expect more from technology and less from each other.* New York, NY: Basic Books.

U.S. Senate Special Committee on Aging. (2002). *Faces of aging: Personal struggles to confront the long-term care crisis.* Retrieved from https://www.aging.senate.gov/hearings/bfaces-of-aging-personal-struggles-to-confront-the-long-term-care-crisis/b

von Bertalanffy, L. (1968). *General systems theory: Foundations, development, applications.* New York, NY: Braziller.

von Bertalanffy, L. (1975). *Perspectives on general system theory: Scientific–philosophical studies.* New York, NY: Braziller.

von Foerster, H. (1984). Principles of self-organization—in a socio-managerial context. In H. Ulrich & G. J. B. Probst (Eds.), *Self-organization and management of social systems: Insights, promises, doubts, and questions* (pp. 2–24). http://dx.doi.org/10.1007/978-3-642-69762-3_1

Walsh, F. (2006). *Strengthening family resilience* (2nd ed.). New York, NY: Guilford Press.

Walsh, F. (2009). *Spiritual resources in family therapy.* New York, NY: Guilford Press.

Walsh, F., & McGoldrick, M. (2004). Loss and the family: A systemic perspective. In F. Walsh & M. McGoldrick (Eds.), *Living beyond loss: Death in the family* (2nd ed., pp. 3–26). New York, NY: Norton.

Watts-Jones, T. D. (2010). Location of self: Opening the door to dialogue on intersectionality in the therapy process. *Family Process, 49*, 405–420. http://dx.doi.org/10.1111/j.1545-5300.2010.01330.x

Watzlawick, P. (1977). *How real is real? Confusion, disinformation, communication.* New York, NY: Vintage Books.

Watzlawick, P., Bavelas, J. B., & Jackson, D. D. (1967). *Pragmatics of human communication: A study of interactional patterns, pathologies, and paradoxes.* New York, NY: Norton.

Watzlawick, P., Weakland, J. H., & Fisch, R. (1974). *Change: Principles of problem formation and problem resolution.* Oxford, England: Norton.

Weinberg, R. S., & Gould, D. (2014). *Foundations of sport and exercise psychology* (6th ed.). Champaign, IL: Human Kinetics.

Whiffen, V. E. (2003). What attachment theory can offer marital and family therapists. In S. M. Johnson & V. E. Whiffen (Eds.), *Attachment processes in couple and family therapy* (pp. 389–398). New York, NY: Guilford Press.

White, M., & Epston, D. (1990). *Narrative means to therapeutic ends.* New York, NY: Norton.

White, M., & Epston, D. (2004). Externalizing the problem. In C. Malone, L. Forbat, M. Robb, & J. Seden (Eds.), *Relating experience: Stories from health and social care* (pp. 88–94). London, England: Routledge.

Wiener, N. (1961). *Cybernetics: Or control and communication in the animal and the machine* (2nd ed.). http://dx.doi.org/10.1037/13140-000

Wile, D. B. (2002). Collaborative couple therapy. In A. S. Gurman & N. S. Jacobson (Eds.), *Clinical handbook of couple therapy* (3rd ed., pp. 281–307). New York, NY: Guilford Press.

Winnicott, D. W. (1962). The theory of the parent–infant relationship: Further remarks. *International Journal of Psychoanalysis, 43*, 238–239. http://dx.doi.org/10.1093/med:psych/9780190271381.003.0059

Wolpe, J., & Lazarus, A. A. (1966). *Behavior therapy techniques: A guide to the treatment of neuroses.* Elmsford, NY: Pergamon Press.

Wood, B. (1985). Proximity and hierarchy: Orthogonal dimensions of family interconnectedness. *Family Process, 24*, 487–507. http://dx.doi.org/10.1111/j.1545-5300.1985.00487.x

World Health Organization. (2002). *World Health Report 2002—Reducing risks, promoting healthy life.* Retrieved from http://www.who.int/whr/2002/en/

World Health Organization. (2016). *International statistical classification of diseases and related health problems* (10th rev.). Retrieved from http://apps.who.int/classifications/icd10/browse/2016/en

Wynne, L. C. (1984). The epigenesis of relational systems: A model for understanding family development. *Family Process, 23,* 297–318. http://dx.doi.org/10.1111/j.1545-5300.1984.00297.x

Zilbergeld, B. (1999). *The new male sexuality.* New York, NY: Bantam Books.

Zinbarg, R. E., Lee, J. E., & Yoon, K. L. (2007). Dyadic predictors of outcome in a cognitive–behavioral program for patients with generalized anxiety disorder in committed relationships: A "spoonful of sugar" and a dose of non-hostile criticism may help. *Behaviour Research and Therapy, 45,* 699–713. http://dx.doi.org/10.1016/j.brat.2006.06.005

INDEX

ABOUT THE AUTHORS

William M. Pinsof, PhD, LMFT, ABPP, clinical psychologist, family therapist, and clinical professor of psychology at Northwestern University, joined the Family Institute of Chicago in 1975. Directing the Institute from 1986 until 2016, he oversaw its affiliation with Northwestern and renaming as The Family Institute at Northwestern. An advocate of psychotherapy integration, Dr. Pinsof has focused on integrating family systems thinking and practice into a general and comprehensive psychotherapy. In 2016, he founded Pinsof Family Systems, an organization that strengthens and heals complex family systems.

Douglas C. Breunlin, MSSA, LMFT, LCSW, is a clinical professor of psychology and program director for the Master of Science in Marriage and Family Therapy at The Family Institute at Northwestern University. His previous works include *Metaframeworks: Transcending the Models of Family Therapy* (with R. C. Schwartz and B. Mac Kune-Karrer) and *The Handbook of Family Therapy Training and Supervision* (coedited with H. A. Liddle and R. C. Schwartz). He has authored over 60 articles and served on the editorial boards of four journals. Mr. Breunlin has served as secretary, treasurer, and board member of the American Family Therapy Academy and is a clinical fellow of the American Association for Marriage and Family Therapy.

William P. Russell, MSW, LCSW, LMFT, is a clinical assistant professor of psychology and core faculty director of the Master of Science in Marriage and Family Therapy at The Family Institute at Northwestern University. He has practiced, taught, and supervised systemic, integrative therapy for over 30 years and has held leadership positions in academic and clinical programs. Mr. Russell is an approved supervisor in the American Association for Marriage and Family Therapy and a board-certified diplomate in Clinical Social Work. He has authored articles and book chapters on integrative systemic therapy.

Jay L. Lebow, PhD, ABPP, LMFT, is editor-in-chief of *Family Process*. He is a clinical professor of psychology and a senior therapist at The Family Institute at Northwestern and Northwestern University. He is author or editor of nine books, including the recent *Couple and Family Therapy*, *Clinical Handbook of Couple Therapy*, and *Handbook of Family Therapy*. He has engaged in clinical practice, supervision, and research on couple and family therapy for over 30 years. Dr. Lebow served as president of the Society for Couple and Family Psychology and has received the Society's Family Psychologist of the Year award as well as the American Family Therapy Academy Lifetime Achievement Award.

Cheryl Rampage, PhD, serves in the role of senior academic and clinical advisor at The Family Institute at Northwestern University. She was the founding director of the Master of Science in Marriage and Family Therapy at Northwestern and was vice president of the Family Institute from 2002 until 2015. Dr. Rampage is a clinical psychologist and author of numerous articles and book chapters on intimacy and gender issues in couple therapy. She is a clinical associate professor at Northwestern and teaches a course on intimate relationships. In addition, she maintains an active clinical practice, focused on couple therapy.

Anthony L. Chambers, PhD, ABPP, is the chief academic officer of The Family Institute at Northwestern University, the director of the Center for Applied Psychological and Family Studies, and a clinical professor of psychology at Northwestern University. He is also the past president and a fellow of the American Psychological Association's Society for Couple and Family Psychology (Division 43). Dr. Chambers completed his PhD in clinical psychology at the University of Virginia and completed his internship at Harvard Medical School and Massachusetts General Hospital, specializing in couple therapy.